FOOD
ALLERGIES
—— and ——
FOOD
INTOLERANCE

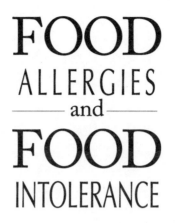

FOOD
ALLERGIES
— and —
FOOD
INTOLERANCE

The Complete Guide to
Their Identification and Treatment

JONATHAN BROSTOFF, M.D.
LINDA GAMLIN

Healing Arts Press
Rochester, Vermont

Healing Arts Press
One Park Street
Rochester, Vermont 05767
www.InnerTraditions.com

Healing Arts Press is a division of Inner Traditions International

*Note to the reader: This book is intended as an informational guide. The remedies,
approaches, and techniques described herein are meant to supplement, and not to be
a substitute for, professional medical care or treatment. They should not be used to treat
a serious ailment without prior consultation with a qualified health care professional.*

LIBRARY OF CONGRESS CATALOGING-IN-PUBLICATION DATA
Brostoff, Jonathan.
    [Complete guide to food allergy and intolerance]
    Food allergies and food intolerance : the complete guide to their identifica-
tion and treatment / Jonathan Brostoff and Linda Gamlin.
        p.   cm.
    Originally published: The complete guide to food allergy and intolerance.
3rd ed. London : Bloomsbury, 1998.
    Includes index.
    ISBN 0-89281-875-1 (alk. paper)
    1. Food allergy—Popular works. I. Gamlin, Linda. II. Title.

RC596 .B76 1999
616.97'5—dc21   99-056018

Printed and bound in Canada

10 9 8 7 6 5 4 3 2 1

Text design and layout by Kristin Camp
This book was typeset in Adobe Caslon and Optima

Contents

Acknowledgments

The authors would like to thank Dr. Michael Radcliffe for his many helpful comments on the manuscript. We are also grateful to Dr. Katherine Sloper, Dr. Jonathan Maberly, Dr. Stephen Davies, Dr. David Freed, Dr. Hugh Cox, Dr. Gail Darlington, Dr. David Pearson, Dr. David Bender, Dr. Robert Gardner, Dr. Celia Gibb, Dr. Ronald Finn, Dr. Len McEwan, Dr. Ian Menzies, Dr. John Hunter, Dr. William Bynum, Dr. Ellen Grant, Dr. Joseph Miller, Dr. Theron G. Randolph, Dr. John Mansfield, Dr. Harry Morrow-Brown, Dr. Ronald Williams, Dr. Jeff Reardon, Sheila Burnie, Maureen Minchin, Moira Mole, and Brian Hammond, who gave us their help, comments, and advice at various times during the preparation of this book. Special thanks are due to David Burnie for his considerable help in preparing the manuscript, and to Marella Buckley for her help with updating the book for its third edition.

Authors' Note

This book is designed to be read by two different types of readers—those who like to read straight through from beginning to end, and those who prefer to dip into topics that interest them. With the second group in mind, we have included numerous page references to point the way to related topics or explanations of technical terms. Those reading straight through should ignore these cross-references. We hope that everyone, including the dippers in, will read chapter 1, as this sets the scene for the rest of the book.

We have had to use some technical terms in writing this book, but all these are explained, and the index can be used to find the place in the text where the explanation is given.

Note to the Third Edition

When the first edition was published, no one was quite sure if the world was waiting with bated breath for a detailed, comprehensive book about food and chemical sensitivity, or whether the slim volumes already available were what readers preferred. The many very positive reactions we received have reassured us that people do find it useful to have all this informaton packed into one book, are not intimidated by scientific data, and like to hear both sides of the controversial isues. It has been enouraging to discover how many readers have been helped by the book. "It saved my life . . ." was one reaction, from a reader whose case history appears in this new edition.

As before, thanks are due to many doctors and other professional people for their help, but we would particularly like to mention Dr. John Hunter and Sheila Burnie for their expert advice, David Reading of the Anaphylaxis Campaign, Anne Muñoz-Furlong of the Food Allergy Network, Scott Adams for advice on gluten-free foods, and Mary Radley for her pithy review of an earlier edition.

Another Man's Poison

What is food allergy, and what is food intolerance? How do the two differ? The best way to answer this question is to tell the stories of Jane and Susan.

Jane's Story

Jane's health problems began as a baby. She had colic and vomited often, and at the age of three months developed eczema on her face and arms. Her mother had hay fever every summer, and her father had suffered from asthma as a child—both complaints are common allergies. Even before Jane was born, their family doctor was well aware that they were an **atopic** family—in other words, they were prone to allergies. As Jane grew older she developed asthma and hay fever, although only mildly. Her asthma seemed to get worse when there was a cat in the room. Using extracts of grass pollen and cat dander, and inserting minute amounts of them under her skin (a **skin-prick test**), the doctor found that she was indeed allergic to both these substances—her arm had a red, itchy bump where the extract had entered the skin.

Once or twice during her early years Jane's mouth and tongue swelled up enormously after eating, and she had to be rushed to the hospital. After thinking carefully about what she had eaten on these occasions, Jane's mother concluded that it was peanuts that had caused this alarming reaction. The doctor used skin-prick tests again, and they confirmed that Jane had a food allergy—she was extremely sensitive to peanuts. Other skin-prick tests were negative, so it seemed that she could eat most foods safely.

Even though Jane avoided peanuts carefully from then on, there were occasional problems. One day when Jane was about eight and her parents were holding a party, she handed a bowl of nuts around to the guests. Later she rubbed her eyelids, and they soon began to swell and itch furiously. Although her hay fever and asthma subsided as Jane grew older, her sensitivity to peanuts remained the same.

As an adult, Jane had a successful career that involved a great deal of traveling and eating out. Wherever she ate she had to be careful to avoid anything with peanuts—even the slightest trace of them. All was well until Jane, by now in her thirties, ordered some cheesecake in a restaurant. She had asked the waiter if the brown powder on the surface of the cheesecake contained any nuts, and he assured her that it was pure chocolate. Usually it was—but the chef had run out of chocolate that day and been forced to use something else. Unfortunately for Jane, that something else was finely grated nuts, including some peanuts.

Within seconds of taking her first mouthful of cheesecake, Jane's mouth was itching. Her tongue began to swell, and her breathing became difficult. She could no longer speak, and, as the swelling blocked her windpipe, she began to turn blue. Within minutes she had collapsed on the floor.

The colleagues she was dining with were horrified and had no idea what to do, but a stranger at the next table intervened. By an extraordinary, and lucky, chance, he was a doctor. Grabbing a spoon from the table, he pushed the handle over the back of her tongue and managed to open up the blocked windpipe. As he did so Jane gradually turned from blue to pink, but she was still in a state of collapse (known as **anaphylactic shock**), and her face was still horribly swollen. Meanwhile, someone had telephoned the hospital, and another doctor arrived with the lifesaving medicines that Jane needed. When these were injected, she slowly regained consciousness.

Thereafter, Jane was even more careful about avoiding peanuts in her food. She realized that she could easily have died had it not been for the presence of a doctor. By scrupulously avoiding peanuts, though, she has remained well. She also carries an emergency kit with a syringe of epinephrine that can be used to treat such attacks should she ever eat peanut by accident again.

Susan's Story

Susan is about the same age as Jane. She was reasonably well as a child, apart from frequent colds and chest infections. At the age of twenty-one, however, she suffered a bad bout of diarrhea when traveling abroad. Although she recovered from this, her bowels never really returned to normal: A mild form of diarrhea stayed with her so that she needed to go several times a day, often at the most inconvenient moment. As the years passed this problem gradually worsened, and unpleasant pains began in the lower part of her stomach. When she finally consulted her doctor about this problem, she was told that it was **irritable bowel syndrome**, or **IBS**, and that she should try to relax more.

For many years Susan also suffered headaches, but thought little of them—she simply took aspirin when she felt one coming on. One day, just after her twenty-eighth birthday, she experienced a strange sort of headache that was on the left side of her head only. She took some aspirin, but the pain did not go away—indeed, it became more intense, and she began to feel slightly sick. Eventually she had to draw the curtains and go to bed because she could not bear the light. There were more of these attacks over the next few months and Susan went to see her doctor again. He told her that these were migraines, and again recommended that she should try to worry less and learn to relax. Although she followed his suggestions, the migraines continued, and so did her bowel problems.

Over the next few years Susan had to give up alcohol and chocolate, as these always seemed to bring the migraine attacks on. But despite avoiding these items, her migraines continued to become more frequent. She also felt excessively tired, especially first thing in the morning, and she sometimes felt lightheaded and confused, or very edgy and irritable. To add to these problems, she began to get odd little pains in her knees. These gradually grew worse, and by the time she was thirty-four she could no longer run up the stairs without pain; she was forced to give up jogging and riding a bicycle, too, because these activities made her knees so much worse. The pains spread to some of her other joints and she began to feel that there was something seriously wrong, because she was ill most of the time.

Susan had previously accepted her doctor's diagnosis that most of her problems were due to her "nerves," but at this point she began to have doubts. She was now married, and had a good job that she enjoyed. Apart from her health problems she had few worries—indeed she felt more settled and happy than at any time in her life—so why was her health getting worse instead of better? She went to see her doctor again, and he gave her a thorough examination but could find nothing wrong. He repeated his earlier diagnosis, and suggested that her joint pains were also psychosomatic.

A few months later Susan read a magazine article about something called "food allergy," which seemed to cause the sort of symptoms she had. She asked her doctor's opinion about this and found he was very dismissive of the idea—as far as he could see, her symptoms were nothing like those of food allergy. Another year went past in which Susan became steadily worse. Then a new doctor joined the practice, and when she next called for an appointment, it was suggested that she see him instead, as he had a special interest in patients like herself. When Susan went to see the new doctor, he explained that symptoms such as hers could sometimes be caused by food, although there were other potential causes as well. He went on to explain why his colleague had dismissed the idea of her having food allergy—the condition he treated was quite different, and he preferred to use the name **food intolerance**. While he could not guarantee that this was her problem, it was certainly a possibility. He suggested that she try a special diet that avoided all the foods she normally ate. Susan began the diet on a Monday with high hopes, but by Tuesday she felt very ill indeed. Her tiredness was far worse, and she experienced a severe migraine attack—the worst one she had ever suffered—that lasted through Wednesday as well. On Thursday she felt completely washed out from the migraine, and Friday was little better. In desperation, she rang the doctor, but he told her that this sort of reaction often occurred—in fact it was a positive sign that foods were the source of the problem, so she should persevere with the diet.

On Saturday Susan woke up quite early, before her alarm clock went off—which was most unusual, because she normally had great difficulty waking up. As she got out of bed, she noticed that her knees did not give their customary painful twinge. She tried walking downstairs and then running up them again. To her amazement, she found that the pains she had endured for two years had suddenly vanished.

As the day went on she realized that she felt altogether different—she was no longer tired, her head felt clearer, and there was no headache or migraine, unlike most weekends. Indeed, she felt better than she had for many years. Over the next few days it became obvious that her bowels were also a great deal better.

When she returned to the doctor, Susan was jubilant—she simply couldn't believe how much better she felt. Even her irritability, which she had thought was just part of her personality, had now vanished. The doctor explained that she must now reintroduce foods, one at a time, to see what effect they had. Over the next two months, she tried out all the foods she normally ate. Some of these had no effect, but others made her very ill—milk, wheat, rye, barley, yeast, oranges, lemons, beef, and tomatoes were the main culprits. By avoiding all these foods, and adding some other, more unusual foods into her diet instead, Susan remained well. Migraines, which had previously afflicted her once or twice a week, were now a thing of the past.

After eight months, the doctor suggested that she try out some of the incriminated foods, to see what effect they had. She found that she still reacted to milk, but was fine on the other foods. The doctor advised her not to eat them more than once every four days. A year later Susan discovered that she could now drink milk again without ill effects. Interestingly, she discovered that she could also drink alcohol, in moderation, and eat chocolate, as they no longer seemed to trigger migraines. By this stage she had begun to forget what a migraine felt like!

Allergy and Intolerance

Both Jane and Susan were clearly being made ill by the food they ate. But their symptoms were very different—and so was the treatment they received from the medical profession. Food allergy—which caused Jane's dramatic illness—is a recognized complaint whose underlying mechanism is fairly well understood. Food intolerance, on the other hand, is not regarded as a sound diagnosis by the majority of doctors. Most would agree that there is such a thing as food intolerance (although they might use a different name for it), but they would argue that it affects relatively few people. Like Susan's doctor, they would regard the majority of patients with vague, multiple symptoms, including headache or migraine, fatigue, and diarrhea, as suffering from emotional and mental problems that express themselves in ill health.

This book deals with both food allergy (Jane's problem) and food intolerance (Susan's problem), but it concentrates most attention on food intolerance, since this is the area that has been sadly neglected by conventional medicine. (The reasons for this neglect, and for the continuing controversy over food intolerance, will be examined later, in chapter 6.)

The Meaning of *Allergy*

The medical controversy about adverse reactions to food is compounded by a long-running dispute over the meaning of *allergy*. For a word that is scarcely more than eighty years old, it has had a very checkered career. A Viennese doctor, Baron Clemens von Pirquet, first used it in 1906 to mean "altered reactivity." Von Pirquet was a pediatrician, and he felt the need for a new medical term to describe certain reactions in his young patients. These changed reactions included the development of immunity to infection on the one hand, and marked reactions to certain foods, pollen, or insect stings on the other. He was principally concerned with reactions involving the **immune system,** the set of cells that protect our bodies from infection. But he apparently intended his newly coined word to refer to any altered response to the environment. In this context, *environment* means all the external things that can affect the body, whether in food or water, in the air we breathe, or in things that come into contact with our skin. Von Pirquet also introduced the word *allergen* to describe the substances that brought about these changed reactions.

At that stage very little was known about how some of these reactions might arise. The following decades brought greater understanding, and the meaning of the term *allergies* was narrowed down— the development of immunity to disease was dropped from the definition, because it was obviously something quite different from adverse reactions to food, pollen, or bee stings.

In 1925 the definition of *allergy* was narrowed down still further. Experiments had shown that many adverse reactions to pollen or food could be transferred from one person to another by injecting a small amount of blood serum into the skin. The area around the injection site became very sensitive to the allergen. This, and other evidence, indicated that the immune system really was at work in these cases, as von Pirquet seems to have suspected. Most of those working in the field decided to limit the definition. Henceforth, a disease could only be described as an allergy if the immune system was demonstrably involved.

The way to demonstrate immune system involvement was by a **skin-prick test.** This involved making a purified extract of the allergen. A small amount of the extract was then inserted under the skin, by scratching or pricking it. If the area came up in a bump with a large area of red, itchy skin around it, then an **immune reaction** had occurred.

It had become clear that patients with certain diseases were likely to give positive skin-prick tests. These diseases were **hay fever, asthma** (breathlessness with wheezing episodes), and **nonseasonal** or **perennial rhinitis** (constant runny or congested nose). Also linked with positive skin-prick tests, although to a lesser extent, were **urticaria** or **hives** (a rash that resembles nettle stings) and one type of **eczema** (areas of red, itchy, flaky skin). Moreover, these five disorders often seemed to go together, either in individuals or in families.

These became the only legitimate subjects for study as far as orthodox allergists were concerned, and they are still described as the **classical allergic disorders**. Included in their ranks was a type of reaction to food that was very violent and came on rapidly after eating the allergen, often within minutes. The symptoms produced included swelling of the lips, mouth, and tongue; urticaria (hives); vomiting; and, in severe cases, collapse or anaphylactic shock—the reaction that Jane experienced when she ate peanuts in the restaurant cheesecake. In these cases, too, there was almost always a positive reaction to a skin-prick test with the suspect food.

Not everyone was happy with the change in the definition of *allergy*. At the time this change was made, several doctors in the United States were already studying what they called *delayed* or *masked* food allergies. In these cases the symptoms were much more varied. They also took far longer to materialize and were generally less severe. Because such patients rarely gave positive skin-prick tests, their reactions to food could not be included in the new definition of *allergy*.

While the doctors concerned with *masked food allergy* protested at the redefinition of *allergy* announced by their colleagues, they lost out to the newly arisen orthodoxy. There was pressure on them to conform, both from the medical establishment and, in some cases, from large food manufacturers who were funding research and were alarmed at the idea of whole sections of the populace discovering they could not eat wheat or milk—the two most common culprits as identified by the alternative allergists. There are very few processed foods that do not contain wheat or milk.

Some of the doctors involved in such unpopular research were highly respected medical scientists, with promising research careers ahead of them. But all this pressure eventually forced them out of the medical mainstream and into private practice, where they continued to use the term *allergy* in their own way—to mean simply "altered reactivity." This tradition has continued in the United States, and many American doctors working in this field still use *allergy* in this much broader sense.

Other doctors, especially in Britain, prefer the less controversial terms *food intolerance* or *food sensitivity.*

We favor the use of these terms in the interests of achieving a constructive dialogue with orthodox allergists and eventually gaining recognition for food intolerance by the medical mainstream. This would create access to treatment for patients as a whole (not just the intelligent and resourceful few who go looking for answers to their health problems) and improve the health status of a great many people worldwide. Such objectives are, in our opinion, more important than fighting about the meanings of words.

Competing uses of the term *food allergy* have also created much confusion among patients. Some with true IgE-mediated food allergy have been misled into thinking that the procedures recommended for patients with food intolerance—such as testing foods by eating a normal portion—are appropriate for them, when in fact they could be extremely dangerous. Patients with food intolerance who think that they have "food allergy" may get the impression that they need to be as ultracautious as those with true food allergy, avoiding even tiny traces of the culprit food. This would be a huge waste of time and effort and be very disruptive for anyone intolerant of several foods.

Enter IgE

A major advance in classical allergy research—and one that helped widen the rift with the unorthodox food allergists—was the discovery of im-**munoglobulin E,** or **IgE,** in the 1960s. This type of immunoglobulin, or antibody, is the main villain in the classical allergic conditions. How it works will be considered in some detail in the next chapter, but it is worth describing briefly here.

An **antibody** is a protein molecule made by the body to help combat disease-causing bacteria and viruses. The antibody binds to a specific target, known as its **antigen.** This target is usually a chemical located on the virus or bacterium, so the net result is that the antibody binds to the invader. The bound antibodies are rather like accusing fingers, pointing at the invading microbe—their presence rouses the body's defensive cells (the **immune cells**) to attack the microbe.

What goes wrong in allergy is that the body makes IgE antibodies in response to an innocuous antigen, such as a food molecule. IgE antibodies are usually found on the surface of special immune cells known as

mast cells, which occur in tissues throughout the body.

If the IgE molecules on the surface of a mast cell bind to their specific antigen, they stimulate the mast cell to release several chemical messengers. The normal purpose of these chemicals is to organize a more effective immune response, but in sufficient quantities they can produce the damaging symptoms of allergy. The antigen that causes such a reaction (a food molecule, for example) is known as an **allergen.**

The discovery of IgE was a breakthrough for classical allergists. Laboratory tests showed raised levels of total IgE in most patients displaying classical allergic symptoms. If the patient knew what allergen caused their symptoms, then a **radioallergosorbent test** or **RAST** (described on page 111) could be applied to measure IgE for that specific allergen. The RAST result almost invariably confirmed that there was an excessive amount of IgE antibody for the incriminated allergen. In a very short space of time, IgE became the touchstone of respectability for classical allergists. Some even changed the definition of *allergy,* yet again, to exclude reactions not involving IgE. This definition is still used by a few allergists.

When immunologists tried RASTs on patients diagnosed as food allergic, they found a basic division. Those like Jane with immediate, violent reactions, even to a very small amount of the offending food, almost always had high levels of IgE for that food, confirming the status of such reactions as classical allergies. Those like Susan with delayed reactions to foods rarely produced positive RAST results for their culprit foods. More recently, some studies have shown that a small IgE reaction in the gut wall could be a contributing factor in people like Susan, but IgE is certainly not the major cause of the problem.

A Battle of Words

"When I use a word it means just what I choose it to mean...," Humpty Dumpty declared in Lewis Carroll's *Through the Looking Glass.* This sort of verbal anarchy should not be encouraged, but there is so little agreement over terms such as *food allergy, food intolerance,* and *food sensitivity,* (not to mention *food idiosyncrasy, false food allergy, pseudo–food allergy,* and *food hypersensitivity*) that anyone writing about this subject is forced to take Humpty Dumpty's tack. There is no option but to select a set of suitable words and state clearly at the outset what is meant by them.

Food allergy is used in this book to mean "any adverse reaction to food in which the immune system is demonstrably involved." A positive skin-prick test, as described above, is usually taken as adequate proof of immune-system involvement, although this should be backed up by a RAST or other laboratory tests, where possible. When skin-prick tests or RAST results are negative, this does not necessarily mean that the immune system is not involved. Although reactions involving IgE are the principal cause of such allergies, there are other possible mechanisms, some of which will be considered in chapter 5. Different kinds of tests are needed for non-IgE allergies.

False food allergy here denotes a special type of nonimmunological reaction, seen with particular foods, in which a substance in the food triggers the mast cells directly. The reaction is not really an allergy at all: the immune system is not at fault, and the body does not overproduce IgE. But because the end result (the mast cells releasing their chemical messengers) is the same, the symptoms are exactly like those of food allergy.

Food intolerance, as used in this book, means "any adverse reaction to food, other than false food allergy or psychogenic reactions, in which the involvement of the immune system is uncertain because skin-prick tests and other tests for allergy are negative." This does not exclude the possibility of immune reactions being involved in some way, but they are unlikely to be the major factor producing the symptoms.

Food sensitivity is employed as an umbrella term for food allergy, food intolerance, and other adverse reactions to food, except where these are purely psychological in origin. As will become obvious, the dividing line between food allergy and food intolerance is sometimes blurred, so there is a need for a term that covers both.

Food aversion—the only noncontroversial term in this list—means "dislike and avoidance of a particular food for purely psychological reasons."

These definitions are ones that the majority of mainstream doctors practicing in this field would feel reasonably happy with. But bear in mind, if comparing this book with other books or articles, that the same words may be used in an entirely different way. It is also important to remember that they are theoretical definitions, and there is a sizable gap between theory and practice when it comes to diagnosing individual patients. In practice the designation of an illness as food allergy or food intolerance would not depend so much on skin-prick or other tests as on the type of symptoms that the patient shows. If the symptoms are among those traditionally associated with allergy, such as asthma or atopic eczema, and if foods are shown to be responsible, then the condition will probably be labeled as food allergy, even if skin-prick tests are negative, as they often are in such cases. If, on the other hand, the symptoms are not of the allergic kind—as in Susan's case—then the label food intolerance will be used. Skin-prick tests will not normally be carried out because they are very unlikely to give a positive result, so they will not contribute much to the diagnosis.

In theory, then, the distinction between *allergy* and *intolerance* is based on causes. In the doctor's office, however, the distinction is likely to be based on symptoms, because it is known that asthma or eczema are probably true allergic reactions, while migraine or depression are not. With a symptom such as diarrhea in a baby, the cause might be an allergic reaction, an intolerant one, or something else entirely. In such cases special tests would be needed to make a diagnosis of food allergy.

Where patients show a collection of symptoms that include, say, asthma and migraine, the diagnosis is more difficult. If all these symptoms clear up at once when certain foods are avoided, is it allergy or is it intolerance? This is not a question that can be easily answered at present, and for the purposes of this book we will use the umbrella term *food sensitivity* to cover such situations.

A final word about definitions. On page 8 we argued for compromise over the meaning of *food allergy*. By contrast, we would urge patients and doctors alike to resist attempts to narrow the meaning of *food intolerance*, a worrying trend that is evident in the latest pronouncements from organizations representing the most conservative and orthodox view of allergy. Rather than defining *food intolerance*, it seems, such organizations simply give an example—just one example—that of lactose intolerance (see page 259). Because the mechanism behind lactose intolerance is understood, and has nothing whatever to do with the immune system, this makes it a comfortable example for orthodox allergists. It is a clever way of ignoring the many other well-documented forms of food intolerance that are much less easily explained. These include cases of food-sensitive patients with both allergic-type and intolerant-type symptoms (asthma, bowel problems, and migraine, for example, or rhinitis, glue ear, and hyperkinetic syndrome) all of which clear up on an elimination diet. The mechanism involved in such cases is not understood, but their very existence hints at unexplained links between food intolerance and true food allergy.

Danny

For a young man of twenty-two, Danny had a surprising number of health problems. Afraid of losing his job as a trainee hotel manager, he pretended not to be as unwell as he really was. He only consulted the doctor when the red, itchy bumps that covered his skin (also called urticaria or hives) became unbearable. It was with great reluctance that he admitted his other symptoms—regular bouts of indigestion and diarrhea, aches in his joints, headaches, and extreme fatigue. There was also some eczema and hay fever, both of which he had suffered from as a child. Skin-prick tests showed that he was sensitive to grass pollen and cat dander, but not to any foods. Nevertheless, the doctor decided to try Danny on an elimination diet, excluding most of the foods that he usually ate. Within six days he returned to the officed looking very pleased. He reported that his hives were gone, along with his headaches, joint pains, and digestive problems. He felt far more fit and energetic as well. Under the doctor's supervision, he then reintroduced foods one at a time. Wheat, milk, eggs, tomatoes, and oranges, it turned out, caused the problems. These brought on urticaria within a few hours, with tiredness, headache, and aching joints later. Danny can avoid these foods most of the time and has remained well. His eczema also cleared up after a while, and his hay fever is less troublesome than before.

This sort of case is interesting because the diet apparently helps with symptoms that are thought to be due to allergic reactions, such as urticaria and eczema, as well as clearing up symptoms like headache, diarrhea, and joint pain. There are many cases of this type on record, making it difficult to draw a sharp dividing line between food allergy and food intolerance.

Another useful term is also now the target of an attempted redefinition by the more orthodox allergists. This time it is **elimination diet**—a well-established description for the diagnostic diet used to detect food intolerance. Recently, allergists have begun using this term to describe any diet where particular food(s) are avoided indefinitely as a treatment for food-induced disease. The widely used term for these is *avoidance diets*. It is vitally important that the difference between the two remains clear.

Changing Ideas about Food Allergy

Until fairly recently, most conventional allergists believed that the sort of symptoms seen in a patient depended largely on the type of allergen involved: the part of the body affected would be the part that first encountered the allergen. Thus, allergens that fell on the skin or brushed against it, called **contactants,** would tend to produce skin reactions such as eczema. Inhaled allergens, or **inhalants,** such as pollen or dust, would produce symptoms in the nose and airways. Food allergens, obviously, would produce symptoms in the lips, mouth, stomach, and gut. It was all very logical.

Among the patients treated by allergists, there were always some whose allergens could not be identified. With these unfortunate patients, it was assumed that some other nonallergic mechanism was producing the symptoms. Asthma patients, for example, were given the diagnosis *intrinsic asthma* if no allergen could be pinpointed. Like many of the labels used in medicine, this is just a clever way of saying that no one has any idea what is causing the disease. These insoluble cases were an indication that something was wrong with the traditional concept of allergies, although few doctors realized this at the time.

In the past twenty years the traditional picture of allergies has changed substantially, as conventional allergists have recognized that things are much less neat and logical than they originally seemed. Allergens do not necessarily cause their major symptoms at the place where they first encounter the body. They can enter the body by one route and then cause symptoms somewhere else entirely, because they are carried to that point in the blood. Thus foods *can* cause asthma or eczema—although they are likely to share the blame with inhalants or contactants, respectively. Inhaled allergens can also cause skin reactions, because they enter the bloodstream through the membranes of the nose or lungs and are carried by the blood to the skin.

It has taken a long time—forty years or more—for these new ideas about allergy to be accepted by orthodox allergists. This is largely because the discoveries were first made by the clinical ecologists in America and their counterparts elsewhere—who tended to attract those patients who had been declared incurable by more conventional doctors. Because of the long-running controversy over clinical ecology, the traditional allergists at first regarded their findings with great suspicion.

Even today there are vestiges of the old ideas about allergy in the way conventional allergists think about food. The traditional concept of a food allergy is of a severe reaction to food that is almost always immediate. The types of symptoms produced are fairly well defined and limited in number—the sort of symptoms seen in Jane's case. Although most conventional allergists now accept that foods may produce slower and less violent reactions, with more varied symptoms, such as asthma and eczema, these are not what spring to mind when the words *food allergy* are used. The same tends to be true of family doctors, and this is sometimes a contributing factor in the disagreements and misunderstandings over food allergy.

Food Intolerance

Jane could fairly be described as a typical case of food allergy. But Susan is not a typical case of food intolerance, because there is no such thing. Food intolerance cannot lay claim to any single set of symptoms. Every patient is different, both in the cluster of symptoms displayed and in the foods that cause these symptoms. Nor is there a single, clear-cut mechanism underlying the symptoms, as there is with food allergy. The available evidence indicates that there may be half a dozen or more different factors that contribute to the illness. In other words, food intolerance is a complex subject, and few generalizations can be made.

Nevertheless, there are certain features that characterize this type of food sensitivity and distinguish it from food allergy. Whereas food-allergy reactions are usually immediate, food-intolerance reactions tend to be much slower. The culprits in food intolerance are foods that are eaten very regularly, especially items such as wheat and milk that are consumed at almost every meal. The slowness of the reaction, combined with the fact that the foods are eaten so often, contributes to the masking effect observed by the first doctors to study these reactions—the link between food and symptoms is unlikely to be made when the body is subjected to a constant bombardment with the food.

Whereas food-allergy reactions can be provoked by quite small amounts of the food—a smear of the food from a badly washed saucepan for some highly allergic individuals—much larger quantities are needed to provoke the symptoms of food intolerance. Food intolerance is also far more insidious than food allergy: it is often difficult to say when it began, because the symptoms are very mild at first but gradually get worse. There are exceptions to this rule however, for in some cases a

Main symptoms of food intolerance

Headache
Migraine
Fatigue
Depression/Anxiety
Hyperactivity (children)

Recurrent mouth ulders

Aching muscles

Vomiting
Nausea
Stomach ulcers
Duodenal ulders

Diarrhea
Irritable bowel syndrome
Constipation
Flatulence, bloating
Crohn's disease

Joint pain
Rheumatoid arthritis

Edema (water retention)

bad bout of influenza or diarrhea can spark food intolerance. As in Susan's case, those with food intolerance tend to collect more and more new symptoms as the years go by, and become intolerant of more and more foods.

Food allergy—at least in adults and older children—usually persists for many years, often for a lifetime, even though the food is scrupulously avoided. Food intolerance, on the other hand, may well disappear if the food is not eaten for a few months. But it will tend to recur if the food is ever eaten regularly again.

The symptoms of food intolerance are extraordinarily varied and affect almost every body system. The illustration above summarizes the major symptoms that are generally agreed upon. Most doctors working in this field would probably wish to add various other symptoms to this list, and there is intense debate over symptoms that might or might not be attributed to food. Some of these controversial areas are considered in chapter 7, where the symptoms of food intolerance are described in more detail.

An important aspect of food intolerance is that the symptoms are not constant—they tend to come and go and to vary in severity. Non-food factors may play an important part, particularly stress, which can greatly exacerbate the symptoms. One of the most curious facets of food intolerance is that the person concerned often has a craving for the particular food or foods that cause the problem. In such cases—which account for as many as 50 percent of food-intolerant patients—eating the food initially gives a sense of great well-being. A possible explanation for this bizarre feature of the disease has now been discovered and is described in chapter 12.

Diagnosing Food Intolerance

Skin-prick tests do not work in the case of food intolerance, as we have already seen, and sadly there are no other simple tests to take their place. The only reliable way to discover if a food is causing illness is to eliminate it from the diet, then reintroduce it and observe what happens. This is not as easy as it sounds, because few people are sensitive to just one food, and eliminating different foods one at a time rarely has any substantial effect. All the offending foods have to be cut out simultaneously for an improvement in health to occur. Without such a return to health, the effect of individual foods cannot be tested, simply because the symptoms vary so much from day to day anyway.

The standard test used for diagnosing food intolerance is the **elimination diet**, in which all or most of the commonly eaten foods are avoided for a period of one to three weeks. If an improvement in health occurs, then foods are reintroduced individually and their effects assessed. Every doctor working in this field has a slightly different approach to the elimination diet—some begin with a complete fast, others allow anything from two to fifty foods in the initial stage—but the results show a remarkable consistency. The patient often feels a great deal worse initially, then recovers fairly spectacularly on day six or seven. Occasionally the process takes a little longer, but if there is no improvement after about three weeks then the diet should be abandoned. Detailed advice on how to carry out an elimination diet, how to prepare for it, and what to do afterward, is given in chapters 14 and 15.

The elimination diet is a fairly lengthy and tiresome procedure, and sometimes the results are not entirely clear-cut. But it is the only diagnostic process that can be recommended. Some of the alternatives offered by both doctors and fringe practitioners are considered on pages 137–41, and readers are urged to look carefully at this section before wasting time and money on bogus diagnostic tests.

Food for Thought

All of us, patients and doctors alike, are conditioned to think about food and other aspects of our environment in a particular way. As civilized inhabitants of temperate climes, we can indulge in the luxury of regarding nature as safe and welcoming, and of thinking of food as entirely wholesome and beneficial. These attitudes are part of our culture, another luxury that we simply take for granted, such as armchairs or automobiles. If we are to understand food intolerance, some of these accepted ideas need to be challenged.

Much of the medical prejudice against food intolerance is rooted in the idea that food—as long as it is part of a balanced diet—cannot be bad for you. What is often forgotten is that our foods were not designed specifically for human consumption, but were drawn from a pool of wild plants and animals that were domesticated by the first farmers.

In the wild, most food items are reluctant food items. They do not want to be eaten, and their efforts to stay off the menu are part of what Charles Darwin called the "struggle for existence." Most animals can run away, or fight back, but plants do not have this option.

Their defense is based partly on thorns and prickles, but far more important than these is the array of invisible chemical weapons that pervade almost all plant tissues. Some of these simply taste bad; others cause vomiting or other ill effects. A few even mimic the hormones of insects or mammals and thus disrupt their growth or sexual development.

Plant-eating animals have, in the course of their evolution, simply adapted to these chemicals in their food. They can detoxify them sufficiently to be able to feed on their chosen food or foods, and the plants can ward them off sufficiently to stay alive. It is rather like the situation between criminals and the police, where each side becomes increasingly cunning, better armed, and more ruthless, but neither side ever wins and obliterates the other. The term *biological arms race* aptly describes this situation.

Fruits and Nuts

Although most foods do not want to be eaten, there are exceptions to the rule in the form of fruits and nuts. These contain the seeds of the plant, and they rely on animals eating them to disperse the seeds. The wild version of a fruit such as an apricot consists of a juicy, sweetish layer on the outside with which the plant tempts birds and other animals. Inside is the seed, which is protected by a hard kernel or pit. The idea is that the animal eats the fruit, but that the seed passes through its gut to the outside and is voided with the animal's droppings, some distance away from the parent plant.

The seed itself is highly nutritious—it contains all the food the young seedling will need to become established—so the plant must guard its seeds well. Animals that might be tempted to break the apricot pit open and eat the seed as well are deterred by toxins, principally cyanides (the chemicals that give almonds and apricot kernels their characteristic smell and flavor). As a final safeguard, the parent plant adds a chemical to the outer skin of the fruit that affects the animal's gut. It speeds up the movements of the gut, making it void the stone more rapidly, so that the damage done by the digestive juices is minimized. This is why so many fruits have a laxative effect.

Nuts are rather more generous to their animal partners. They rely on animals such as squirrels that hoard food for the winter months, and they operate a "planned-loss" strategy whereby a great many of the seeds are actually eaten. The payoff is that the squirrels not only disperse the seeds but also plant them in a suitable spot when creating their winter stores. Since they inevitably forget where some are planted, a proportion of the nuts survive and grow into trees.

Both nuts and fruits have a major problem to contend with, despite these cunning stratagems: there are a great many other living things that would like to eat them without providing any service in return. These range from small animals that might nibble away at the fruit without dispersing it, to bacteria and fungi that would rot the nut as it lies in the soil.

A range of chemicals is present to keep these creatures at bay, many of them selective toxins that affect one type of creature but not another.

The "poisonous" berries of many wild plants are poisonous only to mammals—birds relish them, and are of far more use to the plant in dispersal. The chemicals that stop bacteria and fungi from spoiling the fruit or nut are not always so specific. Although their main effect will be on microscopic life-forms, they may have minor untoward effects on larger animals as well—including human beings.

Clearly, there is a massive chemical arsenal in wild foods, even in the foods that want to be eaten. In the course of our evolution, we have adapted to the challenge of eating these chemicals.

Eating Everything

Being an omnivore—an animal that eats adaptably, taking whatever is available—is a high-risk, high-return strategy in the natural world. It opens up a huge range of foods, but it makes it impossible for the omnivore to adapt to the specific chemical toxins of a single food source. Rats are omnivores, which is why they are so remarkably successful and so very difficult to poison. When a rat encounters a new food, it nibbles at it very cautiously, taking a tiny amount. Then it waits for a day or so. As long as it is not ill, it returns to eat some more.

At one time the human approach to eating out would have been very similar. Until about ten thousand years ago our ancestors were hunter-gatherers whose food consisted of wild plants and animals. Like the rat, they generally would have approached new foods with extreme caution. They also would have been endowed, as we are today, with the best type of equipment for breaking down food toxins. That equipment resides in the liver in the form of chemical compounds called **enzymes** that can break down foreign molecules. A powerful set of detoxification enzymes is something every good omnivore needs.

We are still omnivores today, although we do not rely much on wild foods. Farming changed our way of eating fundamentally, but it was not a change that happened overnight. The process took thousands of years, beginning with the collecting of wild grasses where these were growing abundantly. The wealth of food available from this harvest allowed people to settle down in one place, whereas before they had always been nomadic. The grass seeds could be stored and eaten for a large part of the year, but other wild plants and animals were still a major element in the diet.

The transition to farming took place once people realized that they could *plant* some of the stored seeds and thus grow more grasses and increase their food supply. In time they would have started to select the seeds used for planting, choosing those from the best types of grass. The process of domestication and plant improvement had begun.

Staple Crops

All this happened in the Middle East about ten to twelve thousand years ago, when the earliest forms of wheat and barley were domesticated. The same sort of events occurred quite independently in the Far East between about seven thousand and nine thousand years ago, and in Central America over seven thousand years ago. Grass-derived crops, which we now call cereals, were important in both areas. In the Far East rice became the main crop (or staple), while in the Americas it was corn. In Africa domestication probably took place rather later, and the main cereal crops were millet and sorghum. Southeast Asian farmers differed in relying on a root crop, the sweet potato *(Ipomoca batatas)* as their staple, and root crops were also important in other parts of the world where grasses did not grow well. The potato became the main crop of the high Andes, and in tropical Africa another type of sweet potato was grown.

With the growing of these staple crops, foods such as grass seeds and roots that had previously been eaten in fairly small amounts became the mainstay of the diet. Some people today believe this was a bad thing for human health, because we were not adapted to eat large quantities of starch, but that is a debatable point. What may be more important is the fact that we are eating large quantities of the particular chemical "armaments" found in these crops. Selection and plant breeding have reduced the amounts of these armaments substantially, of course, which is why our crop plants lack the bitterness of their wild equivalents, such as crab apples or sloes. But it is possible that some chemicals with more insidious effects may remain, and that relying so heavily on a staple crop may expose us to excessive amounts of those chemicals.

A possible suspect in this regard is wheat. Certain people, known as **celiacs,** are made seriously ill by wheat (see page 104). The tendency to develop celiac disease is inherited, which suggests that there are genetic differences making some people better able to cope with a wheat-based diet than others. This was confirmed by experiments in which very large amounts of wheat protein were given to healthy volunteers. The relatives of celiacs were made ill by these large amounts of wheat protein— so were normal people to some extent, but the relatives of celiacs suffered much more.

Enzymes

Enzymes are specialized molecules found only in living things (the ones in biological laundry detergents are derived from living things). They are absolutely essential to life, because they make specific chemical reactions happen. For example, they join other molecules together to build up the cells that make up living bodies. They also break down food (digestive enzymes) so that the energy it contains can be utilized, and break down toxins (detoxification enzymes) to make them harmless. They transform surplus food into fat stores, or break down the fat to yield energy when food is short.

Although they cannot be seen, even under a microscope, there are hundreds of thousands of different enzymes in the human body. Each has a very specific job to do: most of them control only one reaction, although others are slightly more versatile. For example, some of the digestive enzymes can break down a variety of food molecules of the same general type. Enzymes themselves are controlled by smaller molecules, which can turn a particular enzyme on or off.

Enzymes are just one type of **protein** molecule. Like all proteins, enzymes are made according to an inherited pattern that is passed on from parent to child. This pattern is stored in the genetic material, the DNA. In fact, DNA acts as a template from which all enzymes and other protein molecules are made. If there is a change in the DNA—a **mutation**—then the enzyme that is coded for that part of the DNA will be altered. Usually these changes are for the worse, and the new enzyme does not work as well as the original version. What sort of effect this enzyme defect has will depend on how important the enzyme is, what sort of reaction it controls, and how badly it has been affected. Defective enzymes may play a part in food intolerance—they will be considered in more detail in chapter 12.

It looks very much as if celiacs are unfortunate casualties of the slow adaptation process between the human race and wheat. Wheat, after all, is a relatively new food—we have only had ten thousand years to get used to it, which is the blinking of an eye in evolutionary terms. Although natural selection should gradually eliminate any genes that make human beings susceptible to wheat (at least among wheat-eating populations), it seems to be a process that has not had time to run to completion. There is some evidence for this, in that wheat proteins reduce the absorption of starch in most people. (Starch, if unabsorbed, goes to feed bacteria in the gut, and could perhaps cause an overgrowth of unwanted bacteria.)

If this theory is correct, then it is possible that some nonceliacs are adversely affected (though not as seriously) by defensive chemicals found in wheat. Not just affected by very large amounts, as in the experiment described above, but affected by a normal, everyday intake of wheat. Natural selection works more slowly on a gene that has mild ill effects than on one with serious ill effects, such as celiac disease. So it is even more likely that *minor* problems with a new food would persist for thousands of years.

This could explain why wheat sensitivity is so common, although there are other equally plausible explanations. Wheat, along with milk, is the most commonly eaten food in Western countries, and may appear in every meal and snack of the day. There is little doubt that a food consumed frequently is far more likely to cause food intolerance (although no one knows precisely why); this alone could account for wheat's bad record.

Other foods, besides cereals, are a possible source of toxic or damaging chemicals. Some are known to cause false food allergy in susceptible individuals (page 109), and a few can cause cancer. Others, such as coffee, have a druglike (**pharmacological**) action on the body, which means that they produce marked physiological effects even though they are eaten in very small amounts. Some of these are looked at more closely on pages 113 and 212.

History Lessons

Another of our cultural myths is that the past is a perfect guide to what we should eat. Hence the common criticism of ideas about food intolerance: "Surely foods that have been eaten for thousands of years can't cause serious health problems—if they did, it would have been noticed before." In fact, experience shows that human beings are rather bad at identifying foods that cause nonacute, long-term illness. The rat, remember, waits only a day to see if a new food makes it ill. Like rats, we are programmed to notice short-term effects only.

The best illustration of this is the failure to identify wheat as a factor in celiac disease until the 1940s. It took a famine in Holland at the end of World War II to remove wheat from the diet, and an observant doctor to recognize that his celiac patients had been miraculously cured. Similarly, the islanders of Guam traditionally used the seeds of the false sago palm, a type of cycad, as food. Although they suffered from a high incidence of senile dementia, no one made any connection between this and the cycad seeds. But in the 1950s an epidemic of dementia began, which continues to this day. Scientists have traced it back to the war years when Guam was occupied by the Japanese, food was desperately scarce, and the islanders had to rely heavily on false sago palm as a result. A constituent of the seeds has proved responsible for degeneration of the nerves and brain.

A third example comes from China, where a cancer survey showed an unusually high level of esophageal cancer in one province (the esophagus is the tube that leads from the mouth to the stomach). The local tradition of making pickled vegetables in huge vats that were left to mature for months proved to be the cause. The thick layer of mold that grew on the pickles was producing **carcinogens** (cancer-producing compounds), which seeped into the pickles. Even though the mold was scraped off before the pickles were eaten, enough carcinogens were there to give susceptible people cancer.

The moral of these stories is not that food in general can cause fatal diseases—the cycad seeds and moldy pickles are extreme in that respect. The important lesson to be learned here is that history is sometimes a poor guide to diet.

Digesting the Facts
To add to the myths about food, there are some long-standing misconceptions about human digestion that fuel the arguments over food sensitivity. The most important one is that food is broken down into very small molecules before any of it is absorbed. Every high school biology student is taught: that the enzymes in the mouth, stomach, and small intestine break down food into its basic constituents. Starches (complex carbohydrates) are broken down into sugars, and proteins are broken down into amino acids. These very small molecules are then absorbed and enter the bloodstream, but larger molecules are excluded by the gut wall—or so the story goes. If this were true, food could not cause allergic reactions in the skin or airways: the molecules that got through the gut wall would be too small to provoke any reaction by immune cells in the blood, which only respond to fairly large molecules, not to simple sugars or amino acids.

Research carried out in the past twenty to thirty years has shown that this picture of digestion is very simplistic and misleading, but the news has been a long time getting through. In one study, healthy adults were given potato starch dispersed in water to drink. After fifteen to thirty minutes, blood samples contained up to three hundred starch grains per milliliter of blood.

After a meal, a small number of undigested or partially digested food molecules are found in the bloodstream, so it is clear that the gut wall is not as impregnable as was once thought. In fact, specialized areas of the gut wall actually sample the gut contents, actively taking up droplets of liquid that contain intact food molecules. How this is achieved is explained on pages 289–91.

TWO

Food Allergy, Mast Cells, and IgE

According to the most widely accepted definition, an *allergy* is any "id-iosyncratic reaction in which the immune system is clearly involved." However, the main agent of allergy is IgE, and allergists have tradition-ally concentrated on IgE reactions or **type I hypersensitivity**. These form the subject of this chapter and the two that follow. Allergic reactions that have nothing to do with IgE or mast cells are described in chapter 5, along with false food allergies.

The History of Food Allergy

Hippocrates, the father of medicine, was the first to record an allergic reaction to food. He observed that while cheese was a wholesome food for most people, some were made severely ill by eating it, even in very small amounts. Other Greek writers recorded violent reactions in cer-tain individuals to eggs, honey, strawberries, nuts, oysters, or other shell-fish. While some of these cases may have been false food allergy (see page 109) others were probably food allergy proper.

In 1921 two German scientists, Carl Prausnitz and Heinz Kustner, showed that something in the blood could reproduce such reactions. Kustner was sensitive to fish and developed urticaria, or hives, soon after eating it. A small amount of blood serum from Kustner was injected into Prausnitz's arm. The next day fish extract was injected into the skin at the same spot and produced a red, itchy bump. When tested previously, there had been no such reaction. The two scientists gave the name *reagin* to the unknown component in the blood that had caused the reaction in Prausnitz.

Proteins

Proteins make up our skin, hair, and bones. They are major components of the nerves, blood, and all other cells in the body. Specialized proteins in the muscles produce contraction by sliding over each other. Another hardworking protein called hemoglobin carries oxygen around in the blood, while strong, elastic proteins make up our tendons and ligaments. Chemically adept proteins known as enzymes control all the chemical reactions in the body and regulate every living process (see page 21). Antibodies, and many other crucial components of the immune system, are also proteins.

Proteins can do these many different jobs because they are made up of long chains of chemicals called **amino acids.** The types of amino acid present and the order in which they occur are different for each type of protein. Once the chains have been formed, they are folded up in a specific way to give a compact protein molecule, often spherical or sausage shaped. In the case of enzymes, one small area on the surface of the molecule is the **active site,** where the crucial chemical reaction controlled by that enzyme occurs. Similarly, in antibodies, the particular combination and arrangement of amino acids at the **antigen-binding site** (see page 28) decides which antigen it will bind.

There are twenty common types of amino acid, each with its own distinctive chemical properties. Some are attracted to water; others repel it. Some can react with one type of molecule; others do not. It is the different combinations of amino acids that make proteins so different from one another. They give enzymes their impressive range of chemical abilities, and account for the versatility of antibodies.

The test became known as the **Prausnitz-Kustner test, or passive transfer test,** and was at one time used in diagnosing allergies. (The only reason it is no longer used is that there is a risk of transferring viral infections such as hepatitis and AIDS.) Progress thereafter was slow, and it was more than forty years before scientists could say exactly what reagin was. The breakthrough came in the 1960s, the result of painstaking research by a Japanese husband-and-wife team, Kimishige and Teruko Ishizaka, working in the United States. They discovered that reagin is a type of antibody now known as IgE.

Fighting Infections—The Versatile Antibody

Antibodies are special molecules produced by the body to fight off infections. They bind firmly to the bacterium or virus that causes the infection, an action that can block infection in a variety of ways. With viruses, which are extremely small, antibodies may be able to prevent them from invading the body's cells simply by binding to them. With bacteria, however, antibodies alone are ineffectual; they need help to defeat the bacteria. Their job is to act as signals to other cells and molecules in the body that have the power to kill. The antibodies form a coat on the surface of the bacterial cells, and this stimulates the immune system's "assassination teams" to go into action against the bacteria.

Antibodies are protein molecules, as are many of the important, hardworking components of the body (see page 26). Proteins are infinitely variable molecules; this is what makes them so useful. In the case of the antibodies, their versatility is employed in making molecules that bind specifically to a particular target molecule, or antigen, and to no other. The measles virus, for example, is bound by antibodies that specifically recognize proteins in the outer coat of the virus—these being the measles antigens. They do not normally bind to anything else, apart from the measles virus.

Anatomy of an antibody

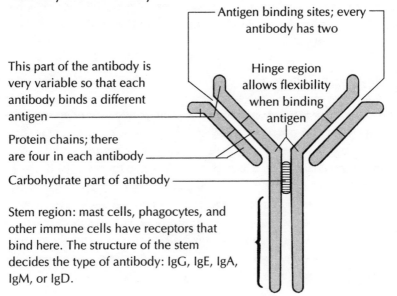

Antigen binding sites; every antibody has two

Hinge region allows flexibility when binding antigen

This part of the antibody is very variable so that each antibody binds a different antigen

Protein chains; there are four in each antibody

Carbohydrate part of antibody

Stem region: mast cells, phagocytes, and other immune cells have receptors that bind here. The structure of the stem decides the type of antibody: IgG, IgE, IgA, IgM, or IgD.

The body produces a vast range of different antibodies—millions of them—so that if it has to combat a new bacterium or virus, it is certain to find an antibody "in stock" that is just right for it. The antibodies are produced by special factory cells called **B cells,** and each B cell produces its own particular form of antibody. When faced with an invading microbe, the body selects a B cell with the right antibody to match that microbe, stimulates the cell to divide, and then instructs all the cells that are descended from it to produce their much-needed antibody. This continues until there is enough of the correct antibody to defeat the infection.

Different Types of Antibody

Antibodies are Y-shaped molecules, as the picture on page 27 shows. At the tip of each arm is an antigen-binding site where the antibody can bind to the particular feature of the antigen that it recognizes. These antigen-binding sites are the most changeable part of the antibody molecule—they vary enormously from one antibody to another. Their chemical structure determines which antigen is bound by that antibody.

The stem of an antibody can also vary, although nothing like as much. There are five basic types of stem, and they produce five different types of antibody, known as **isotypes.** The names of these isotypes (in order of abundance) are: IgG, IgA, IgM, IgD, and IgE. In all cases the letters *Ig* stand for "immunoglobulin"—another name for antibody. Imbalances between the different isotypes of antibody may play a role in food intolerance, and they will appear again in chapter 12.

IgE and Mast Cells

IgE molecules are just as specific for their antigen as other antibody isotypes, but they operate in a rather different way. Their main function is to defend the body against parasites such as ringworms and flukes—these are much larger than bacteria and viruses, so the body has different strategies for killing them. In the Tropics, where parasites are common, quite high levels of IgE may be found even in nonallergic people. Cooler conditions are not as favorable to parasites, and high standards of public hygiene in the West have reduced parasitic worm infections even further, so that they are now very rare. Consequently, in nonallergic people living in temperate climates, the level of IgE is usually very low.

Like other antibodies, IgE molecules are produced by B cells. But once they have been produced, the IgE molecules behave differently from most other antibodies in that they attach themselves to **mast cells** and **basophils.** These two types of cell look slightly different under the microscope, and whereas basophils are found floating in the blood, mast cells are embedded in the solid tissues of the body. Mast cells are better known and understood, so we will conveniently ignore the basophils from here onward: the two types of cell probably work in much the same way.

Although the stem of the IgE molecule is attached to the mast cell, the antigen-binding sites are still free. So when the right antigen comes along, it will bind to the IgE molecules. This is the signal the mast cell has been waiting for. Packets of chemicals inside the cell are suddenly released to the outside, where they act as messengers, causing major changes in the cells and tissues around them. One of the main chemicals to be released is called **histamine**—hence the use of drugs that counteract its effects, **antihistamines,** in the treatment of allergies. The packets of chemicals inside the resting mast cell look like small granules under the microscope, so the process of releasing the chemicals is called degranulation.

Histamine and other chemicals released by mast cells are called **mediators** because they bring about, or mediate, changes in the body. A powerful cocktail of mediators, containing ten or more separate substances, spills out of a degranulating mast cell. Each mediator has its own particular effect on the body—some make the blood vessels open out; others make them leakier so that blood escapes through the vessel wall. Several mediators make smooth muscles (also called involuntary muscles) contract—these are muscles that operate our lungs, stomach, intestine, and bladder. When they contract sharply, air may be expelled from the tubes leading to our lungs, or semidigested food from our bowels.

This is bad news for parasites, which may be directly affected by the mediators themselves, and then assaulted by the body's reaction to the mediators. In the case of parasites in the gut, for example, the direct effect of the mediators may make the parasites loosen their grip, and the diarrhea that follows flushes them out of the body. For parasites in the blood, the expansion and leakiness of blood vessels produces the redness and swelling that we describe as inflammation. One feature of inflammation is that all-purpose defensive cells called

The Ubiquitous Mast Cell

Mast cells are found embedded in our tissues throughout the body. They are especially common around the tubes leading to the lung (the **bronchi**), in the nose, and in the gut—in other words, they are well positioned to guard the body's vulnerable entrance points from parasites. Each mast cell can have as many as a hundred thousand IgE molecules on its surface. These will not all be from the same B cell, so they will respond to different antigens.

The chemical mediators that do so much damage to allergic individuals are stored in tiny membrane-bound packets inside the mast cell. These give the cell a granular appearance under the microscope. For the mast cell to release its packets of mediators—to **degranulate**—an antigen must bind more than one IgE molecule on the cell surface. The crucial signal for degranulation is the cross-linking of two or more IgEs by an antigen.

Although this is the main way of making mast cells degranulate, there are other methods as well. Some foods contain substances that trigger mast cells directly, causing false food allergies in certain people (see page 109). Some bacteria produce toxins that can trigger mast cells directly. It may even be possible for the body to trigger mast cells itself, in response to an irritant substance in food, for example. These different methods of firing the mast cells make the diagnosis of allergy a complex business.

phagocytes (which simply means "eating cells") are attracted to the site of the invasion. Phagocytes can engulf and destroy the unwanted invaders, as shown on pages 292–93.

One group of phagocytes, the **macrophages** (big eaters) have the role of perpetuating the inflammation reaction. They produce an enzyme (see page 21) called **phospholipase** or **PLA**. What PLA then does is cut up certain fat molecules—the **phospholipids**—found in the membranes of all our body cells. The fragments released from the phospholipids by PLA are then worked on by other enzymes, which turn them into potent chemical mediators, known as **prostaglandins**.

There are at least twenty different types of prostaglandin and they have a variety of effects on the body, but all are involved in regulating the immune response, and particularly the inflammation response. Some

How a mast cell is triggered into action

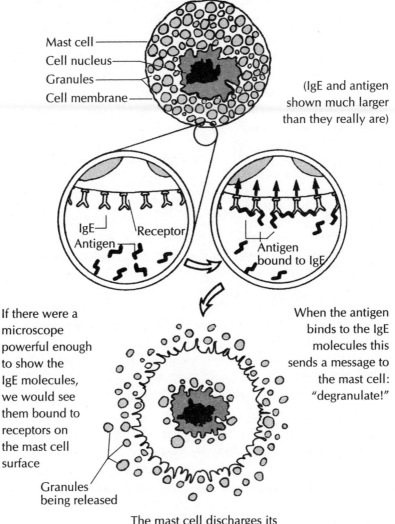

Mast cell
Cell nucleus
Granules
Cell membrane

(IgE and antigen
shown much larger
than they really are)

IgE
Antigen
Receptor

Antigen
bound to IgE

If there were a
microscope
powerful enough
to show the
IgE molecules,
we would see
them bound to
receptors on
the mast cell
surface

When the antigen
binds to the IgE
molecules this
sends a message to
the mast cell:
"degranulate!"

Granules
being released

The mast cell discharges its
granules, which then break
open to release histamine and
other mediators

prostaglandins have opposite effects on the body from others, so it appears that they work together, one modifying the actions of the other. In this way, they can fine-tune the body's response to damage or danger.

The prostaglandins produced in the aftermath of a mast-cell reaction are responsible for keeping up the attack on the invader. So it is no coincidence that they have an effect on the body similar to histamine's: they make smooth muscles contract and promote inflammation. They help produce the late-phase reactions seen in allergic individuals, which are considered in more detail on page 48.

Mast-cell reactions are not the only source of prostaglandins in the body, and these ubiquitous messengers also play a role in diseases such as rheumatoid arthritis (see pages 164–66). Prostaglandins can be made by almost any body cell. Indeed, they are made all the time, and constantly destroyed before they can have any effect (a common type of control mechanism in living organisms). The effect of the macrophages, attracted by the mast cells, is simply to boost production of prostaglandins so that they are made faster than they are destroyed. Several other types of cell can boost prostaglandin manufacture in the same way.

How IgE Produces Allergies

Anyone who lives in a town or city will have been kept awake, at some time or another, by the sound of a burglar alarm ringing endlessly in an empty shop or house. The alarm is meant to ring only if someone breaks in, but it can be triggered by some other quite innocent event, such as a strong wind or the vibrations of a passing truck. This is more or less what happens in the case of allergies. The mast cells, which are meant to respond to invasion by parasites, are triggered by an innocuous substance such as eggs or cow's milk. But why should this happen?

The answer is that the body misguidedly makes IgE antibodies that fit the antigens in these substances. A very complex and intricate set of controls normally prevent the body from making IgE in response to such harmless materials, but in the allergic individual something goes awry and the control mechanisms break down.

In the case of Jane, her body had mistakenly made IgE antibodies to a protein antigen in peanuts. The strange symptoms that she experienced upon eating peanuts were all produced by mediators released from her mast cells. Mast cells in the tissues of the mouth were triggered as soon as the food came into contact with them, producing symptoms almost immediately. Her lips and tongue swelled up because tiny blood vessels inside them became leaky, allowing fluid to seep out into the surrounding tissues.

The cause of Jane's collapse (**anaphylactic shock**) when she ate peanuts again was a sudden drop in blood pressure, likewise produced by the mediators. This time, it seems, more IgE was present and far more mediators released. By making the blood vessels all over her body expand and become leakier, the mediators left her without enough blood pressure to keep the vital organs functioning.

In the case of asthma, it is the effect of histamine on the smooth muscles of the bronchi and bronchioles (the smaller airways) that produces the symptoms. These vital tubes, which carry air to the lungs, go into a spasmodic contraction. How the allergens reach the airways, and the types of allergens involved, will be dealt with in chapter 3. The way in which mast cells cause other allergic reactions, such as hay fever and perennial rhinitis, will also be described there.

As you might expect, people with these allergic disorders tend to have a higher level of IgE in their blood than others. But there are a few whose IgE levels are normal. Conversely, there are quite a large number of people who have high levels of IgE and give positive skin-prick tests to common allergens (see box on pages 34–35), but who display no symptoms. Perhaps these symptom-free individuals have fewer, or less accessible, mast cells than others, making them less susceptible to high IgE levels. Or perhaps the mechanisms behind allergy are more complex than they appear, and IgE is only part of the story.

Antigens and Allergens

Are antigens and allergens fundamentally different from each other? This is a question that causes a lot of confusion and it is worth spending some time looking at what these two words actually mean.

An **antigen** is any molecule that can provoke the body into producing antibodies to it. To do this the molecule must be above a certain size, because the B cells and their colleagues in the immune system are programmed to ignore very small molecules. So simple chemical molecules, such as water or salt, cannot act as antigens. However, some quite small molecules, which are too small to act as antigens on their own, may combine with proteins in the body, thus producing molecules that are large enough to be recognized by the immune system. Small molecules of this sort are called **haptens**.

Living organisms are composed of a great variety of chemical compounds, and some make more effective antigens than others. The important point about an antigen is that it should have at least one distinctive chemical structure on its surface—a chemical "handle" that the antibody can grab

---

Skin-Prick Tests

The standard test for allergy is the skin-prick test, which looks at how the skin reacts to allergens. These tests may also be called: prick/puncture skin tests (PSTs), prick-skin tests, scratch tests, or prick-scratch tests. (Note that skin-prick tests are not the same as patch tests—see page 108; the skin tests used to assess the dose for neutralization therapy, see page 360; or intradermal tests, a traditional test for allergy, rarely used in the United States now because of the risk of anaphylactic shock.)

Allergen extracts are used; these are prepared from pure samples of foods, pollens, house dust mite, and so on. A drop of the extract is placed on the arm, and a prick or scratch made in the skin below the drop. A minute amount of the allergen enters the skin, and if the patient is sensitive to the allergen there will be a marked reaction, known as a **wheal-and-flare** response.

Skin-prick tests work well for some types of allergen, particularly inhalants, but are never 100 percent accurate. Where the allergen is found in food, they are generally much less useful. First, of course, they will be negative in cases of non-IgE food allergies (see page 95) and in food intolerance. Additionally, there are often positive skin responses to foods in atopic individuals, despite the fact that there are no actual symptoms when the foods are eaten (a false positive).

With immediate reactions food, false negative results—negative blood and skin tests despite a genuine reaction to the food—are rarer, at least in adults and older children, but are often seen in babies under one year. If you give a false negative result, most allergists will conclude that you are not allergic to that food, but this is not always correct, and if you are convinced that you react to that food, ask for a double-blind placebo-controlled food challenge to be performed. Check that there are no other reasons why the result might be falsely negative (see below).

With delayed reactions to food involving asthma or atopic eczema, skin-prick tests are not particularly useful. False negatives are

hold of. This structure, which the antibody recognizes, is called the **epitope**.

One major group of antigen is the proteins, which are widespread in all living things (see page 26). The chemical variety of proteins makes them good antigens—there are plenty of distinctive handles for an antibody (itself a protein) to seize. Some other chemicals found in living things

particularly common in babies with atopic eczema, and false positives also occur (see page 108).

Not all false reactions to skin-prick tests can be explained, and very little research has been done on this. However, research has shown that sometimes skin-prick tests give false negatives simply because the reaction is localized—in the gut, nose, or wherever. IgE antibodies can often be found in the part of the body that is affected, but they have clearly not entered the bloodstream, which is why they are not present in the skin.

There can also be faults in the test procedure that give false negatives. Taking antihistamines will decrease your response, and you should stop these drugs several days before the test—the time varies depending on the particular antihistamine, so check with your doctor. Treatment with steroids, either as creams or tablets, can also diminish the reaction. Commerical allergen extracts do not work well for fruit and vegetable allergies, because the allergenic proteins are unstable. A good allergist will repeat the test with fresh juice extracted from the food. This may also be appropriate for a nonvegetable food where you have had clear-cut reactions to eating it but the test is negative.

Patients may be offered a choice between skin-prick tests and RAST blood tests for IgE (see page 111) for diagnosis. The latter are more expensive, and not significantly more accurate than the humble skin test. Reasons to choose RAST rather than skin-prick tests include:

- extreme sensitivity to foods, when a skin-prick test can produce a severe reaction; these are unpleasant but very rarely fatal
- severe skin disease affecting most of the body, which makes skin testing difficult
- dermatographism—scratching the skin or touching it roughly produces hives where touched
- difficulty in stopping antihistamines

are less distinctive chemically and they do not readily act as antigens—fats and oils, for example. Complex carbohydrates—which are made up of chains of sugar molecules—can act as antigens, although the sort that we eat in quantity (such as the starch found in potatoes and bread) are very dull chemically and unlikely to be antigenic. These foods also contain proteins, however, and it is mainly these that act as antigens.

The other potential source of antigens in food, apart from the proteins, are small molecules such as phenols, amines, and carotenoids. Some of these give the food its color and flavor; others are there to deter animals from feeding on that food, or prevent it being attacked by bacteria and fungi. The majority of these small molecules are natural compounds, but artificial colors, flavors, and preservatives greatly increase the number present in modern food.

Most of these molecules are too small to be antigens in their own right, but can act as haptens. To do this they must combine with proteins in the food itself, or with proteins in our bodies—something they may do quite easily, as they tend to be very reactive. The extent to which these small molecules can act as haptens is somewhat controversial, and the issue is clouded by the fact that many of these compounds also have toxic or pharmacological (druglike) effects on the body.

An **allergen** is essentially the same thing as an antigen, except that it happens to cause an allergic reaction in a particular person. The proteins in cow's milk, for example, are antigens to most of us, but for the child with cow's-milk allergy, they are allergens. *The main difference between an antigen and an allergen is not in the molecule itself but in the way the individual's immune system reacts to it.*

Having said that, some foods are more allergenic—more likely to cause allergies—than others. It seems that either the food antigens themselves, or some other item found in the same food, stimulates the immune system to respond more aggressively. One group of natural substances that might do this are the lectins. These are protein molecules, found in many foods, which are not usually allergens themselves, but which bind to human cells. They cling to cells in the gut, and they may also be able to pass through the gut wall into the bloodstream, thus reaching every part of the body. Some lectins are known to affect the immune response, and a few promote the formation of IgE at the expense of other antibodies, especially in people prone to allergies. Many of the foods that commonly feature in food allergy, such as peanuts, are particularly rich in lectins. Perhaps the peanut lectins make the body more inclined to form IgE—so producing allergies to the other constituents of peanut.

The foods that most commonly cause food allergy are cow's milk, egg, wheat, soy, peanuts, tree nuts, shellfish, and fish, with items such as sesame seed and poppy seed in the second rank. Many fruits and vegetables also cause allergic reactions, usually through cross-reaction from another allergen (see pages 376–78), but the symptoms are usually limited to the mouth (Oral Allergy Syndrome).

Just because certain foods are more commonly implicated in allergy than others, it does not mean that allergy to other foods is ruled out. Pretty much any food can cause an allergic reaction, judging by the reports in medical journals. If you have an allergy to something unusual, such as garlic, buckwheat, chamomile tea, or fenugreek, you may be told that this is "impossible"—even physicians are known to make this mistake, unfortunately.

Another misconception—this time confined to patients—needs mentioning here. There is no simple link between particular foods and particular symptoms in either IgE-mediated food allergy or food intolerance. Some sufferers get the idea that one food causes anaphylaxis, another causes hives, another asthma. It doesn't work like that. Although there are some tendencies—peanuts have a strong tendency to cause anaphylaxis, for example—there are no tight food-symptom links. Many other foods can cause anaphylaxis, and peanuts can evoke other symptoms.

The Allergic Family

Classical allergic disorders, such as hay fever, perennial rhinitis, asthma, and urticaria, tend to run in the family: parents who suffer from them are much more likely than others to produce children with allergies. And if both parents have allergic problems, then the children have an even higher chance of being affected. Not that the child and the parent will necessarily suffer from the same disorder. The parent may have severe rhinitis while the child suffers from asthma and eczema—or vice versa. Indeed, the child may begin with eczema in babyhood, lose the symptoms at two or three years of age, but then develop asthma instead. These facts all suggest an underlying predisposition to allergy that manifests itself in different ways.

Doctors describe this constellation of symptoms as **atopy,** a word whose derivation and meaning are difficult to pin down. It comes from the Greek and is variously defined as meaning "no place," "out of place," or "another place." It is generally understood to mean that there is a deep-rooted problem that may produce symptoms in various places on the body, not just in one place as with most diseases. Patients with any of these classical allergic symptoms tend to be described as atopic, especially if other members of their family have allergies. They almost always show a positive reaction to the skin-prick test (see page 34) when tested with a variety of common allergens.

Although atopics have more IgE in their blood than the average person, if the offending allergen can be eliminated—by avoiding a particular food, for example—their IgE levels often return to normal. So it seems possible that the root cause of the problem is a failure to suppress IgE production to particular substances.

Clearly the genes responsible for these control mechanisms are not operating normally, but why the controls are so specific for particular substances is not known. It is especially puzzling in individuals who are violently allergic to just one substance. Other, less fortunate, individuals are allergic to a wide range of substances and readily develop new allergic reactions. In such cases it would seem that there is a more generalized fault in the IgE control mechanism.

All in the Genes?

If atopy is inherited, then the genetic information that is passed on from parent to child must in some way be faulty. Studies of atopic families have led to some understanding of the genetic mechanisms involved, and they help explain some puzzling features of the problem.

By looking at seven families with asthma and allergic rhinitis, researchers in Oxford, England, identified a single gene that they believe is largely responsible for allergies. This discovery, published in 1989, was a surprise to doctors and research workers, who had previously thought that several genes must be involved. (Some still suspect that this really is the case.)

Everyone carrying this gene shows some positive reactions to skin-prick tests, or to laboratory tests for IgE. However, 15 percent of those carrying the gene have no symptoms. And among the other 85 percent, the severity of the symptoms varies greatly. All this suggests that other factors are at work. They may be minor genes that modify the effects of the main one, or they could simply be environmental factors, such as breathing polluted air, a damp or dusty home, infections, or diet.

It is definitely the case that the environment affects the likelihood of developing allergic responses. Identical twins—who carry exactly the same genes—can differ in terms of allergy. One may be afflicted and the other not, showing that something in the environment, which only one has experienced (probably an infection), is also important. It is interesting that Scandinavian babies born in the spring, when birch pollen is in the air, are more likely to develop hay fever later in life. And in the case of food, early exposure to potential allergens is risky for the children of atopic parents (see pages 307–9).

It is clear then, that the allergy gene creates a tendency to allergy, and environmental factors, especially early in life, may then push the individual into expressing that potential. The question remains whether these factors alone can explain why 15 percent with the crucial gene have no symptoms, or whether minor genes might also be involved.

The fact that parents with no obvious symptoms and no atopic relatives can still produce an atopic child suggests the existence of minor genes. Either the mother or the father is probably carrying the main gene for allergy, but its effects are masked by more beneficial genes. When all the parental genes are reshuffled to produce eggs and sperm, and then combined with genes from the other parent, a different genetic setting is produced. In this setting the main allergy gene is no longer masked.

Allergy and Age

If defective genes lead to allergy, then we would expect most allergies to begin early in life, as indeed they do. Symptoms cannot be produced the first time a person is exposed to an allergen, however. Although the body already has the capacity to produce antibodies to the allergen concerned (in the form of as-yet-unactivated B cells), the antibody itself is not there. An initial exposure is required to enable the body to find the right B cell from its extensive stock and multiply it up to useful levels. Once this has happened, a second exposure to the allergen can stimulate antibody (IgE) production. The allergen can then trigger IgE-coated mast cells—with devastating results.

Despite this, babies may react to a food allergen the first time they eat it, because molecules of the food may have reached them by other means. One such route is breast milk, which contains molecules from the foods the mother herself is eating—only a few, of course, but enough to sensitize a highly atopic baby. Some babies may even be sensitized before birth by food molecules in the mother's blood that pass into the fetus's blood. So it is important for atopic mothers-to-be to think about their diet. Chapter 13 suggests practical steps that can be taken by parents to reduce the risk of sensitizing their children.

As children get older, their early symptoms often disappear or at least diminish. Allergies to milk, egg, and soy are those most likely to disappear with age, while allergies to peanuts, nuts, and fish tend to persist into adult life.

For some children the initial symptoms of the allergy, such as eczema, may disappear only to be replaced by other symptoms, such as asthma. Others apparently lose their allergic reaction entirely, but may succumb to other health problems in adult life that turn out to be food related. There has never been any systematic study of such patients, so it is difficult to know whether their childhood illness has in any way influenced their health later. But some doctors who specialize in treating food allergy believe that the child's allergic reaction to foods does not disappear but is simply suppressed by the body, only to recur in adult life, often in a different form. Pediatricians say that children grow out of their allergies, but perhaps they only grow out of their pediatricians!

If this theory is correct, it might be better to investigate their allergic problems more closely in childhood and, in the case of food allergens, to eliminate the incriminated foods from their diet, rather than simply waiting for them to "grow out of it." Experience shows that cutting out allergenic foods for a period of time—a few months, a year, or sometimes longer—can often eliminate the sensitivity in the long term, as well as providing more immediate relief from the child's symptoms. But there are a variety of other factors to consider—some of which will be discussed in more detail later.

Although most allergies (particularly the acute types of food allergy) first appear in childhood, there are a few adults who suddenly develop an allergy for no obvious reason. Dr. A. W. Frankland, formerly of St. Mary's Hospital in London, describes the case of a woman of fifty who suddenly became allergic to sesame seeds, which she had previously eaten without difficulty. One day while eating a cookie containing sesame, her mouth and throat began to tingle, and hives developed on her skin. These symptoms disappeared after an hour. When she ate another such cookie two weeks later, the reaction was far more severe. Her lips and eyelids swelled, hives developed all over her body, and she collapsed unconscious on the floor. Only prompt medical attention saved her life. This is an unusual, but not isolated, case, and it is difficult to explain in terms of what we now know about allergies as inherited disorders.

THREE

The Classical Allergic Diseases

The classical allergic diseases are hay fever, perennial rhinitis, asthma, urticaria, atopic eczema (atopic dermatitis), and immediate-onset food allergy. The way in which IgE produces these problems—by stimulating mast cells and basophils to release damaging chemical mediators—is described in chapter 2. This chapter looks at each disease in more detail, and considers the relative roles of different types of allergen.

Multiple Causes

Allergens can be conveniently divided into four groups: those we eat, the **food allergens** or **ingestants**; those we breathe in, the **inhalants**; those that come into contact with our skin, the **contactants**; and those that are injected, such as insect stings or antibiotics, the **injectants**. Airborne allergens, such as pollen and dust, can act in two ways: as inhalants, when they are breathed in, and as contactants, when they land on the skin or eyes.

At one time doctors thought that the type of allergic reaction depended solely on the sort of allergen involved—inhalants would only cause problems in the nose and lungs, contactants would only cause problems on the skin, and food would only cause problems in the mouth and gut. The demise of this simplistic view of allergies has been described on page 13.

In any one allergic disease, there may be two or more allergens at work, some airborne, others ingested. Dr. Harry Morrow-Brown describes the case of a two-year-old boy whose atopic eczema improved considerably after milk and beef were excluded from his diet. However, he did not lose all his symptoms. Some months later his parents took him on vacation, and to their surprise the child recovered completely while away. On the journey home they picked up their pet dog from the boarding kennel; before they reached home the child was scratching as much as ever. It turned out that the particles of skin (dander) produced by the dog were a contributory cause of the eczema, aggravating the symptoms produced by milk and beef. With the dog banished and the house thoroughly cleaned, the boy's skin healed completely.

As this example shows, considerable detective work is often necessary to track down the many contributing causes of an allergic reaction. With problems such as asthma and rhinitis, particularly, it is essential to understand the part that airborne allergens play before trying to assess the role of food. Although this book is, strictly speaking, about food allergy, we must also consider the role of inhalants and contactants in these allergic diseases.

Hay Fever

Pollen, produced by plants and carried on the wind, is the most notorious of the airborne allergens—it causes the symptoms known to doctors as **seasonal allergic rhinitis and conjunctivitis** and to the rest of the world as hay fever. Not all hay-fever sufferers respond to the same pollen, and the timing of the symptoms will depend on which pollen is the culprit (see page 85).

Mast cells in the nose and eyes respond to the proteins in the outer coat of the pollen grain. The mediators that are released cause inflammation of the delicate membranes, which the hay-fever sufferer experiences as red, itchy, watery eyes and a runny or congested nose. Some people also suffer from itching in the mouth or ears. Irritability and fatigue may accompany these physical symptoms, although whether these occur as a direct effect of the allergens on the nervous system or simply as a secondary effect of the unpleasant physical symptoms is debatable.

Food can probably contribute to hay fever, though pollen is always the major allergen. Some people find that by avoiding particular foods, they reduce their sensitivity to pollen, and a lucky few lose their hay-fever symptoms altogether. Sensitivity to foods can also mimic hay fever if the foods concerned cause rhinitis and are only eaten in the summer, or in much larger amounts then (see page 85).

Perennial Rhinitis—Constant Runny or Congested Nose

Hay-fever sufferers may feel sorry for themselves as the summer months approach, but they are envied by those afflicted with perennial rhinitis, who have to endure similar symptoms year-round. In their case it is usually airborne allergens, such as mold spores or house dust, that trigger mast cells in the nose. If the eyes are also affected, this will cause conjunctivitis. It is almost always airborne allergens that affect the eyes, but the nose is also susceptible to allergens from other sources, including food. For the full range of allergens that can provoke rhinitis, see pages 84–89.

Problems Caused by Rhinitis

The nose is intimately linked to several other organs, and problems here are likely to have effects elsewhere. Because the nose is connected to the middle part of the ear by a tube (the **Eustachian tube**), perennial rhinitis can affect the ears as well. The Eustachian tube's function is to drain any fluid from the ear and allow air to get in so that the pressure on either side of the eardrum is equalized. If the tube becomes blocked with mucus from the nose, air can no longer reach the middle ear; the air already there may also be replaced by a thick, sticky secretion produced by the ear itself. This mucus sticks to the delicate bones that play a vital role in our hearing, and thus causes deafness. The condition is known as **chronic**

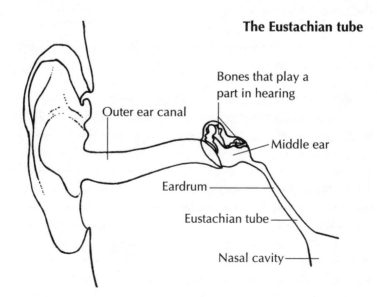

The Eustachian tube

Bones that play a part in hearing

Outer ear canal

Middle ear

Eardrum

Eustachian tube

Nasal cavity

Chris

Chris had been fascinated by aircraft since he was a small boy, and he loved his job as a pilot, flying helicopters out to oil rigs. Unfortunately, he suffered badly with what he called hay fever, although it affected him for most of the year. He had to take antihistamines to ease his streaming nose and eyes, but these made him drowsy, and soon his job was at risk. His doctor tried a battery of skin-prick tests with common allergens such as pollen, house dust, feathers, and cat dander, but there was no positive response to any of these. She then tried more direct forms of testing in which house dust and other allergens were sprayed into the nose. These tests were also negative. Since so much depended on curing Chris's rhinitis, his doctor talked to him in detail about his lifestyle, in the hope of getting a clue to what might be the problem. Chris was sure that he lived a very healthy life—in fact, he was something of a health fanatic, who took lots of exercise and was keen on weight training. He was also very careful about what he ate, and took yeast tablets every day for extra vitamins. The doctor asked him, as an experiment, to cut these tablets out for a while. She was aware of some people having allergic reactions to yeast, and while she thought it unlikely that yeast could cause Chris's symptoms, anything was worth a try. To her surprise—and Chris's—his nose was completely clear within four days. When he tried taking the tablets again, his rhinitis promptly returned. Later he discovered that he would get a milder form of rhinitis from drinking large amounts of beer, or eating a lot of bread, but in general he has had no further problems.

secretory otitis media (CSOM) or glue ear, and although it may be caused in other ways, allergy (particularly to house dust mite) is undoubtedly an important one. The problem is particularly common in children.

Recently doctors have discovered that glue ear is related to passive smoking—a child living among cigarette smokers. It has long been known that tobacco smoke prevents the lungs from keeping themselves clear of particles, by paralyzing the tiny hairs that sweep them clean, and it now seems that tobacco smoke has the same sort of effect inside the ear.

Children suffering from glue ear are likely to complain of popping or itching in the ears, or say that their ears feel "blocked up." The first signs of deafness are sometimes mistaken for disobedience, because the children fail to do as they are told. In younger children there may be little outward sign of the problem, although some shake their head in a characteristic way or repeatedly scratch at their ears. Deafness may result in a child being slow to begin speaking—often the first indication that anything is wrong. Needless to say, there are a great many other reasons for delayed speech, and it would be a mistake to jump to conclusions on this basis alone.

The airways

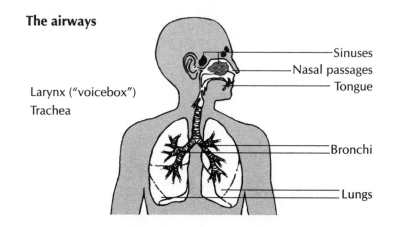

Larynx ("voicebox")
Trachea

Sinuses
Nasal passages
Tongue
Bronchi
Lungs

Other problems that can follow from rhinitis are allergic sinusitis and nasal polyps. The sinuses are air-filled cavities in the skull that are lined with delicate membranes linked with those lining the nose. Most cases of **sinusitis**—inflammation of these membranes—result from an infection in the nose that spreads outward. But allergic reactions can also occur here. The main symptoms of sinusitis are a severely blocked nose, with a headache over the eyes if the frontal sinuses are affected or an ache in the cheeks if the maxillary sinuses are inflamed.

Prolonged irritation to the membranes of the nose and sinuses can result in swelling, and this may eventually produce **nasal polyps** in some people—small grapelike protrusions of the membrane. The polyps are usually harmless, but they may obstruct the nasal passage, making breathing difficult. The sense of smell can also be lost, and there may be symptoms similar to sinusitis if the opening between a sinus cavity and the nose becomes blocked. The polyps can be removed surgically if they do cause discomfort. For some inexplicable reason, many cases of nasal polyps are seen in people who are sensitive to aspirin (see page 78).

One final problem that should be mentioned in connection with rhinitis is **postnasal drip** (sometimes known by the general name catarrh).

Excess mucus from the nose trickles down the back of the throat and thus into the **trachea**—the main tube leading to the lungs—to be coughed up later. Postnasal drip can follow various infections, but it is sometimes allergic in origin.

Asthma

The inhalants that cause rhinitis can also cause asthma, the target organs in this case being the tubes (or **airways**) leading from the trachea into the lungs, known as the bronchi and bronchioles. A variety of airborne allergens may be responsible; see pages 84–89.

When these allergens trigger mast cells in the airways, they cause

---

Helen

Helen had atopic eczema as a baby and began to have asthma attacks when she was about six. These got a great deal worse when she was eight years old, and on close questioning the doctor discovered that her parents had recently built an aviary inside the conservatory that was attached to their house. Skin-prick tests showed that Helen had a strong reaction to feathers, and when the birds were removed from the house her asthma settled down to its previous level. In the hope of getting rid of it completely, her parents replaced all feather pillows and cushions with foam-filled ones. Although this seemed to help a little, Helen still had asthma attacks once or twice a month. These frequently came on after parties or outings, and the doctor suggested that it might just be excitement triggering the attacks. Then her asthma started to become more frequent again, and as the attacks often took place at school, it was interfering with her studies. Helen's mother began to wonder if foods that Helen only had at parties or at school, during breaks, were responsible. Potato chips, soft drinks, and other food containing additives were obvious suspects, because Helen was not given this sort of food at home. She agreed to go without these foods for a month to see if this had any effect. Within a few days her attacks virtually disappeared, and tests with different types of additives showed that artificial colorings and sulfites could bring on an attack within a few hours. As long as she avoids junk food, Helen is now free of asthma.

Late-Phase Reactions

If an allergic patient is given a skin-prick test (see page 34), there will be a strong response—known as a wheal-and-flare reaction—almost immediately. This redness and itching subsides after some time, but then a different sort of reaction can set in, producing a larger, less itchy, but more painful lump. This is known as the **late-phase reaction,** and it is produced by the messenger substances called prostaglandins (see page 30) that play an important role in producing it.

When a person encounters allergens in everyday life, late-phase reactions are more difficult to discern, especially if there is frequent exposure to the allergen. But such a reaction can sometimes be observed in asthmatic patients, for example. Brief exposure to their allergen will produce an acute reaction almost immediately, followed by recovery, followed by a more insidious return of the asthma between four and twelve hours after the exposure. The late-phase reaction has usually exhausted itself by the next day.

Late-phase reactions are important, because they probably contribute substantially to the development of chronic allergic reactions—a long-term condition in which the patient is scarcely ever free of symptoms, although the severity of the symptoms may fluctuate. During late-phase reactions, the affected organ (such as the airways or the skin) tends to be more sensitive to nonspecific irritants, so the symptoms may be sparked again very easily, even if the allergen has been removed. A succession of late-phase reactions can easily lead to a situation where the organ is constantly overreacting to minor irritants.

Certain drugs block late-phase reactions by preventing cell membranes from releasing the phospholipid molecules that would normally be used to make prostaglandins. The drugs that do this are corticosteroids (prednisolone, for example), which mimic the action of hormones produced by the body. The fact that corticosteroids are so useful in controlling asthmatic symptoms shows what an important role late-phase reactions can have in allergic illness.

Corticosteroids are not simply used for allergy treatment—they suppress inflammation generally because prostaglandins are widespread messengers, produced in a variety of ways. They therefore find a use in diseases such as rheumatoid arthritis where inflammation needs to be controlled.

inflammation of the membranes lining the tubes, which become thicker and produce more mucus. This restricts the free passage of air and sets the stage for a full-blown asthma attack. Such an attack occurs when sufficient mediators are released by the mast cells to make the smooth muscles of the airways contract. The airways suddenly become much narrower. Stale air inside the lung cannot easily escape, so the lungs have difficulty drawing in fresh air with its life-giving oxygen. The air whistling through the constricted openings makes the characteristic wheezing sound.

While most asthmatics conform to the general pattern described above, there are also milder forms of the disease in which there is no wheezing and no asthma attack as such. In such cases the predominant symptom is breathlessness. Some asthmatics have a persistent cough as their main symptom.

Although inhalants are the major culprits in asthma, foods also play a part in about 80 percent of cases. Often there is more than one allergen involved (see page 85).

Asthma without Allergens
When asthma begins for the first time in adulthood, allergies are frequently not involved. No comprehensive studies have been made of the causes of asthma in adults, but cigarette smoke and other irritants in the air, especially at work, are often to blame. Sometimes asthma goes hand-in-hand with other damage to the lungs from such sources, creating a condition known as Chronic Obstructive Pulmonary Disease (COPD). Asthma that begins in childhood is almost always linked to allergies. Despite this, nonallegic factors can contribute substantially to attacks.

Asthmatics who are constantly exposed to their allergen—as is the case with house-dust sensitivity—are likely to have airways that are highly irritable, because of the inflammation in the membranous linings. The late-phase reaction, described in the box opposite, plays a large part in producing this state of chronic sensitivity. Once it has developed, all sorts of irritating stimuli can then spark an asthma attack. Common irritants include smoke (cigarettes, bonfires, and the like), factory fumes, ozone, colds and chest infections, cold air, and sulfur dioxide (given off by various foods and drinks; see appendix 1).

Becoming emotional or afraid can have the same effect as these airborne irritants, as can laughing, crying, excitement, or strenuous exercise.

It was the ability of the emotions to bring on an asthmatic attack that led to the mistaken notion of asthma being largely psychosomatic.

Hives and Edema

There can be several different causes for urticaria (also called hives or nettle rash), of which allergic reactions are just one. Where allergy is at the root of urticaria, it is probably the mast cells found in the lower layers of the skin that cause the problem. When they degranulate, the mediators released have a powerful effect on the tiny blood vessels, or **capillaries**, that lie all around them in the skin. These capillaries become leakier, allowing **serum** (the watery part of the blood) to seep out into the skin itself. This produces the characteristic swellings and itchiness of urticaria.

Where there is a great deal of seepage from the blood vessels, the tissues below the skin may also become filled with watery fluid. This produces a puffiness that doctors describe as **localized angioedema** (or **edema**). About 50 percent of people who are afflicted with urticaria also get angioedema, and some people have angioedema without any urticaria. However, there are a large number of other disorders that can produce angioedema, some of them very serious. They should all be eliminated by a full medical examination, before the possible role of allergy is investigated. (See also pages 100–101.)

There are two forms of urticaria, which differ in their timing. The type that troubled Kustner (see page 25) is **acute urticaria,** which comes on very rapidly and usually clears within twenty-four hours. It is usually accompanied by other symptoms, such as feverishness, faintness, or nausea and can be the first sign of anaphylactic shock (see page 33). **Chronic urticaria,** the other form, is a persistent rash, or one that appears for several hours every day or comes and goes over a much longer period of time. The official definition is hives that last longer than six weeks.

The blame for acute urticaria can usually be pinned on a food that was eaten just before the attack began, although there are other causes of acute urticaria, including insect stings, drugs (notably penicillin), and, more rarely, something that was applied to the skin. Whatever the cause, the reaction is usually so prompt and unequivocal that the patient easily makes the correct diagnosis.

With chronic urticaria, things are not so simple. This is a symptom that can be caused in dozens of different ways. Release of histamine from mast cells deep in the skin produces the symptoms, but the triggers that activate the mast cells vary enormously. The common triggers include:

- cold
- heat
- pressure or vibration
- exercise
- water
- light or UV light
- a long-term unrecognized infection elsewhere in the body
- a reaction to a food additive or to alcohol; these may act by triggering mast cells directly as in false food allergy (see page 109)
- drug sensitivity (often aspirin or related drugs, but it can also be antibiotics, sulfonamides, morphine, and other narcotics) sensitivity to histamine (found naturally in food, or produced by bacteria in the gut)
- gut flora imbalance (possibly, but controversially, including *Candida*)
- a reaction to preservatives (often parabens) used in creams and ointments
- sensitivity to food (a relatively uncommon cause)
- reactions to pollen (an uncommon cause)
- contact with latex, pets, or other items to which there is sensitivity (a relatively uncommon cause)
- premenstrual changes in hormones
- chemical sensitivity
- an autoimmune disease; in some cases the body produces antibodies against IgE, or against the receptors for IgE, both of which can activate mast cells
- a cancer (the least likely explanation)
- a rare hereditary defect
- a rare disease called mastocytosis in which the number of mast cells in the skin is greatly increased

The first six items are collectively described as *physical urticarias.* They are widely accepted by the medical profession, as are the last four causes listed. Varying degrees of controversy surround most of the other items (see pages 114–17). Several different causes may contribute to chronic urticaria, and in some cases, two or more factors have to be present at the same time to produce symptoms. This can make diagnosis of causes very difficult.

While atopic people are somewhat more likely to develop chronic urticaria than nonatopics there is no strong link with true allergy. Even where a particular food additive, food, or drug is responsible for the chronic urticaria, no allergy antibodies (IgE) are found to the offending item so skin-prick tests are not generally used in diagnosis.

Chronic urticaria is dealt with again in chapter 5, and treatment is described on page 114.

Atopic Eczema (Atopic Dermatitis)

Eczema is a term that is often used rather loosely for a variety of skin conditions. Strictly speaking, it means a red, itchy rash that tends to flake and then ooze or "weep" as it progresses. The disease is far more common in children, who usually compound the damage by constant scratching. Bacteria, fungi, or other microorganisms may infect the oozing skin and make matters still worse, while prolonged scratching will cause bleeding.

In adults, oozing does not generally occur, and the skin tends to become thickened instead. Some doctors feel that these symptoms should not be described as eczema, although they are undoubtedly the counterpart of childhood eczema. They therefore use the term *atopic dermatitis* as a general description of both types of disease. In this book we will use *eczema* for both children and adults, since this is the most widely understood term.

There are several different kinds of eczema, but what concerns us here is the variety known as **atopic eczema,** which is seen mainly in atopic individuals. What distinguishes it from other forms of eczema is the pattern of distribution over the body. The red itchy patches usually start on the face, particularly on convex areas such as the cheeks and chin. In time the skin on the face heals, and for some children this will be the end of their eczema. But for others the rash appears on the body, eventually settling in the folds of skin at the buttocks, knees, ankles, elbows, and wrists. In severe cases the rash may cover the whole body.

Atopic eczema is mainly a disease of childhood, although there are rare instances of it first appearing in adult life. About three-quarters of

---

Richard

Richard had suffered from eczema since he was just two months old, and when he was eight he still needed twice-daily applications of hydrocortisone cream to keep the itching under control. Since he did not seem to be growing out of his eczema, his mother asked the doctor if she could try changing his diet to see what effect that had. She was told to avoid eggs, milk, and all milk products as a first step, which she did. Within a week Richard's eczema had cleared up, and even when the cream was stopped it did not return. When milk was reintroduced into his diet, Richard was fine, but twenty-four hours after eating eggs he began to scratch furiously. By avoiding eggs he has remained free of eczema.

---

children affected develop the disease before they are a year old, and most in the first six months of life. The disease tends to come and go thereafter, and usually disappears by the age of fifteen. Because this type of eczema is so common in the children of atopic parents, and because it is usually followed (or accompanied) by hay fever or asthma, it is considered an allergic disease. However, this is not a typical allergic reaction; although IgE may be involved, mast cells play no part (see page 109).

Several different types of allergen can cause atopic eczema: allergens that are eaten (which affect about a third of children with atopic eczema), allergens that are inhaled, and allergens that contact the skin directly, either settling on the skin from the air, or contained in clothing, laundry detergents, or cosmetics.

However, allergens are often only part of the problem. General irritants, such as detergents, are also thought to be important, and these can bring on eczema in the sensitive individual.

Allergies to Food

The medical profession's original, rather limited concept of food allergy, as described on page 6, was of an immediate, violent reaction to food. Jane's reaction to peanuts was a textbook example of such an allergy. General advice on how to cope with such food allergies is given on pages 56–69.

Not all allergic reactions to food occur immediately after eating it, however. There is a rare form of food allergy in which the allergen is not an intact food molecule but one of the products of partial digestion. Eating the food produces no ill effects at first, but violent symptoms begin several hours afterward, as the food begins to break down in the stomach.

Delayed reactions are also seen when food contributes to allergic symptoms such as asthma, rhinitis, eczema, or chronic urticaria. It may be several hours or even days between the food being eaten and the symptoms appearing. With symptoms of this sort, it may also be necessary to eat quite large amounts of the food, or to eat it for several days in succession. If the food is one that is eaten regularly—as is often the case—the link between cause and effect is likely to be obscure, and food allergies of this type often go unrecognized. An elimination diet, of the kind described in chapter 14, may be necessary to work out what is causing the problem.

The idea of food producing symptoms in distant parts of the body, such as the nose or bronchi, may at first sight seem implausible, but research shows that allergens can be absorbed into the bloodstream intact (see page 23) and these must then be carried to all parts of the body. It is thought that these bloodborne allergens can react with mast cells in any susceptible organ. If the allergen were to interact with mast cells in blood vessels around the bronchi, for example, the mediators released by the mast cells would affect the nearby bronchial linings and the bronchial muscles—exactly the same effect as for airborne allergens. Not surprisingly, if a food produces asthma it usually produces other symptoms as well, because the allergen is being carried throughout the body.

In the case of rhinitis, the allergen can be carried to the nasal membranes in the bloodstream, producing symptoms six to ten hours after the meal or even later—up to twenty-four hours in some patients. Alternatively, the action of chewing food in the mouth may transmit allergens into the nasal cavity, thus provoking a response in the nose directly. Similarly, asthmatics can react to minute food particles that are inhaled while eating. Those with an exceptional sensitivity to peanuts have even been affected by someone else eating peanuts or peanut butter nearby.

Without doubt most sufferers from rhinitis, asthma, and associated problems are responding to airborne allergens alone. But a significant proportion suffer from food sensitivities that contribute to their symptoms, *and food may be the sole cause of the problem in some cases.* Until fairly recently, most doctors did not appreciate the importance of food in producing such symptoms; many children were diagnosed as having what was called "intrinsic asthma"—that is, asthma with no obvious external cause—when their wheezing may have been due to food. Similarly, atopic eczema has usually been treated with corticosteroid creams, which are successful for some but not the most severely affected. Trying to identify potential food triggers may be a better approach for such children.

Food Allergy in Babies

Food allergy usually shows itself in childhood, and the most common problem is a reaction to cow's milk among babies and young children. Babies who are bottle fed are obviously at greater risk of developing a sensitivity to cow's milk, but atopic babies who are breast fed can react badly to foods that the mother is eating, because minute quantities get into the breast milk. Again, cow's milk is a common problem, but it is certainly not the only one—any food that the mother eats may act as an allergen for the breast-fed baby, especially if eaten in large quantities.

Babies may react immediately to their allergen, with symptoms such as vomiting, urticaria, and swelling of the lips, face, and eyes. In such cases there is usually a positive skin-prick test. Once the allergen has been identified it must be avoided, for a while at least (see chapter 11). Some babies grow out of the allergic reaction in time.

Not all babies react to their allergen immediately. Some have a delayed reaction, with symptoms such as eczema, diarrhea, asthma, or rhinitis. Irritability, restlessness, and crying are also reported, although most doctors would not accept these as allergic symptoms. Infants with delayed symptoms often fail to give a positive skin-prick test, and the link with food may not be at all obvious, either to the mother or the doctor. Diarrhea in babies is dealt with more fully on pages 263–64. General guidelines for dealing with food sensitivity in babies and young children are described in chapter 11.

A few babies suffer recurrent pneumonia as a result of allergy to cow's milk. They will also have diarrhea or vomiting, show little appetite, and may have asthma or a runny nose as well. It seems likely that some milk is inhaled during feeding, and this causes an allergic reaction in the lungs.

If a baby is anemic, then allergy to cow's milk should be suspected, because this can cause bleeding from the digestive tract, which in turn leads to a shortage of iron. Sometimes the bleeding goes unrecognized, so that anemia is the first noticeable sign of the baby's food allergy.

FOUR

Treating Classical Allergies and Identifying Food Allergens

Allergies are well-recognized conditions, and those suffering from true food allergy are far more likely to receive adequate medical treatment than those with food intolerance. Even so, well-informed patients can make a significant contribution to their own treatment.

The patient who understands something about allergies may be able to help the doctor in unraveling the complexities of cause and effect. But it is important to stress that self-help should only be an adjunct to proper medical treatment, never a substitute. Some allergic conditions can be life threatening; others can deteriorate to the point where they produce irreversible damage to health. No one should attempt to treat them without medical supervision.

Options in Allergy Treatment

Because the mechanism behind true or classical allergies is well understood, the potential for treating them with drugs or with allergy shots is very good. The drugs used include **corticosteroids** (sometimes referred to simply as steroids, although they are not the same as the steroid drugs used by athletes), which have a general suppressive effect on inflammation; **antihistamines**, which counteract the effect of the mediator histamine; and leukotriene antagonists for use in asthma. (For more details on these drugs and how they work, see pages 431–43.) Although at one time there were serious side effects associated with many anti-allergy drugs, the modern formulations have overcome most of these problems. The drug treatments now available are both safe and effective.

Allergy shots usually consist of a series of weekly injections, spread over a period of months, beginning with a very low dose of the allergen and gradually increasing the dose. When successful, this treatment re-educates the immune system so that it no longer mounts an all-out reaction to the allergen. Hay fever is the most suitable candidate for treatment with allergy shots, and they may also be useful against perennial rhinitis. Physicians are more cautious, and rightly so, about using allergy shots for asthma, because the risks of a severe and potentially fatal reaction to the shots is higher. But, with care, asthmatics can also benefit from allergy shots.

Allergy shots do not seem to help with atopic eczema, probably because the immune reaction involved is different. Sometimes eczema symptoms actually get worse during such treatment, even though other allergic symptoms improve. (Some doctors report that enzyme potentiated desensitization [EPD]—see page 362—which seems to work in a different way from traditional allergy shots, is useful for atopic eczema, but there have been no scientific trials of this.)

Those with allergies to foods cannot, at present, be treated with allergy shots (see page 73) although this may change, and new vaccine-type treatments are being developed which could become available in the next few years (see page 73). Drugs, too, are of limited use in true food allergy.

This lack of treatment options means that, for those with a classic IgE-mediated reaction to food (the kind that comes on immediately with swelling or itching in the mouth, and sometimes progresses to a severe whole-body reaction and collapse) there is no option but to avoid the food completely (see page 58). However, there are other treatments which may help to make life-threatening food allergies less worrisome, by reducing sensitivity (see pages 71–72). The food still has to be avoided, but there is much less risk of dying from eating a trace of it in some concealed form.

Those rare and complex cases involving multiple IgE-mediated food allergies and delayed reactions such as diarrhea (which may be reactions to digestion products of the food, see page 54) can often be eased with additional treatments (see pages 71–72). Food avoidance is still needed, but the reactions to accidental ingestion are less severe, and the risk of developing new food allergies may also be reduced.

For those with asthma or atopic eczema in which food-reactions play a part, there is a choice between avoiding the offending food to alleviate symptoms, or controlling the symptoms with drugs.

Before embarking on an elimination diet for asthma or eczema, it is important to weigh the costs and benefits of dietary treatment. In cases where the symptoms are relatively mild, it may be better to rely on drugs alone. The decision involves a great many personal considerations, including, for example, the relative importance of food to the person concerned, this person's perseverance and willpower, and the number of meals that have to be eaten away from home. Nutritional needs also have to be taken into account. It is a decision that can only be made by the individual patient (or by the parents, in the case of a small child) in consultation with the doctor concerned.

What to Do about Immediate Allergic Reactions to Food

This is the one area where tracking down the source of the problem is unlikely to be difficult—except when reactions are not consistent (see page 65) and in the case of babies and small children, where some detective work may be necessary (see chapter 11).

What is hard is living with such an allergy. In the vast majority of cases, a food allergy of this type is lifelong and irreversible, and for highly sensitive individuals it can be life threatening. Assuming that you know which food or foods you are allergic to, the best policy is to avoid them scrupulously. Anyone who has had a severe reaction to food in the past should be aware that a further exposure can sometimes precipitate a worse reaction. If you have ever experienced swelling of the tongue and lips, difficulty in breathing, or generalized urticaria, then you should be *very cautious* indeed about trying the food again. If you have ever collapsed after eating a food (anaphylactic shock), then under no circumstances should you eat it again, however small the amount. Even a relatively mild reaction, such as vomiting and hives in response to a food, can be the foretaste of something much more serious, and it is vital that such warnings are heeded. A study published in 1998 revealed that one hundred fatal cases of food allergy occur in the United States each year.

Asthmatics are at particular risk, because a general anaphylactic reaction will induce a severe asthma attack at the same time, and this in itself can be fatal. Anyone with a true allergy to food who is also taking the drugs known as beta-blockers (used mainly for heart conditions; see page 63) should be aware that they increase the risk of a severe anaphylactic reaction, and make it more difficult to treat.

An initial test that can be done at home is to apply a small amount of the food to the face, making sure that none of it goes anywhere near the mouth. If this produces a rash, then the food should certainly not be eaten. If it does not, then it is worth approaching your doctor to see about skin-prick testing. A positive skin-prick test shows that the food is *not* safe to eat, but the reverse is not necessarily true, so foods that give a negative skin test must be eaten in tiny amounts at first, preferably with medical supervision in case there is a severe reaction. Once the offending food is identified for sure, you may want to keep it out of the house entirely, so that there is no risk of a small amount contaminating the food of the allergic person. A few peanut-allergic children are so sensitive to peanut allergens that they can be affected by the molecules of peanut butter that escape into the air while being eaten by others, or simply by a jar of peanut butter being opened.

Passengers on airlines have been affected by other passengers nearby opening packages of peanuts, and at least two airlines—British Airways and Air 2000—are now willing to eliminate peanuts on a particular flight if a highly peanut-sensitive person is traveling. One boy suffered a severe anaphylactic shock when a relative who had been eating peanuts kissed him—almost the kiss of death, except that he had an adrenaline injection kit (see page 62) and a mother who knew how to use it effectively and unhesitatingly.

Those with a serious food allergy, or the parents of food-allergic children, should have a comprehensive knowledge of the dishes and processed food products that are likely to contain their problem food. The lists on pages 383–99 can be a useful starting point: you may want to photocopy the relevant list and add your own discoveries of potentially risky items to this. The Food Allergy Network (see page 451) publishes this type of information regularly and will help in keeping you up to date. Most supermarkets and some food manufacturers now supply lists relating to their own products. You can also call the manufacturers with questions about specific foods.

Those who are highly allergic to certain foods should take note of the labels *spice, natural flavor,* and *artificial flavor.* These can include wheat, milk, corn, or potato in trace amounts—only a problem for the extremely sensitive individual. Spice can also include garlic oil, which is an allergen for a tiny minority. Pressure is being exerted on the Food and Drug Administration at present to make these labels more accurate and informative.

Incidental additives (such as wheat flour used to dust processing lines or prevent dried fruits from sticking together) do not need to be declared at all if they serve no function in the final product and are present in amounts that are considered insignificant by the manufacturer—a few parts per million seems to be the rule of thumb. Certainly, the vast majority of those with food allergy will survive eating such miniscule traces, but a few ultrasensitive individuals may not.

Any food-allergic person must be very cautious about eating in restaurants and cafés, and religiously read the labels on packaged food. Labels can be deceptive, however, because they often use unfamiliar words to describe a potentially allergenic food component—such as *lactalbumin* for one of the proteins found in cow's milk. For a full list of such synonyms, see appendix 3.

Another pitfall for label readers traveling outside of the United States is the "25 percent rule" on composite ingredients. In most of Europe, for example, when an ingredient such as sausage or salami is included in a product, it can be listed simply as "sausage" or "salami" as long as it constitutes less than 25 percent of the product. The individual ingredients of the sausage do not have to be listed. If the sausage contains soy meal, dried egg, milk powder, or wheat flour, as it could very well, this may cause serious problems. Avoid such products rather than take a potentially fatal risk. Even if you have eaten a packaged food safely in the past, you should look at the label every time you buy it because manufacturers can change the recipe.

Peanut-sensitive individuals should watch out for a new product— peanuts that have been stripped of their original flavor by chemical treatment, reflavored as almonds or other more expensive nuts, and molded to the appropriate shape. The packages will have to declare their ingredients, of course, but the bowl of nuts on a bar or party table may not be quite what it seems. There are also now available pretzels and cocktail balls with a peanut paste filling that is quite unexpected, and therefore potentially dangerous.

Never try to pick out the offending food from a dish that has already been prepared, and then eat what is left. Some unseen molecules of the food will have seeped into the mixture, and you may be sufficiently sensitive to react to them.

The biggest problem is eating out. In a recent American study, re-

Genetic Engineering and Food Allergy

There has been much concern expressed about the effects of genetic engineering on food allergy sufferers. It is reassuring to see that the concern is shared among government officials and those involved in the industry, and as a result there is probably little risk to consumers at present.

Regulatory agencies such as the FDA seem to be thoroughly aware of the risks and are prepared to be vigilant. In its 1992 biotechnology policy statement it stated that "a protein copied by genetic engineering from a food commonly known to cause an allergic reaction is presumed to be allergenic unless clearly proven otherwise. Any food product of biotechnology that contains such proteins must list the allergen on the label."

Biotechnology companies also seem to be taking allergies seriously. When Professor Steve Taylor of the University of Nebraska heard news of the transfer of a gene from Brazil nuts into soybeans, he raised the alarm. The new variety of soy was only intended for use as animal feed, but as Professor Taylor pointed out, once harvested one soybean looks much like another—some could easily find their way into human food, with potentially fatal consequences for a nut-allergic person. The company concerned took the point and withdrew their new variety immediately.

searchers looked into seven deaths from violent allergic reactions to foods and found that six of these occurred when eating away from home. One of these unfortunate victims ate chili in a restaurant, quite reasonably expecting it to contain meat, beans, chiles, and vegetables. It turned out that the cook had used peanut butter to thicken the sauce, and the man was highly allergic to peanuts. Peanuts or peanut butter may also be used in the glaze on roast meat, or inconspicuously in cakes, cookies, and candies. Some Chinese restaurants use peanut butter to stick down the ends of egg rolls or to add flavor to noodles. Some peanut-allergic individuals simply avoid Chinese restaurants altogether. Those with milk allergy or egg allergy have to be equally vigilant. Egg may be present but unseen, for example, in meatballs, where it is sometimes used to bind the other ingredients together.

Sandwiches can also be a hazard. In August 1999, a British athlete died after a few bites of a sandwich. Although the filling was described as "coronation chicken," it actually contained some peanut.

One obvious strategy when eating in a restaurant is to choose plain food, such as grilled fish or meat, where "what you get is what you see." This is not always possible and, if such foods are not available, you will have to make sure you know what is in the food you are eating. Try to speak to the chef directly if you can, but accept that this may not always be possible. (In many restaurants now there is no chef; the food is prepared in a factory and delivered in prepacked portions.) Waiters and waitresses are often too busy to really take the trouble to find out what is in the food, and if they don't understand the seriousness of food allergy, they may not bother. Most of the cautionary tales about allergic reactions in restaurants have as their villain the waiter or waitress who *said* they'd checked with the chef but hadn't.

One way around this problem is to telephone the restaurant in advance and discuss the problem with them—say that you need to know exactly what is in the food you are eating. You should be able to judge how helpful they are prepared to be from this initial contact. For the person who is sensitive to milk, Chinese or Japanese food is a good bet, because there is no tradition of using milk in Asian cuisine. However, this does not apply to packaged Asian food and ready-made meals from supermarkets, where milk products are often added by Western manufacturers—always read the labels.

Autoinjectors and Emergency Room Treatment

For those who have had a severe reaction to food, it may be advisable to carry a syringe kit or an autoinjector (brand names include AnaKit and EpiPen) containing emergency medication, in case the food is inadvertently eaten again. The syringe can be used only once and contains epinephrine (adrenaline), which counteracts the effects of the mast-cell mediators by causing the blood vessels to contract.

Knowing exactly how to use the injector is of vital importance, so make sure you are shown by an expert. An alarming Canadian study published in 1999 showed that 75 percent of health professionals got some part of the technique wrong when showing patients how to use an autoinjector. Pharmacists were the most likely to give accurate instructions. There are dummy injectors available for training purposes; these help enormously and most pharmacies have them.

You may also be given antihistamines in a liquid or chewable form, for use in an emergency, but never make the mistake of thinking that they are a substitute for the injector. In anaphylaxis they are a minor secondary treatment of uncertain value. Asthmatics may also be issued with an epinephrine inhaler, and this is more likely to help; you can use it in addition to the injector as long as you do not have a heart condition.

Even with this powerful rescue medication available, it is still necessary to avoid the food, of course—the epinephrine will only be effective if a very small amount has been eaten. Do not delay in using the syringe if you begin to experience a severe reaction to the food. In this situation, a wait-and-see attitude could be disastrous. The sooner you use the epinephrine, the more effective it will be, and you will avoid the possibility of lasting, irreversible damage to sensitive parts of the body.

Having used the syringe, contact your doctor or go to a hospital quickly, because you may need further doses of epinephrine. The dose should be repeated every fifteen to twenty minutes until you are fully recovered. Tell the doctor if you have been taking corticosteroids, as these may suppress your body's normal ability to produce its own corticosteroids, which are needed in this crisis situation. You may require a dose of corticosteroid, as well as epinephrine, to counteract the effect. Anyone who is taking ACE inhibitors or beta-blockers (prescribed for angina, high blood pressure, abnormal heart rhythms, and severe anxiety) may be resistant to the effects of injected epinephrine. Check with your doctor if you are taking either of these long-term medications: it is not unknown for patients to be given an epinephrine injection kit despite the fact that it will not work for them.

Not all anaphylactic reactions come on immediately. They can sometimes take an hour or even two hours to develop. There are usually some initial signs that things are amiss, such as itching or swelling in the mouth, nausea, and stomach pains. If the food is affecting the throat, hoarseness or a lump-in-the-throat sensation may be the first signs.

Should these be followed by more generalized feelings, such as itching all over, sneezing, runny nose, diarrhea, and weakness, then a serious anaphylactic reaction may be developing. Other odd sensations that may accompany this stage are a feeling of warmth and a sense of dread or apprehension. Incontinence, disorientation, and abdominal pains may also be experienced.

If there are any signs such as these, *do not delay getting medical help*. Go to an emergency room if you can, and make sure you are seen quickly—don't sit quietly waiting your turn. Tell the doctor if you have been taking corticosteroid drugs.

On rare occasions, a severe reaction to food will seem to be over, but the symptoms then recur between four and eight hours later. You should be given corticosteroids to reduce the chance of this happening and kept in the hospital for several hours just in case. Sometimes, however, patients are discharged prematurely, and occasionally there have been deaths as a result. If it is a long journey from your home to the emergency room, and you have been discharged less than eight hours after the original reaction, consider staying in the waiting area, or somewhere nearby, until this danger period has passed.

Anyone who has had a severe reaction in the past should consider wearing a medical information bracelet with the relevant information on it. If you were to eat your culprit food by mistake while away from home and were found unconscious, it could save your life. Without it, you might not get the correct medical help. The address for MedicAlert, which supplies these bracelets, is given on page 454.

It is a good idea to work out a crisis plan for handling an emergency. You could ask your family doctor or specialist to help with this. Write down the plan, so that everyone in the family knows the details, and leave it posted prominently in the kitchen. In the case of allergic children, give a copy to their teachers as well as to grandparents, baby-sitters, and the parents of friends whose houses the children visit. Make sure everyone knows where the epinephrine injection kit is kept and how to use it. The plan should include details of what type of emergency medical service (EMS) to call. In some states, only paramedics carry epinephrine, while in others those with basic or intermediate certification also carry it. Additional shots of epinephrine may be needed on the way to the hospital, so calling the right ambulance service is crucial. Contact the Food Allergy Network (see page 451) for details of EMS arrangements in each state.

Most patients who have had a severe allergic reaction will automatically be referred to an allergy specialist. If your doctor has not done this, request a referral. This is especially important if you have asthma, or if you experienced an asthma attack or general breathing difficulties, during the allergic reaction. Some experts suggest that any child with a true allergy to cow's milk or egg should not be given peanuts, tree nuts, fish, or shellfish until three years of age.

Mislabeled Food

Do not ignore warning signs on the basis that you have not eaten any of the offending food: there is always the possibility of contamination when processed food is produced in factories making several different products. In a two-week period in February 1997, for instance, one British supermarket chain had to recall all its own-brand chocolate spreads after these were found to be contaminated with hazelnut; another supermarket chain found that its delivery of own-brand toffee yogurts actually contained hazelnut yogurts, and walnut pieces were discovered in the blueberry muffins in a third shop. In two out of these three incidents, the contamination caused a serious allergic reaction in a susceptible person.

In the United States, there have been problems with boxed fruit drinks being contaminated with milk because the same production lines were used for milk drinks. Some tofu desserts are made in ice-cream factories and can therefore be contaminated. Such minute traces of a food will only affect the most highly sensitive individuals.

Ready-made meals are also vulnerable to mislabeling (in one incident a vegetable lasagne package actually contained a vegetable bake, which includes nuts) and to contamination (a nut-sensitive patient wound up in the hospital after eating a ready-made Italian meal, in which the pesto sauce had acquired traces of walnut oil from processing machinery). All the large supermarket chains now seem to be much more aware of such problems, and these incidents should become increasingly rare. So there is no point in being paranoid about any packaged or ready-made food, but it is just as well to be aware of the possibility of contamination so that you do not ignore the warning signs of an allergic reaction should one occur.

Puzzling or Inconsistent Allergic Reactions to Food

If you have had an immediate, violent reaction to food but are not sure which food component is responsible, then you are in a more difficult position. It is important to identify your allergen so that you can eat safely with the minimum of dietary restrictions. A little intelligent detective work may help you to guess the identity of the culprit, and your doctor should be able to arrange for a skin-prick test to check your conclusions.

One possibility you should consider is that you are reacting to an additive rather than a food. If you consistently react to commercial ice cream, for example, but not to milk, cream, or homemade ice cream, then you may be allergic to polysorbates, which are used as stabilizers in ice cream manufacture. Careful reading of labels and some cautious experimentation with suspect additives should help you to identify the source of the problem. Appendix 6 gives more details on food additives and identifies "families" of additives that are chemically similar to each other—if you are allergic to one, you may also react to others with a related chemical structure.

Another possibility is that you are allergic to a digestion product of the food rather than the food itself (see page 54). Vomiting and diarrhea begin some hours after eating, and anaphylactic shock is a possibility. This sort of allergy is thought to be very rare.

Immediate, violent reactions are particularly common with shellfish, but are often inconsistent—a person will react severely on one occasion but not at all on another. One reason for this is that shellfish are actually comprised of two separate animal groups (see page 375). Another is that the shellfish themselves vary, depending on what they have been eating. They tend to accumulate various chemical compounds, including toxins, from the creatures that they eat. These are passed on intact to the human consumer. The adverse reaction that follows may be an allergic one, or it may be a false food allergy (see page 109) or simply a straightforward case of poisoning by toxins that the shellfish have accumulated. With increasing pollution of coastal waters by raw sewage, there is also the very real possibility of infection by bacteria or viruses, which may further confuse the picture.

To add to the complexities, shellfish are often treated with preservatives known as benzoates after they are caught. A few people are allergic to these widely used additives, and while they will certainly react to various other foods as well, the reaction to shellfish is likely to be more marked because of the prodigious quantities of benzoate used. The amount will vary tremendously from one batch of shellfish to another, and this may explain the variable reactions seen in a small proportion of those sensitive to shellfish.

Fish can also cause inconsistent allergic reactions, and again it can be a contaminant, not the fish itself, that causes the problem. The offending substance in this case is produced by a parasitic worm called *Anisakis simplex* that infests the fish. In earlier times, when fish were gutted onboard ship immediately after being caught, these worms were removed with the gut contents, but modern streamlined fishing practices have changed all that. The fish are often brought back to shore before being gutted, which gives the worms time to migrate out of the gut and into the flesh of the fish. If it is not thoroughly cooked, infected fish can pass on the worm. Fortunately, the infection is quickly thrown off by most people, and rarely lasts more than a few days. But the stage may have been set for allergic reactions later.

Allergic reactions occur when a worm-infested fish is eaten by someone who has previously had such an infection and recovered. The worms do not need to be alive to produce the allergic response—they still carry their characteristic antigens, even if they have been killed by cooking. The immune system, which was previously required to fend off the living worms, sees the antigens as signs of a new attack and responds accordingly: this can produce a massive allergic reaction, leading to collapse in some cases. Researchers believe that there are probably far more of these allergic reactions from eating fish than anyone realizes, but that most doctors are unaware of the problem and so the cases are not identified and recorded. The original worm infestation may have seemed like nothing more than a mild dose of food poisoning or an upset stomach, so the patient often has no idea that it occurred.

Catherine

Catherine had suffered from asthma since childhood—she could not remember a time when these attacks of breathlessness and wheezing did not set in once or twice a week. Skin testing had always been negative and she had simply learned to live with the problem, controlling her symptoms with drugs. Then, in her forties, Catherine began to suffer from frequent headaches and felt very tired. Her doctor could find nothing wrong and suggested that she might like to try an elimination diet to see if this was of any help. Catherine cut out milk, eggs, wheat, and citrus fruits, and found that she felt a great deal better. When she retested milk, this brought on a headache within an hour, followed by a severe attack of asthma. On a diet with no milk or milk products, her headaches are few and far between. To her great surprise, she is also free of asthma attacks for the first time in her adult life.

No one knows how many people react to this parasitic worm, but one recent research paper identified twenty-eight cases. Needless to say, an allergic reaction to fish itself is far more common than allergy to the *Anisakis* worm, but in cases of fish allergy the reaction to fish tends to be consistent.

Another possibility that should be considered, in puzzling cases of food allergy, is sensitivity to antibiotics. Because these are added to animal feeds, they can turn up in trace amounts in meat, eggs, and milk. Someone who is extremely sensitive to a particular antibiotic may react to the tiny amounts found in such foods.

Other foods can also be present as contaminants if processing machinery has not been cleaned thoroughly when switching from one product to another. Once again, peanuts cause more trouble than any other food. A factory producing both peanut butter and almond butter caused a serious allergic response in a peanut-sensitive individual by contaminating the almond butter with peanuts. Candies can suffer the same problem. With growing awareness of the potential hazards, manufacturers are now taking more care. If you are ever doubtful about a food, proceed cautiously, taking a very small amount at first. You can also apply some to your face first, as described on page 59.

Those with an allergy to latex (rubber), usually acquired at work, may react to traces of latex from gloves worn by food-processing workers. Such cases are very rare, but the reaction can be severe.

Finally, there are some food-allergic individuals who only produce symptoms if they take strenuous exercise after eating the food. Exactly why this should occur is unknown, but changes in the state of the blood vessels that occur naturally during exercise must somehow trigger adverse reactions in the mast cells. This type of reaction can lead to collapse (**exercise-induced anaphylaxis**), which can sometimes be fatal. (Some people react in this way not as a response to specific foods, but to any food. This is not an allergic reaction.)

Allergic Reactions to a New Food

In theory, you should not experience an allergic reaction to a food you have never eaten before: you need at least one prior exposure to become sensitized. In practice, people do sometimes suffer allergic symptoms on their first exposure to a food, and this is due to cross-reactions.

In one unusual and alarming case, a boy with a mugwort allergy collapsed and almost died upon drinking a cup of chamomile tea. Both mugwort and chamomile are members of the daisy family, the Compositae, as is ragweed, a plant with highly allergenic pollen. Sunflowers also belong to this family, and their seeds may cause a reaction. When such reactions happen there are usually warning signs, such as tingling of the mouth and lips, which should be heeded immediately.

Honey may contain pollens of many different kinds, and this can occasionally produce an allergic reaction when eaten. Knowing about potential cross-reactions may be useful in case you suffer an unexpected response of this type.

A few of those who are allergic to birch pollen cannot eat hazelnuts. This is not particularly surprising, since birch and hazel belong to the same plant family. What is unexpected is the cross-reaction seen between birch pollen and apple—a very high proportion of those with birch hay fever are allergic to apples. It is thought that this is due to proteins that are widely distributed in plant products. Peaches, pears, plums, cherries, and even potatoes are also reported as affecting a few people with birch-pollen allergy. However, apple sensitivity is the most common.

There are other odd cross-reactions between different fruits and vegetables that may be explained in the same way. Ragweed pollen seems to share some antigens with melons and bananas, while mugwort pollen shares antigens with celery. Some people react to a cluster of allergens: mugwort pollen, celery, and spices. For a full list of pollen-food cross-reactions, see page 377. Note that house dust mite and latex may both cross-react with certain foods. Latex cross-reacts with a wide range of fruits, particularly bananas, avocados, chestnuts, and figs. The shared allergen is a natural substance that protects against attacks by insects.

Dealing with Cross-Reactions from Pollen

If you suspect you have suffered a cross-reaction from a pollen to a food, how should you proceed? Obviously, if it is a violent reaction such as the one to chamomile tea described above, complete avoidance is the only course. Sensitivity to foods can sometimes be so pronounced that they do not have to be eaten to produce symptoms. For example, some patients with birch-pollen hay fever cannot even peel or scrub potatoes without reacting to them. One woman with grass-pollen hay fever suffered an asthma attack, red eyes, and a streaming nose at the smell of boiling Swiss chard. However, for the majority of hay-fever sufferers, cross-reactions from pollen to foods are very mild, do not get significantly worse, and affect the mouth only. Regard these symptoms as a warning and avoid the food as much as possible, but don't worry too much. The only causes for serious concern are:

- If the food concerned is celery, since this is particularly likely to produce a swelling in the throat that can lead to suffocation.
- If the food concerned is peanuts.
- If the symptoms experienced on eating the food have been getting steadily worse.
- If you have ever experienced swelling of the lips, tongue, or throat; difficulty in breathing; urticaria (hives) all over the body; or collapse.
- If you have asthma: this can be very dangerous. If you are asthmatic and begin to feel odd after eating a food (with tingling or itching in the mouth or lips, for example), then stay close to a telephone for at least an hour so that you can summon help if necessary. In most cases the symptoms will wear off and nothing further will happen; simply avoid eating that food in the future. Should any further symptoms appear, do not hesitate to seek medical help.

Very often the allergen in the food is destroyed by cooking, or even by storage, so it is worth some cautious experimentation with cooked, canned, or frozen and defrosted versions of the culprit food. Cooked apples are almost always tolerated by apple-sensitive people. You can always apply some of the food to your skin first, before eating it, to see if it produces a rash—this will warn if a severe reaction is likely.

Treatment of hay-fever symptoms is rarely of any help in clearing up responses to food.

Multiple Food Allergies

Most people with true food allergies are affected by only one or two foods. In rare cases, however, multiple food allergies develop, often with a quite complex pattern of symptoms. One food may produce the classic set of symptoms, starting in the mouth and throat, while other foods produce hives, or severe diarrhea or vomiting, often with stomach pains.

Some of these reactions may not occur immediately after eating the food. Note that we are talking here about true food allergies, mediated by IgE, and almost always giving positive skin-prick tests and RAST blood tests. It is important not to confuse such cases with food intolerance, where multiple foods are often involved and symptoms are delayed, but where skin-prick tests and RAST are negative showing that IgE is unlikely to be involved. The symptoms of food intolerance are almost always less violent than those of food allergy, and most are unlikely to be life-threatening.

If you have immediate violent reactions to a variety of foods but negative tests, consider the possibility that you are eating traces of a problem food (such as milk or egg) without realizing it. Read pages 58-62 and get into the habit of studying food labels (see page 369) and regarding all ready-made food with suspicion.

Anyone who truly has multiple IgE-mediated food allergies faces serious difficulties and, to make matters worse, there is a tendency to develop new allergies over time. There has been no systematic study of such individuals, as they form a very small minority of patients, but the impression given by their case-histories is that something else may be going on besides the straightforward IgE-mediated reactions. Exactly what that is remains a mystery.

The cornerstone of treatment is careful avoidance of all the offending foods, but supplementary treatments may help to make life easier. Among the options worth considering are:

- Cromolyn sodium, a drug that blocks the reaction of mast cells (see page 30) to allergen. Used mainly in an inhaler or as nose or eye drops, for asthma and hay fever, cromolyn sodium can also be taken in capsules to block food-allergic reactions. It is no miracle cure, however. Offending foods must still be avoided, but the effects of eating a little by mistake are generally less severe, as several research studies testify. This drug also seems to help those who still have symptoms despite avoiding foods carefully. Although there is no evidence on this point, it seems plausible that using cromolyn sodium would also reduce the rate at which new food allergies develop. It is essential to take a sufficient dose of the drug. At least 400 mg, and possibly 800 mg or more, is needed, before each meal (or before any meal where all the ingredients are not known for sure). Increasing amounts of the drug may be needed in time, and while this drug is extremely safe and side effects are rare, taking huge and ever increasing doses is clearly undesirable. Our preferred strategy is to reserve this drug for special occasions and social events.

• Enzyme potentiated desensitization or EPD (see page 362) may reduce sensitivity sufficiently to allow the occasional eating accident to pass without such severe reactions. In the hands of an expert, it is considered a safe treatment, even for those who have suffered life-threatening reactions to foods, but it would be wise to have resuscitation equipment at hand. Remember that food avoidance will still be necessary.

• Some patients seem to respond well to treatment with antifungal drugs and a no-yeast, no-sugar diet (see page 244). This is just an impression gained by working with patients and has not been scientifically validated. There is no explanation for this response, but it might suggest that an overgrowth of yeast in the gut (see chapter 10) contributes to the tendency to develop new food allergies, perhaps by priming the immune system, or by increasing the permeability of the gut wall. However, there could be some other mechanism at work here that is not understood at present.

• Taking a bacterial replacer (see page 250) may also help to reduce sensitivity to food allergens according to some recent research. This treatment is probably worth trying, although there is no guarantee that it will help.

Treatments of this kind are rarely offered by the more orthodox allergists in the United States. In seeking out a specialist who can offer such treatment, bear in mind that many offer a mixed bag of tested and untested remedies. If you are offered any therapy other than that listed above, request references describing its use, question the doctor about his reasons for using the method, and ask how many other doctors use it. Be discriminating about which treatments you accept. Skepticism is warranted where a practitioner claims that the treatments offered are bound to succeed, or will work for innumerable ills, not just allergic reactions. Enthusiasm is not necessarily an indication of medical skill.

Any new allergist whom you consult may well want to repeat your skin-prick tests, just to check. Be aware that, with reactions of this type, avoiding the offending foods carefully for several years can change some of your skin-prick tests to negative, but this does not necessarily mean that your sensitivity to the food has disappeared. Test the food carefully, with a very small amount at first, to avoid a serious reaction.

Immunotherapy for Food Allergy

Allergy shots—the traditional series of injections for hay fever—are occasionally suggested for food allergies. In practice these are not actually used because of the risks of a violent allergic reaction occurring as a reaction to the treatment, and because the protection obtained by this method is never 100 percent reliable, even for hay fever. Doctors do use this treatment for those with severe life-threatening anaphylactic reactions to bee stings or wasp stings, since it is impossible for anyone to be sure of avoiding angry insects, and in such patients the treatment is very successful. But in the case of food allergy, it is considered wiser for people to avoid eating peanuts or milk or shellfish than for doctors to try (and perhaps fail) to desensitize them.

At least two different research teams are trying to develop a completely different kind of vaccine for food allergies. The vaccine is intended to block all allergic reactions by preventing mast cells (see pages 28–32) from firing. Initial trials of this vaccine are promising, but many more years of research and development are needed before it will be available. This situation may change in the next ten years. Some researchers believe that, by purifying the allergens more thoroughly, identifying the parts that induce allergic reactions, and producing chemically modified allergens tailored to individual patients, they will be able to desensitize food-allergic patients safely. Even if the new vaccines prove safer and more reliable than the existing allergy shots, it is unlikely that they will allow allergy sufferers to eat large helpings of the offending food with normal frequency. No one yet knows how effective these vaccines will be in patients with severe, potentially fatal reactions. It seems probable that they will only be useful as a fail-safe, to prevent life-threatening reactions to unanticipated traces of the food.

Prevention of Peanut Allergy

Cases of peanut allergy are increasing steadily, year by year. Some doctors believe this is due to the increasing consumption of peanut butter, especially by young children. They suggest that children should not be given peanut butter or other sources of peanut until they are at least a year old, and preferably not before their third birthday. Breast-feeding mothers have sometimes been advised not to eat any peanut-containing food, and some doctors have suggested that women at high risk of allergy should avoid peanuts while pregnant. This is probably good advice although there is no really good evidence to back it up.

Something that probably is worth doing, and involves far less trouble, is avoiding nipple creams and other skin creams that contain **arachis oil**—this is simply peanut oil by another name. Breast-feeding babies probably get a minute dose of peanut allergen from such nipple creams, and a newborn is highly vulnerable to becoming sensitized, especially to allergens absorbed in very small amounts.

Some creams prescribed for eczema contain arachis oil, and there is a suspicion that these could sensitize a young child to peanuts. Your doctor should be able to find out the exact contents of any cream prescribed and identify a peanut-free alternative. Many over-the-counter creams used for skin problems such as cradle cap and diaper rash also contain arachis oil. Ask the pharmacist to recommend a peanut-free product. If you need further information or assistance, you could contact the Food Allergy Network (see page 451 for the address).

Do children grow out of food allergies? There is no simple answer to this question—some do, some don't. Generally speaking, most babies who are allergic to cow's milk will grow out of the allergy within a few years, but a few will still be allergic to it in their teens. Likewise for small children who are allergic to egg. But an allergy to peanuts is far more likely to be lifelong. For more general advice on allergy prevention, see chapter 13.

What to Do about Asthma

A balanced approach is advisable in the case of asthma. First, medicinal drugs may be necessary to control the immediate symptoms and make life bearable for the patient. The drugs currently in use are described in appendix 8. Second, an effort should be made to identify airborne allergens. Some careful detective work, using the list of allergens on pages 83–89, may help pinpoint the culprits. Skin-prick tests can also be useful here, although they are not always accurate. Once airborne antigens have been identified, they can be eliminated as far as possible from the home, using the methods described on pages 91–94.

Coping with an asthma attack

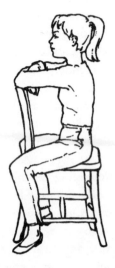

The most important thing to remember during an asthma attack is to stay calm. Sitting upright with your elbows resting on the back of a chair can be helpful. If the back of the chair is not high enough, add a pillow or two. Sitting in this position lifts your rib cage and reduces the amount of muscular effort needed to breathe. Fresh air is valuable, so open a window as long as it is not too cold. A large group of onlookers tend to increase the asthmatic's anxiety and thus make matters worse.

Allergy shots are also an option, especially when the allergen is difficult to avoid. Note that they are used only for inhaled allergens, not for any food allergens that might be involved in your asthma. Asthmatics taking allergy shots should be aware of the dangers and take steps to protect themselves—most of those dying from allergy shots are asthmatics whose airways tighten up sharply due to an allergic reaction to the shot. Your peak flow should be measured before the injection and again before you leave the doctor's office. Never have a shot if you are experiencing asthma symptoms, or if your peak flow is less than 70 percent of your best reading. The shortest safe waiting time after each shot for someone with asthma is thirty minutes, and ideally you should wait an hour or more—if your doctor suggests anything less, look for someone with a more cautious approach. Ask if the doctor has resuscitation equipment and where it is kept. You could need very prompt resuscitation treatment in an emergency. If you are taking beta-blockers (see page 63) or have a heart condition, discuss the safety issues with your doctor at the outset.

Serious reactions can even begin some hours after the injection, so stay within reach of a phone for about twenty-four hours. If you do experience any effects, remember to tell the doctor before the next injection, because the dose must be adjusted. Also inform the doctor if you have an infection of any kind, as this can alter your reaction.

There are other desensitization treatments that are much safer for asthmatics than traditional allergy shots (see pages 360–62) and these can tackle food allergens as well as inhaled allergens. They have not been as thoroughly tested as conventional allergy shots, but there have been a few trials showing that they work for some patients at least.

If something in the workplace is responsible for the asthma, either as an allergen or an irritant, every effort should be made to change to a different working environment as soon as possible. The asthma will almost certainly get worse as the months go by. Although as the asthma tends to clear up when away from the workplace, eventually it becomes *persistent and irreversible.* Occupational asthma, as it is known, can be severely disabling, and no financial compensation can recompense anyone for such serious ill health.

After six to eight weeks, the effect of eliminating airborne allergens and irritants can be assessed. If there are still serious symptoms then it may be worth trying an elimination diet but only if you have other symptoms, such as digestive problems, diarrhea, or headaches, suggesting food sensitivity (see chapter 7). Continue with the basic measures for avoiding airborne allergens while the diet is in progress. Where foods provoke asthma, skin-prick tests are not all that useful in identifying the problem food. So a diet—such as that described in chapter 14—is the only reliable means of diagnosis. In the case of babies and young children, see chapter 11. Remember that children should not be put on an elimination diet without medical supervision.

Medical care during the elimination diet is particularly important for anyone who has ever had a severe attack of asthma, whether an adult or a child, because there is a risk of death if a serious reaction occurs when a food is reintroduced. If you are testing foods at home, your doctor should be able to give you a supply of suitable medicine (such as an epinephrine autoinjector) for use in a severe asthma attack.

Where asthma is brought on by food, the reaction is sometimes dependent on some other factor being present at the same time, such as alcohol, aspirin, cold drinks, or exercise just after the meal. In such cases it can be quite difficult to pinpoint the exact causes of asthma attacks. Aspirin or aspirinlike drugs can also be a direct cause of asthma attacks, and these can be severe or even fatal. Careful avoidance of aspirin is vital—see page 78.

If foods do turn out to be instrumental in the asthmatic attacks, then avoiding those foods entirely is the simplest solution. Where this proves too difficult or dull, then the drug cromolyn sodium, taken by mouth, may be of benefit (see pages 432–34).

Asthma is a complex disease that may not be entirely due to allergy. For this reason, not all asthmatics will be able to track down the source of their problems using the methods described; some will have to rely mainly on drugs to control their symptoms. For this group, and indeed for all asthmatics, avoiding exposure to irritants such as smoke and fumes will help greatly. Certain jobs carry a very high risk of asthma, because they involve exposure to particular chemicals—these are described on pages 88–89. All those with a history of asthma, even if they have been free of symptoms for many years, should try to avoid such occupations and should never take up smoking, because of the likelihood of precipitating asthmatic attacks once more.

There are ways in which food might actually help combat asthma. Various studies have suggested a protective effect for asthmatics from a diet which is low in salt, and rich in antioxidants such as vitamin C (fruit and raw or lightly cooked vegetables), vitamin E (sunflower oil, seeds, or margarine are the best), and beta-carotene (carrots and mangoes are the top sources). Eating tomatoes, including juice and tomato paste, also seems to help, probably due to an antioxidant called lycopene. Fats, particularly saturated fats, may make asthma worse.

Asthmatics keen on a healthy diet should be cautious, however, about taking supplements of omega-3 fish oils (those containing EPA and DHA). Recent studies show that asthmatics who are sensitive to aspirin (see pages 78–79) may deteriorate while taking these supplements, probably because of differences in the metabolism of prostaglandins (see page 30). The link here is that omega-3 oils are turned into prostaglandins by a complex series of reactions in the body, and one of the effects of aspirin is to interfere with prostaglandin manufacture. Those with aspirin sensitivity are thought to have a slightly different body chemistry when it comes to making and transforming prostaglandins, turning this common drug into a potential killer. For some people, this metabolic abnormality seems to produce a bad reaction to high doses of omega-3 oils as well, although the response is neither so sudden nor so severe—it's just that the inflammation in their airways gets worse. One study suggests that eating large amounts of oily sea-going fish (the source of omega-3s) could have the same effect, which would seem logical, but the evidence on this point is far from certain.

What to Do about Rhinitis and Associated Problems

Rhinitis has quite a lot in common with asthma—indeed, the two conditions often go hand in hand, and patients who can avoid the allergens that trigger their asthmatic attacks tend to find that their rhinitis clears up as well. So the approach to dealing with rhinitis is much the same as that for asthma, described above. The same goes for associated conditions such as allergic sinusitis.

The first step should be an attempt to identify airborne allergens, using the list on pages 84–89. Skin-prick tests are useful in pinpointing the inhalants that trigger rhinitis, but of little use for foods. Efforts to eliminate airborne allergens should continue for some months to allow a fair assessment of the effects. It is best to begin in the winter, because pollen and outdoor mold spores are at their lowest levels then—their presence may mask any good effects achieved by eliminating pets or reducing levels of house dust mites, and this can be very discouraging. If such cleanup measures do produce an improvement, continue them through the summer months to see if the symptoms recur.

At the end of this process, it should be clear whether any airborne allergens are involved, and which ones they are. Where it is difficult to avoid such allergens, allergy shots or other desensitization treatments may be worth considering—see pages 361–63.

If the symptoms persist despite all these measures, then an elimination diet could be used to assess the role of food—see chapter 14 for the detailed procedure. For babies and young children, see chapter 11. Where the rhinitis is fairly mild, using drugs to control it may be a more practical solution. The drugs that can be prescribed are detailed in appendix 8.

One particular set of symptoms calls for a special mention here. In the case of rhinitis with **nasal polyps**, especially if accompanied by asthma urticaria (hives), sensitivity to aspirin should be a prime suspect. How aspirin produces this cluster of symptoms is only partially understood (see page 76).

Avoiding aspirin and aspirinlike drugs is the best treatment. Remember that the following synonyms for aspirin may be used: *salicylate, salicylic acid,* and *acetylsalicylic acid.*

If avoiding aspirin and related drugs proves ineffective, then some doctors suggest that restricting the diet may be worthwhile. Aspirinlike compounds (salicylates) occur in various plants; the drug was originally extracted from the bark of willow trees. Certain fruits, nuts, vegetables, and spices are rich in salicylates; a complete list is given in appendix 2. If you are sure that aspirin aggravates your symptoms but are still not well despite avoiding aspirin drugs, then you could consider trying a low-salicylate diet to see if you improve.

All the aspirinlike drugs that need to be avoided are known as non-steroidal anti-inflammatory drugs (NSAIDs). These are used for pain relief (for example, in headache and backache remedies), for the treatment of arthritis, and for several other inflammatory diseases. Unfortunately, you will not see the words *nonsteroidal anti-inflammatory drug* on the package.

There are twenty-five or more distinct drugs to be avoided, and many are sold under several different brand names, with new drugs and brands being introduced all the time. We suggest that you protect yourself as follows:

- Whenever you are prescribed any new drug, remind the physician that you are sensitive to aspirin (or, if you only have nasal polyps at present, mention this). If you are at all concerned about what you have been given, double-check with the pharmacist.
- Whenever you buy any painkillers, headache or migraine tablets, or cold and flu remedies, always buy them from a pharmacy and check with the pharmacist that they do not contain aspirin or aspirinlike drugs. Never take drugs of this kind unless you bought them yourself.
- You should also be cautious about anything flavored with peppermint, mint, or menthol as some with aspirin sensitivity react to these. Painkillers that do not contain aspirin generally contain acetaminophen. While most will be able to tolerate this, about 5 percent of people who are sensitive to aspirin also react to acetaminophen.

What to Do about Eczema

First, see a doctor and make sure it really is atopic eczema. Other possibilities, particularly dermatitis herpetiformis (see page 104) should be ruled out before making any dietary changes. In general, atopic eczema is a mild disease that disappears in time, and most cases are probably best treated with creams or other medication (see page 441–43). It is certainly not fair to an eczematous child to deny the relief that these medications can bring while attempting to sort out the problem with dietary investigations. A balanced approach using drugs, diet, and other investigations is required. Where there is a secondary bacterial infection, then a course of antibiotics may be necessary. With dry, uninfected eczema, there is a promising new form of drug treatment based on traditional Chinese herbal remedies. The herbs are made into a tea, which is drunk once a day. The taste is not at all pleasant, but the beneficial effects are usually worth it—about two-thirds of patients are substantially better, and these are people whose eczema has resisted all the usual forms of treatment. Generally speaking, the herbal treatment works better in adults than in children. At present this treatment is not widely known, but it may soon be available by prescription through your family doctor. Be very cautious about Chinese herbs, especially ointments, that have not been prescribed for you by a doctor of traditional Chinese medicine. Analysis has shown that some preparations contain illicit corticosteroids, often at dangerously high levels at which side effects are common.

Another new, and still highly experimental, treatment for eczema is to give the bacterium *Lactobacillus acidophilus*, which is a natural inhabitant of the gut but can become depleted. This can be taken in capsule form (see page 250). There is probably no harm in trying this approach in addition to other treatments, but check with your doctor first.

For the child (or adult) with severe eczema, life can be misery, and it is certainly worth investigating the possible role of food in the illness. The best response is usually seen in babies less than a year old, and guidelines for investigating their reactions to food are given in chapter 11. For older children, the difficulties of a restrictive diet may outweigh the benefits, although some children are very good at sticking to a diet once they see its results.

The diagnosis of food sensitivities in children with eczema can sometimes be made by a skin-prick test (see page 34), although this method is not foolproof. The diagnosis should be confirmed by eliminating all the suspect foods from the diet and then reintroducing them one at a time. Check that your doctor approves of this procedure before you start.

Elimination Diet for Atopic Eczema

A reaction to food will usually occur within about two hours of eating it, with itching and redness.

A small minority of children with atopic eczema, when testing a food after a period of avoiding it, will suffer a severe immediate reaction, with swelling of the lips and tongue, hives, and sometimes vomiting, asthmatic wheezing, or general anaphylaxis leading to collapse (see page 33). Such reactions could potentially be fatal.

It is difficult to predict with certainty which children will react in this way, but the following may be at greater risk:

- children with asthma as well as eczema
- children with severe allergies from an early age
- babies with a positive skin-prick test for the food concerned
- children with high levels of IgE to the food (this requires a special type of test, not yet widely used, which measures the quantity of a specific IgE in the blood)

Never test a food at home if it has ever caused hives or swelling of the face or mouth.

There may also be warning signs:

- a rash, or reddening, around the mouth after eating the food (before the elimination diet)
- on testing the food after avoidance, an immediate dislike and rejection of the food (but this is not foolproof; some children like the taste)

Ideally, children at high risk should test foods under medical supervision, with resuscitation equipment at hand, but this will be very difficult to arrange for most people. Alternatively, you could be issued an epinephrine autoinjector, which will block a severe reaction for long enough to allow you to get the child to an emergency room, but most doctors will be reluctant to prescribe this.

Whether a child seems to be at high risk or not, proceed very cautiously with food testing. First smear a little of the food on the child's face and rub it in gently—if there is no reaction within an hour, put a tiny drop on the lip and wait another hour. If this is uneventful, then give the child a small portion to eat—about half a teaspoonful. Finally, you can try a normal portion. Don't go beyond the first step if you are in sole care of the child—there should be two adults around to handle any emergency that might arise. Look out for the early signs of a severe response: a swollen mouth, tongue, or face, hives, wheezing, vomiting, or faintness. Make sure that you know in advance how to get the child to the nearest hospital or summon an ambulance. Keep the risks in proportion, because the likelihood of anaphylaxis is extremely small. However, you do need to be prepared, just in case your child is one of the unlucky few.

After the Diet

If, through an elimination diet, you do identify food sensitivities in your child, be sure to see your doctor promptly and ask for a referral to a nutritionist, so that a good diet, adequate for health and growth, can be established. Putting a child on a long-term avoidance diet, without professional advice, can result in serious malnutrition.

Creams and other medication can be used during the diet to alleviate the itching. The strength of medication used should be carefully chosen to reduce the severity of symptoms without eradicating them entirely, so that the response to foods can be assessed.

If skin-prick tests do not indicate any particular foods, then a simple form of elimination diet, avoiding the foods that are most often a problem in eczema, may be tried (see page 281). Again, food testing should be approached cautiously.

Before any dietary investigation is started, however, the possible role of airborne and contact allergens should be considered. This involves a certain amount of detective work, thinking over times when the child is better or much worse, and looking for clues as to what is causing these changes. Bear in mind that eczema is likely to fluctuate considerably anyway, and not every change will be in response to a change in the allergen load. Emotional stress can cause flare-ups. What you should be looking for are major changes that occur regularly in response to a particular event—a marked improvement during vacations, for example, or a deterioration when staying in a particular house. The list of allergens on pages 89–91 can be used as a starting point for your investigations. Researchers are currently working on a patch test that can confirm the role of airborne and contact allergens in atopic eczema. This test should become available in 2000, or soon afterward. Patch tests can also help in diagnosing the role of food in atopic eczema (see page 108).

If you feel that some airborne or contact allergen might be contributing to the eczema, then take whatever steps you can to eliminate it before embarking on dietary investigations. Reducing dust, damp, and molds in the house (see pages 91–94), keeping wool off the skin, avoiding low-temperature detergents (see page 90), and rinsing clothes thoroughly after washing are basic measures that anyone with an eczematous child should try. If there are pets, remove them temporarily or keep them away from the child.

Nonspecific irritants may be even more important than allergens, and these, too, should be eliminated. Simple measures include putting pure cotton clothing next to the skin, not using too much soap, and avoiding contact with chemical preparations as much as possible. Keeping a child's fingernails short reduces the damage done by scratching, and not allowing the house to get too hot is also helpful—heat aggravates the itchiness in the skin.

All these measures may take a little while to have any effect, and you should allow several months to elapse before coming to any conclusions. If the eczema is still troublesome, it may be worth trying an elimination diet.

All those who suffered from eczema as children would be well advised to avoid exposure to irritants in later life, even if their eczema appears to have cleared up. Surveys have shown that such people are far more likely to suffer from irritation to the skin on their hands. **Occupational dermatitis** or **hand dermatitis**—a common complaint of cleaners, beauticians, mechanics, nurses, and laundry workers—is roughly ten times more likely among those who once suffered from eczema. Such jobs should be avoided, and so should the use of cosmetics—sparing use and a regular change of brands is the best policy. Hypoallergenic cosmetics are useful in that they lack perfumes and other potential irritants, but the name is somewhat misleading, because they can provoke allergies if used often enough.

Housework, of course, is a necessary evil that only the lucky few can avoid. The obvious way to prevent trouble is to wear rubber gloves. Unfortunately, rubber itself can be an irritant, especially in the warm, humid conditions that prevail within such gloves. Wear cotton gloves inside the rubber ones to prevent direct contact with the skin, and avoid using very hot water: the cooler the hands are within the gloves, the better. Alternatively, wear PVC gloves.

Identifying Your Allergens

The lists that follow can be used as a starting point in tracking down your allergens. Careful detective work will be needed to identify allergens with any certainty—beware of jumping to conclusions, or you may be burdening yourself and your family with unnecessary avoidance measures. There is one list for asthma and rhinitis, and a second for eczema.

ALLERGENS THAT SHOULD BE SUSPECTED IN ASTHMA AND RHINITIS

General Points

- **Infections:** Infections can trigger asthmatic attacks, so attacks that are worse in the winter do not necessarily point to a particular allergen. In some children, wheezing only occurs during infections, and there is probably no allergen involvement.
- **Salt:** Too much salt in the diet may make asthma more likely—try reducing the amount of salt eaten to see what effect this has.
- **Irritants:** Various airborne irritants can provoke both rhinitis and asthma, including smoke from cigarettes, bonfires, incinerators, and the like; perfume and even strongly scented flowers; and industrial fumes, especially those containing sulfur dioxide. Sulfur dioxide is also given off by some foods and drinks (see appendix 1). Chewing and swallowing quickly can help reduce the amount of sulfur dioxide released, but avoidance is probably a better solution.

  If possible, reduce exposure to these irritants before trying to work out which allergens may be involved. In particular, eliminate cigarette smoke from the environment, as it is bound to make these conditions worse. Once allergens are identified and dealt with, the asthmatic may be able to cope with certain irritants again because the bronchi are less sensitive, but no asthmatics should be expected to tolerate someone else's cigarette smoke in their own homes.
- **Other nonspecific triggers:** Cold air, exercise, fear, anger, and other emotions can also trigger attacks, so you should consider the possible involvement of these factors. However, there is likely to be some other factor that is the primary cause of the asthma. It is only when the bronchi are already sensitized that they respond to triggers such as these.
- **Multiple triggers:** Remember that there may be more than one allergen producing the same symptom—food may be one cause, and inhalants or contactants another. Where foods are involved they may make the bronchi more sensitive, so that an airborne

allergen then triggers an attack. *In such cases the food alone may not bring on an asthmatic attack.*

Potential Allergens

• **Pollen:** Mostly causes seasonal allergic rhinitis (hay fever). The timing of the symptoms will depend on the type of pollen at fault, which varies considerably from region to region. Pollen can also cause asthma. Where there is sensitivity to perennial allergens as well, the rhinitis may persist all year, but get worse in the pollen season. Hay fever that begins in late July or August and continues into the fall may be due to ragweed, but it could also be mold allergy.

Broadly speaking, grass pollen is in the air in early summer, and ragweed pollen from late summer into the fall. Seasons are generally shorter in the northern states of the United States than in the southern states. Parts of Florida, southern Texas, and southern California may have some grass pollen in the air year-round.

Ragweed pollen may also be present year-round in some areas of Florida and California, but counts are generally lower than in the northern states and the midwest, so only the more sensitive hay-fever sufferers will notice. There are a great many other allergenic pollens, each with their own specific seasons: for detailed information on the local pollens, and for diagnostic skin-prick tests, consult an allergist. Pollen count information (see page 454) may also help with diagnosis.

In some people certain foods can heighten sensitivity to pollen (see appendix 4). Foods eaten only in summer (or in greater quantities then) can produce symptoms that may resemble hay fever—suspect summer fruits and ice cream.

• **House dust:** Sheep's wool or other components of dust may be the problem, but more often it is the **house dust mite,** *Dermatophagoides* (the skin eater). This minute animal lives on flakes of human skin shed by all of us in great quantities. It is not an insect, as is often stated, but a mite—a distant relative of the spiders. Still, it is killed by some insecticides. Some people react to the mites themselves, but most are allergic to the fecal pellets (droppings). These are covered with a thin layer of protein produced by the mite, and it is the protein that acts as an allergen. House dust mites thrive in old sofas and armchairs,

House dust mites and pollen

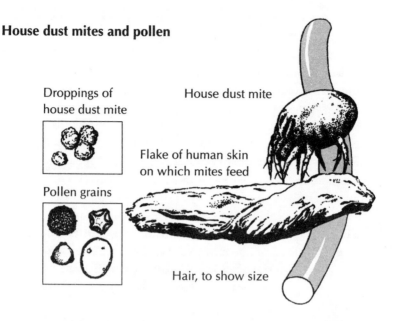

Droppings of
house dust mite

House dust mite

Flake of human skin
on which mites feed

Pollen grains

Hair, to show size

mattresses, and carpets. Sunshine and dry air are the mite's greatest enemies, so it prefers wall-to-wall carpets cleaned with a vacuum cleaner to loose rugs that are taken outside, beaten, and left to hang in the sun for a while. Damp weather favors the mite, so there may be a seasonal variation in the severity of attacks (note that damp also favors molds). Shampooing a carpet can stir up mites and provoke an attack—especially in children playing on a carpet. Sensitivity varies: some people can obtain relief simply by discarding an old mattress or sofa; others require the house to be scrupulously clean and free of all carpeting and upholstery.

- **Molds:** Damp houses and other buildings provoke symptoms. Raking up fallen leaves, handling compost, or spending time in a greenhouse or cellar also tends to make symptoms worse. So does mowing the lawn if the grass clippings were not collected after the last mowing—these will have grown molds that are stirred up by mowing again. House plants, Christmas trees, damp straw or hay, and domestic humidifiers are other possible sources. The symptoms may appear only in midsummer or late summer and autumn—or may worsen at this time.
- **Dogs, cats, rabbits, horses, hamsters, mice, and other pets:** Symptoms may not appear until many months after the pet is

acquired—sometimes as much as a year. In very sensitive individuals, clothing that has been in contact with an animal can trigger an attack. Traces of animal allergens can linger in a house where pets have lived previously, even if carpets are removed. Old horsehair sofas or mattresses can affect someone who is sensitive to horses.

A brief exposure to an animal can cause symptoms that persist for up to a week. The symptoms may be mild and transient when the animal is actually there, with a more severe, delayed reaction that sets in later.

- **Feathers:** Pet birds and feather-filled pillows, comforters, and cushions can all cause symptoms. However, some people who appear to react to feather pillows are actually sensitive to the house dust mite and its waste nestled within the down.

- **Wool, cotton, and other textiles:** Fibers are common in the air of most homes. People working in textile or clothing factories may become sensitized at work.

- **Barn mites in stored grain:** These can cause allergies in farmers and farm workers.

- **Flour, grain dust, sawdust, and other inhaled particles:** Workers in flour mills, sawmills, and food processing plants are most likely to become sensitized. With allergies to wheat flour, eating bread may also provoke symptoms. The dust from castor beans is particularly troublesome, mainly because it contains lectins (see page 36) that act as general irritants—but it can also produce true allergies.

- **Airborne food particles or droplets:** Examples include egg applied by a spraying machine to glaze pies and the spray produced by fish-gutting machinery. Once sensitized, individuals may also react when they eat the same food.

- **Animal urine:** Those working with laboratory animals are the most likely to be affected.

- **Vaccines:** The use of eggs for culturing certain vaccines (such as influenza and measles-mumps-rubella) can lead to problems for those who are highly sensitive to eggs, because a minute amount of egg protein persists in the purified vaccine.

- **Foods:** Any food could, in theory, cause asthma. Other symptoms, such as pain in the abdomen, diarrhea, or headache are likely if food is the cause. It is very rare for asthma to be the sole symptom of food sensitivity. The reaction may occur rapidly in response to a small amount of the food, or it may be delayed by several hours or even days and require a large portion of the food. Some individuals have to eat the food for several days in succession before there is a response. Recent research from the University of Colorado suggests that those with gastro-esophagael reflux (heartburn) may be more likely to develop food sensitivity affecting the airways because droplets from the stomach, containing food molecules, are inhaled and provoke the immune system.

Foods can also cause rhinitis. In addition, hay-fever sufferers, especially those sensitive to birch pollen, may experience an itching mouth and swollen tongue after eating certain fruits or nuts. This is due to a cross-reaction between pollens and certain foods—see pages 69–70. Such symptoms may occur rapidly, but more often the rhinitis begins many hours after the food is eaten.

• **Yeasts:** Alcoholic drinks, overripe fruits, breweries, and bakeries are common sources, but see pages 398–99 for a full list. Mold and yeast sensitivity may sometimes be helped by a no-sugar, no-yeast diet—see page 245.

• **Food additives:** As for foods, although the response time is usually shorter. Colorings used in food may also be present in medicinal drugs.

• **Drugs:** Antibiotics and aspirin are the common culprits, but any drug, in theory, could provoke an allergic response. The highly sensitive individual may respond to trace amounts of antibiotics found in meat, eggs, or milk.

Aspirin (salicylate) can trigger asthma especially in those suffering from nasal polyps.

• **Paints, air fresheners, aerosols, natural gas, and fumes from insulation:** Many household chemicals produce vapor that may act either as an allergen (when combined with a protein) or as an irritant. They can contribute to both asthma and rhinitis. Air fresheners are actually *designed* to fill the air with vapor. They work by supressing the sense of smell, and can have very unpleasant effects on some people. Keeping the house clean and well ventilated is a much better way to combat household smells.

• **Industrial fumes, dust, or other airborne particles in the workplace:** Dust in factories manufacturing antibiotics is often implicated, and may lead to sensitivity to the same antibiotic taken by mouth, whether as a drug or in food. Similar problems affect insulin production.

Fumes released during the smelting of platinum, the spray-painting of automobiles, and the manufacture of plastics, polyurethane foam, varnishes, paints, adhesives, and synthetic fabrics may act either as allergens (when combined with a protein in the body) or as irritants. Isocyanates and phthalic anhydride are common offenders. Fumes released when plastics are heated or burned are also potential triggers. Phenylene diamine, used in the fur industry, and piperazine, a drug used to kill parasites, are other common causes of asthma. Enzyme manufacture, soldering (especially of electronic components), textile dyeing, beauty care, and hairdressing are other high-risk occupations. The disease may begin soon after the first exposure, or it may take several months or years to appear—more than a decade in some cases. The attacks may be delayed and not occur until the evening, when the patient is at home. Symptoms may clear up over weekends, but not in everyone. Once someone has become sensitized, very small amounts—carried on the clothing of another person, for example—may be sufficient to trigger an attack.

• **Latex (rubber):** Those most susceptible are hospital workers and others whose jobs involve wearing latex gloves daily. Children who undergo a large number of surgical operations, such as those with spina bifida, may also be vulnerable. Where such children come from allergy-prone families, special measures need to be taken.

Latex particles in the air from motor vehicles may be a source of allergic reactions, but this has not yet been investigated.

ALLERGENS THAT SHOULD BE SUSPECTED IN ECZEMA
General Points
• **Irritants:** Remember that in eczema, irritants may be more important than allergens in causing the symptoms. Common irritants include detergents, soaps, hair-care products, and household chemicals of all kinds; rough clothing, including wool and synthetic fibers (pure cotton is the least irritating); hard (calcium-rich) water; solvents and other chemicals used in the

workplace; heat; and scratching. Acidic foods may also act as irritants.

Potential Allergens

• **House dust:** See pages 85–86.
• **Molds:** See page 86.
• **Pets:** See pages 86–87.
• **Wool:** Woolen sweaters or wool-mixture garments are the usual sources. Wool may act as a general irritant rather than an allergen.
• **Enzymes:** The enzymes used in laundry detergents are the usual source. The use of enzymes is widespread now; and in general, any detergent designed for use at low temperatures will contain enzymes. For enzyme-free detergents that contain a minimum of potential irritants, try the specialist allergy suppliers listed on pages 459–60.
• **Foods:** Any food can act as an allergen in eczema, but those most often implicated in children are milk, eggs, and citrus fruits (mostly oranges). Chicken, nuts, fish, wheat, peanuts, tomatoes, lamb, and soy are also common offenders. See chapter 14 for details of how to investigate the role of food, or chapter 11 if the patient is a baby or small child. Skin contact during food preparation can also provoke eczema.
• **Food additives:** Coloring and preservatives are frequent culprits, particularly the azo dyes (see page 418) and benzoate preservatives. They may be acting as nonspecific irritants rather than allergens. Colorings used in food may also be present in medicinal drugs, including antihistamine preparations. See page 457 for a pharmacy that can supply colorfree medications.
• **Creams and ointments:** Some ingredients used in skin preparations may, occasionally, be guilty of making atopic eczema worse. Peanut oil (arachis oil) is still used, astonishingly, in some anti-eczema creams, despite the increasing prevalence of peanut allergy. Lanolin can also provoke reactions in some people. Patch tests, on an area of unaffected skin, may help to identify such problems.
• **Drugs:** Eczema is seen in some patients who are sensitive to aspirin (salicylate), although this is not thought to be an allergic reaction to the drug.
• **Pollen:** Pollen grains landing on the skin may contribute to eczema in some children, but they are unlikely to be the sole cause.

- **Grass and other plants:** Direct contact with some plants may provoke eczema in the sensitive individual.
- **Metals:** Nickel, chromium, and cobalt are the most frequent offenders. Women are more likely to be nickel sensitive than men, because inexpensive jewelry frequently has a high nickel content. So do the metal studs in jeans.
- **Cement:** The chromate in cement causes skin irritation in many construction workers.
- **Chemicals in the home and workplace:** Various chemicals can cause skin irritation and eczema, particularly rubber chemicals and plastics. High temperature and humidity make the skin even more sensitive, so wearing rubber gloves can readily produce sensitivity to rubber—see page 83 for suggestions on how to overcome this problem.

ELIMINATING COMMON AIRBORNE ALLERGENS

- **House dust mite:** Many allergy sufferers are primarily affected by the house dust mite allergens in their mattresses and bedding. Any mattress or pillow that is more than a year old will harbor large numbers of mites. Getting into bed or turning over in bed forces out a blast of air from within the mattress—air that carries a heavy load of allergens. This can be prevented by a mattress cover that holds in the mite allergens. The best covers are made of a material that allows water vapor through (suppliers are listed on pages 459–60). Alternatively, the cover can be made of ordinary (impermeable) plastic, such as builder's plastic, but this tends to make the sleeper hot and sweaty.

It is preferable to buy a new mattress and cover it immediately. If you cover your existing mattress, the mites will continue to flourish inside the cover, and when the cover is removed, or if a hole develops, allergens will leak out. Replace your pillows and cover the new ones right away.

Replacing and covering the mattress and pillows is all that some patients need, while others are more sensitive to house dust mite and must therefore take other precautions. If symptoms still occur in bed, or first thing in the morning, try covering your comforter; it should be washed or dry-cleaned first, then thoroughly dried. Blankets should be regularly washed (a temperature of at least 135 degrees Fahrenheit is needed to kill the mites) or dry-cleaned. Air the bed every day, and air the room by opening the window, to reduce moisture levels—humidity favors the mites. The allergy sufferer should not make the bed unless wearing a suitable mask and should stay out of the bedroom for some time after the bed has been made to allow the allergens in the air to settle.

You may also have to treat the bedroom carpet if it is harboring a lot of mite allergens. Thorough vacuum cleaning may help, but most carpets also need mite-killing steam treatment with the temperature at or above 212° F (100° C).

Some highly sensitive people must remove wall-to-wall carpets from the bedroom, along with any unnecessary fabrics, soft toys, clothes, and so on. Rugs, if hung up outside in the sun regularly and beaten to remove dust, harbor far fewer mites. Curtains should be washed regularly.

If symptoms are experienced in other parts of the house, improving the ventilation may be helpful, as this will reduce mite numbers. Should this alone prove ineffective, consider replacing any very elderly armchairs or sofas, since these can often be full of mites.

If symptoms occur within a few hours of vacuuming, mite allergens dispersed into the air by the vacuum cleaner are probably at fault. Special vacuums with true HEPA (high efficiency particulate air) filters retain the allergenic particles. See pages 459–60 for suppliers. Dusting should be done with a damp or electrostatic cloth.

It may be difficult to part a child from his or her favorite teddy, even if this is harboring millions of house dust mites. Should you be faced with this problem, place the teddy in a plastic bag and leave it in a freezer for six hours to kill the mites. Then wash the soft toy as thoroughly as possible and dry it in a tumble dryer. Thereafter, the mites can be kept at bay by repeating the freezer treatment weekly.

• **Molds:** Take all necessary measures to eliminate damp and condensation from the house. Ventilate all rooms, cupboards, and so forth. Electric space heaters are cheap to run and can help to keep a troublesome damp spot dry—do not use fan heaters, though, as these churn up the spores.

Cover pans when cooking to reduce the amount of steam

generated. Fitting an extractor fan in the kitchen can also reduce the amount of moisture in the air, which in turn reduces condensation.

Avoid having vinyl wallpapers, metal window frames, and other household fittings that favor condensation. Take baths rather than showers, because they create less steam.

Check for signs of dampness and mold growth behind furniture and in cupboards, refrigerators, and freezers regularly. The rubber seals on refrigerator doors often harbor black molds.

Throw away any furniture, curtains, carpets, or cushions that have been damp and smell of mildew—even if they are now dry, they still contain mold spores.

Do not leave vegetables and fruits lying around for too long before eating them.

Do not have too many plants in the house. Remove dead leaves and flowers, and do not overwater them. Take off the top layer of soil and replace it from time to time.

Do not use humidifiers.

Heat the whole house well—do not leave some rooms permanently cold and unventilated.

Make sure clothes and shoes are thoroughly dry before putting them away in drawers or cupboards.

Wine corks sometimes have a thick growth of mold that is expelled forcibly and widely dispersed in the air when the cork is pulled from a bottle of wine. To prevent this from happening, thoroughly clean the cork and neck of the bottle under running water before removing the cork.

- **Animal skin (dander) and feathers:** Don't keep furry or feathered pets. If you already have pets that you cannot bear to get rid of, consider housing them outside or in part of the house that the affected person can easily avoid. Do not allow pets into the bedroom of the person affected. If they sleep on furniture or carpets, clean up after them with a vacuum that has an effective allergen filter.

For very sensitive individuals, it may be necessary to avoid people and clothing that have been in contact with animals.

For those sensitive to feathers, eliminate all bedding stuffed with feathers, as well as cushions, armchairs, and sofas. If you are also sensitive to synthetics, then comforters filled with wool or silk are available (see pages 459–60 for suppliers).

For those sensitive to horses, check that you do not have any old items of furniture stuffed with horsehair.

• **Pollen:** This is the most difficult allergen to avoid. Keeping windows closed on warm, sunny days can be helpful. They should remain closed in the evening and during the early hours of the night in large cities. Avoid opening the window when driving because pollen that has risen on warm air currents during the day falls again when the air cools down.

Keep away from meadows, parks, and other grassy areas when it is warm and dry. Wearing sunglasses may help reduce symptoms in the eye.

If you have been outside on a summer's day, there may be a lot of pollen caught in your hair and your clothing. Washing your hair and changing your clothes may help alleviate symptoms during the evening.

For very sensitive individuals, a stay at the beach during the height of the pollen season is recommended—the sea breeze brings in pollen-free air. Alternatively, air filters can be used (see pages 459–60 for suppliers) and are usually effective—as long as the individual stays indoors with the windows closed.

FIVE

Other Forms of Food Allergy

The first part of this chapter covers allergies to food that are not due to IgE. The second part deals with reactions that, strictly speaking, are not allergies at all: false food allergies and problems caused by histamine in foods. This last section is relevant to all types of food sensitivity. Histamine-rich foods can be a problem for people with either food allergy or food intolerance, because both may have gut walls that are abnormally leaky.

Non-IgE Food Allergy

Doctors traditionally recognize four types of reaction in which the immune system responds to an antigen so strongly that unpleasant symptoms are caused. These are called **hypersensitivity reactions**. The reaction caused by mast cells and IgE is the most common and troublesome of the four, and is known as type I hypersensitivity. This is described in chapters 3 and 4. The other three reactions involve different parts of the immune system. Type II hypersensitivity is not relevant here, while type IV hypersensitivity is a very slow immune response produced by a particular group of immune cells called T cells. It may be involved in some reactions in the gut, such as Crohn's disease (see pages 158–61), but it is not generally relevant to food allergy. This section is therefore confined to type III reactions and to reactions that do not fall neatly into any group.

How immune complexes are formed

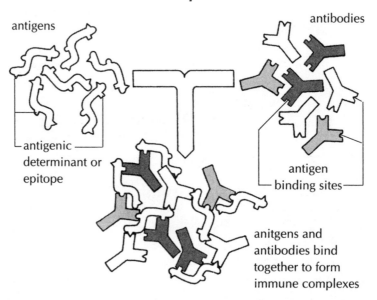

antigens

antibodies

antigenic determinant or epitope

antigen binding sites

anitgens and antibodies bind together to form immune complexes

Type III Reactions

Type III reactions occur when there is a substantial production of antibodies in response to an antigen in the blood. It is the sheer weight of numbers that causes the problem—the antigens and antibodies, bound together in **immune complexes,** are like so much litter going round in the bloodstream.

In the case of food, undigested molecules get into the blood through the gut wall after a meal (see page 24). This is a normal process that occurs in the healthiest of individuals, although in the food-sensitive person it is likely to be more pronounced because the gut wall is leakier. Once the food molecules enter the bloodstream, they encounter antibodies—again a natural, healthy process that leads to the formation of immune complexes when the antibodies and antigens bind together. Immune complexes attract the attention of phagocytes or "eating cells," the vultures of the immune system that clear up any debris, dead cells, and invading bacteria they come across.

Immune complexes form all the time, whenever antibodies encounter their antigen. Normally they are cleared from the blood by the phagocytes within a few hours. But if the immune complexes are both large and numerous, the phagocytes may not be equal to the task. Then the immune complexes accumulate in the blood, and eventually they are deposited in the blood vessels. This is the condition known as **type III hypersensitivity** or **serum sickness**.

Serum sickness happens in autoimmune diseases, such as SLE (systemic lupus erythematosus, or lupus), where there are a great many antibodies to the patient's own proteins circulating in the blood. It is also believed to happen, to a lesser degree, in rare cases of food allergy—in some types of kidney disease, for example, where the disease seems to be induced by food. Although there is no definite proof for this, the circumstantial evidence is quite strong (see pages 99–100).

Inflammation

How immune complexes affect the blood vessels depends very much on what sort of antibodies they contain—there are five different isotypes, as explained on page 28. In the healthy person, the main antibody formed to food is **immunoglobulin A**, or **IgA**, which has special protective properties. Unlike most other antibodies, it does not activate the defensive proteins in the blood known as the **complement system**.

The products of the complement system cause inflammation, a reaction designed to mobilize the body's protective forces. The effects of inflammation are to make the blood vessels in the vicinity leakier and to attract other immune cells into the area—the leaky vessels make it easier for the immune cells to gain access to the surrounding tissues. What appears on the outside as a swollen, red, tender area is in fact a microscopic battleground, where the body's own cells and tissues are unfortunate casualties of the general mayhem.

The purpose of inflammation, in the healthy individual, is to fight off infection. The body assumes that the antibodies have attached themselves to an invading bacterium or virus and sends in the troops. Obviously, the body needs to have control systems that tell it *not* to react when the antibodies are bound to something innocuous—such as a food protein that happens to have wandered into the blood through the gut wall. This is the function of IgA. Because it does not activate the complement system, it can quietly mop up nonharmful antigens for disposal by the phagocytes without setting off a damaging episode of inflammation.

For this system to work, the body must somehow distinguish food from other sorts of antigen. And it must make sure that IgA—rather than IgG, another, more inflammatory type of antibody—is manufactured to fit the food molecules. The details of how the body does this are

---

Tests for IgG—are they worth it?

IgE is not, of course, the only type of antibody (see page 281). Some practitioners, usually those working outside the mainstream, may offer you blood tests for a different type of antibody, IgG. Although these can be raised in food sensitivity, they are not usually specific for particular problem foods. So if you are sensitive to milk, for example, your IgG to milk may be raised, but so may IgGs to other foods. This is possibly because the gut is leakier, and lets more food antigens through into the bloodstream. So these tests are not necessarily diagnostic.

---

still far from clear, but a general picture is emerging from current research, and this is described in chapter 12. The process is known as the **induction of oral tolerance**.

What, if anything, goes wrong with this system? There is only a limited amount of evidence available, but it does seem that the system for producing IgA (rather than IgG) to react to food molecules breaks down in some people. When this occurs, the immune complexes circulating in the blood after a meal will be potentially inflammatory. If they are deposited in a blood vessel, damage to the walls of the vessel will follow.

Such people may also have some IgE in their food-molecule immune complexes, so mast cells could be triggered to add to the inflammation. Whether this actually happens is not clear. But if it does, then there are important implications for the way we think about allergies; the dividing line between type I (IgE) food allergy and type III food allergy may not be as sharp as is often assumed.

Symptoms Produced by Immune-Complex Deposits

Patients with the autoimmune disease SLE (see page 97) illustrate the sort of symptoms that can be produced when immune complexes are deposited in the blood vessels. Among other things, they suffer from skin rashes (including hives in some cases), painful joints, and damage to the kidneys and lungs.

All these symptoms are produced when the deposited immune complexes cause inflammation in tiny blood vessels known as capillaries. In the case of the joints, the capillaries supplying blood to the joints become inflamed, and this causes pain.

In the kidneys, immune complexes can become deposited around the delicate membranes that do the important job of filtering the blood. Their task is to remove excess salts and certain toxic compounds from the blood so that these can be flushed out of the body in the urine. Proteins in the blood are not normally allowed to escape into the urine, but when there is damage to the structure of the kidney, then this can occur. Because the body's much-needed proteins are being lost in the urine, the general state of health will eventually deteriorate—especially in children, who need protein for growth. The failure of the kidneys also means that excess water is retained, so there is puffiness in various parts of the body (edema).

Food and Kidney Disease

The question of whether foods might produce excess immune complexes in the blood, and thus cause the same sort of damage to the kidneys, is a highly controversial one. Two groups of doctors—one working in Japan, the other in Miami—have made a special study of children with kidney disorders, and they believe that food is the source of the problem for some of these children. When put on an elemental diet (a synthetic food mixture that contains a minimum of antigens; see pages 321–22), children with certain types of kidney disease may improve. Those who do recover are then challenged with various foods, and some reproduce their original symptoms—protein loss in the urine, and retention of water leading to puffiness in various parts of the body.

The food most often implicated is cow's milk—the most common allergen of childhood. But the majority of these children appear to be sensitive to several foods, and to various airborne allergens, such as pollen. Some of them also show sensitivity to environmental chemicals, a subject that is dealt with more fully in chapter 9. By putting these children on restricted diets, their symptoms have been fully or partially controlled. There are reports that neutralization treatments (see pages 361–62) are also useful when the food or foods concerned are difficult to avoid.

It must be emphasized that children with such diseases as these are rare, and the vast majority of cases of kidney disease are due to other causes. Nevertheless, it does seem that food allergy can cause kidney damage in some children. Whether it can affect adults in this way is an open question.

Almost all the children affected in this way are atopic—that is, they show one of the classical allergic disorders, such as asthma or eczema. This raises the possibility that IgE and mast cells are somehow involved in the damaging reactions in their kidneys. While this is possible, it does not seem that IgE has a central role. Neither is it entirely certain that deposition of immune complexes is to blame. Some of the available evidence suggests that it is, but other studies point to different forms of immune reaction producing the damage.

Finally, type I allergic reactions to airborne allergens, such as pollen, may sometimes be linked with kidney disorders. Reactions of this type are thought to be extremely rare. It is not known whether IgE and mast cells are responsible for the damage in the kidney or whether some other mechanism is at work.

Inflammation of the Blood Vessels and Spontaneous Bruising

If inflammation occurs in the walls of the blood vessels, the vessels become more permeable, as we have already seen. When the inflammation is not too serious, and mainly affects the tiny blood vessels (capillaries) in the skin, the result is likely to be urticaria (hives) (see pages 50–52). In such circumstances it is mainly fluid that leaks from the blood vessels, with few cells making an escape. (The approach to dealing with this form of urticaria is much the same as that described on pages 114–18.)

If the inflammation is more serious, then the blood vessels can become much leakier and even break open, so that red and white blood cells escape into the surrounding tissue, as well as fluid. This condition is known as **vasculitis,** and it may affect larger blood vessels as well as capillaries.

The first noticeable sign of vasculitis is usually swelling, or edema, due to water leaking from the blood into the surrounding tissues. If there is generalized edema—a reaction that affects the whole body—there will be a marked gain in weight, as much as eleven pounds, in twenty-four hours. There may also be aches and pains, especially in the legs, that tend to come and go.

As the condition gets worse, the blood vessels become leakier and eventually rupture. Red blood cells start to seep into the tissues and are noticeable externally as tiny reddish spots, which then turn purple or black and finally yellowish before disappearing—the same sort of color changes as are seen in a bruise. The condition is known as **purpura.** Larger escapes of blood produce **spontaneous bruising**.

If vasculitis is allowed to continue unchecked, more serious damage to the vessel wall may occur, and this can eventually lead to a vein becoming permanently inflamed or even completely blocked. Such damage is serious and often irreversible, so it is important to treat vasculitis at an early stage.

A Role for Food?

There are various causes for vasculitis and purpura. Infections can precipitate an attack, as can certain drugs. A shortage of **platelets,** the tiny particles in the blood that promote clotting, can also lead to purpura—such a shortage occurs in some autoimmune diseases, where the body attacks its own tissues. If all these possibilities have been eliminated, then it is worth considering allergy as a potential cause. In rare cases, food allergens circulating in the blood can be responsible—these can be identified by an elimination diet of the kind described in chapter 14. There may also be instances of IgE-mediated allergy producing vasculitis. An acute attack of vasculitis and purpura can accompany the sudden collapse (anaphylactic shock) that sometimes occurs upon eating a food allergen.

Many of those suffering from allergic vasculitis show sensitivity to various chemicals, so it is important to eradicate these from the immediate environment before trying an elimination diet. This may be sufficient to clear up the symptoms or at least reduce their severity. Even if it has no apparent effect, avoidance of chemicals should continue during the elimination diet, as there may be dual sensitivity; complete recovery will only occur if both food and chemical factors are eliminated simultaneously.

It has been suggested that immune complexes can cause inflammation in much larger veins and arteries, and even in the heart itself, thus provoking a far greater range of symptoms. These include muscle spasms, irregular heartbeat, severe pain in the legs, loss of circulation to the fingers and toes (in extreme cases to the whole limb, with consequent gangrene), loss of vision, seizures, and paralysis on one side of the body. It should be emphasized that food-allergic patients with symptoms such as these are probably extremely rare, and some doctors would dispute their existence altogether. Most of the reported cases appear to be sensitive to a very large range of foods and chemicals, and they have suffered serious ill health for many years.

Bird-Fancier's Lung

Those who are exposed to large quantities of airborne allergens can develop a serious inflammation of the lungs known as **alveolitis.** In this disorder it is not the tubes leading to the lungs that are affected (as in asthma), but the lungs themselves. Tiny air sacs known as **alveoli** perform the actual work of the lungs in extracting oxygen from the air and passing it to the blood. If an allergic reaction to airborne allergens occurs in the alveoli, the large number of immune complexes produced can be deposited there and cause highly damaging inflammation. The structure of the alveoli begins to break down, causing shortness of breath, tightness in the chest, fever, and a dry cough.

There are several forms of alveolitis, including farmer's lung and mushroom-worker's lung, but the only one likely to have any relevance to food allergy is bird-fancier's lung. In this disorder it is tiny particles from bird droppings that initiate the allergic reaction in the alveoli. The connection with food allergy is a tenuous one, but some doctors claim that eating eggs can exacerbate the symptoms in a few patients. This might occur if the antibodies produced to the antigens in the droppings also bind to antigens from egg proteins carried in the bloodstream. This dual binding, or cross-reactivity, can occur where antigens are chemically similar. Laboratory experiments suggest that there is cross-reactivity between the antigens of chicken's eggs and the antigens found in the droppings of budgies and pigeons.

Allergic Diseases That Are Hard to Classify

Doctors now recognize several forms of non-IgE food allergy (reactions mediated by the immune system, but not involving IgE antibodies as central players) that do not really fit into any of the four hypersensitivity categories (see page 95). This group of misfit diseases has been growing over the years as more research occurs into food reactions. The most common reaction of this type in adults is **celiac disease,** a specific response to gluten. This reaction, along with dermatitis herpetiformis, which is similar in origin, is explained on page 105. To summarize the reaction very briefly, gluten (found in wheat) provokes an autoimmune response by the body which then damages the lining of the intestine. There may be other cases of foods provoking autoimmune antibodies— something similar has been suggested for cow's milk in type 1 diabetes (see page 185).

Several conditions seen in babies are classed as non-IgE food allergy, including **dietary protein enterocolitis syndrome, dietary protein proctitis,** and **dietary protein enteropathy.** The first of these can also affect older children, and a similar condition is seen in adults, usually linked to eating shellfish. Cow's milk is the most common offender in all cases, particularly in babies, but the first two conditions can also be caused by soy, egg, wheat, rice, chicken, fish, and other foods.

Dietary protein proctitis is recognized by blood-streaked stools, with few other symptoms. The symptoms of the other two disorders are more severe and are likely to include vomiting, diarrhea, a bloated abdomen, and poor growth. All these conditions are diagnosed by internal examination using endoscopy and a biopsy (taking a tiny sample of the intestinal lining for viewing under a microscope). There is a typical influx of immune cells visible in the biopsy sample.

The only treatment, in all these disorders, in strict avoidance of the offending food or foods.

Mixed IgE and Non-IgE Allergies

There is yet another group of misfit diseases, with equally daunting names—allergic esoinophilic esophagitis, allergic esoinophilic gastritis, and allergic esoinophilic gastroenteritis. The names make more sense when you realize that all these diseases involve the arrival of hordes of immune cells called *eosinophils* in the walls of the digestive system, hence *eosinophilic*.

When this influx of cells affects the esophagus (the tube leading down to the stomach) it's esophagitis (*-itis* means "inflammation"), when it affects the stomach it's gastritis, and when it hits the intestines it's gastroenteritis. No one knows what gets the eosinophils going, but a reaction to specific foods is definitely involved. Sometimes there is IgE to those foods, but not always. This group of diseases seems to be on the increase.

The symptoms of allergic esoinophilic esophagitis are, principally reflux (regurgitation) of food, occasional vomiting, refusing food, stomach pain, and disturbed sleep. In allergic esoinophilic gastritis there is vomiting, pain, poor appetite, poor growth, and obstruction of the stomach outlet, which may, in rare cases, produce pyloric stenosis. Allergic esoinophilic gastroenteritis looks much the same, but there can be diarrhea as well, and babies may be puffy and irritable. All these conditions are most common in babies, but the first two can continue through childhood, and the third may occur in adults, too. Allergies to several different foods are likely, so the diagnosis usually requires an elemental diet (see pages 321–22). It takes three to eight weeks of avoiding the foods before the symptoms disappear. Food avoidance is the only treatment at present, although some physicians may use steroid tablets for a few weeks to get the inflammation under control.

Celiac Disease and Dermatitis Herpetiformis

Celiac disease (also called celiac sprue) is not usually thought of as a food allergy or intolerance, but in fact it is an adverse reaction to food involving the immune system—so it fits the common definition of food allergy. In practical terms, and for historical reasons, it is treated by gastroenterologists not allergists, but some allergists are now beginning to regard it as a food allergy. We are also aware that our readers include celiacs in search of advice on hidden food ingredients and other topics. What is more, the issue of food intolerance is certainly relevant to celiacs because intolerance of other foods can result from celiac disease (see below).

In celiac disease just one type of food is at fault—a complex group of proteins, usually referred to as gluten, that are found in wheat, barley, and rye. A related but less troublesome protein (avenin) is found in oats. Other names you may hear used for the offending proteins are *gliadin* and *prolamins*.

Celiac disease tends to run in families and those suffering from it have a particular genetic marker. This genetic makeup predisposes them to a series of events leading to celiac disease—first there is an immune attack on part of the gluten proteins, and this attack then develops into an autoimmune reaction directed against the lining of the small intestine.

The symptoms of celiac disease are very specific. In babies they consist of pale, foul-smelling stools, gas, bloating, and poor growth. These symptoms usually develop a few weeks after cereals are introduced into the diet. When celiac disease begins in adulthood, the symptoms are diarrhea, fatty stools that float rather than sink, pain, gas, bloating, weight loss, malaise, and weakness. Irritability can also be a symptom, and recurrent mouth ulcers affect some sufferers. In rare cases, constipation may be the main symptom.

Celiacs suffer a characteristic flattening of the villi—little finger-like projections from the lining of the small intestine, whose role is to actively absorb important nutrients. This damage to the villi leads to malabsorption of nutrients, and so to weight loss and weakness—the untreated celiac is actually suffering from malnutrition. At the same time, paradoxically, there is a leakage of large molecules that should not normally penetrate the intestinal wall. These reach the bloodstream and may cause additional problems (see below).

Celiac-style damage to the villi is so typical that diagnosing celiac disease traditionally relies on a biopsy, in which a small sample is taken from the small intestine lining and examined under a microscope. (The only disease to share this characteristic appearance in the intestine is dermatitis herpetiformis, a skin disease producing an intensely itchy and burning/stinging rash on the buttocks, back, elbows, and knees. This is also caused by an immune reaction to gluten and often affects celiacs or their relatives.)

There are also blood tests for celiac disease, and they can be helpful, but they do not always give an entirely clear-cut answer, unlike a biopsy. A new and more accurate test, which looks for antibodies to an enzyme called transglutaminase, is set to become available in the United States soon.

It is vital that anyone who suspects celiac disease should have a biopsy, blood tests, or both before embarking on a gluten-free diet. Self-diagnosis is a very bad idea in celiac disease, because the test results will not be clear if a gluten-free diet has already begun.

A tiny minority of celiacs have a true IgE-mediated allergy to wheat, as well as celiac disease (which means that they will probably give a positive skin-prick test or RAST to wheat). Their symptoms, if they eat wheat by mistake, are likely to be far more severe as a result.

At the other end of the severity spectrum are those with no obvious symptoms of celiac disease but with characteristic damage to the intestinal lining. Such cases of hidden celiac disease are usually found when close relatives of celiacs are investigated. The fact that there is damage suggests that such people should be following a gluten-free diet (see below). Some celiac children appear to lose their diarrhea and other obvious symptoms by their teens, but the damage to the small intestine may continue, with consequent nutritional problems. Doctors believe that they should continue to follow a gluten-free diet to avoid this condition.

Many experts believe that there are also a great many celiacs with mild to moderate symptoms in the United States who are never diagnosed, or who get the wrong diagnosis for many years. There is far less underdiagnosis in countries such as Italy, which offer routine screening of children for celiac disease, according to a recent report by the United

States National Institutes of Health. The idea that celiac disease is "rare" in the United States is a self-perpetuating myth according to some doctors and researchers working in this field: because it's "rare," it's not tested for, so it's not diagnosed—which keeps it "rare."

At present, the only treatment for celiac disease is to eliminate the foods that contain gluten, that is, any food containing wheat, rye, or barley. Other grains, including corn, rice, sorghum, and millet, are safe. There has been considerable debate recently about oats, and many doctors now believe that small servings (less than 1.75 ounces/50 grams per day) are safe for fit and healthy adults who have been on a strict gluten-free diet for some time and are doing well on that diet. It is vital to obtain oats from a source where they are not likely to be contaminated with wheat during growing, harvesting, storage, or milling. Check with a celiac support group (see pages 452–53) for sources of wheat-free oats.

The studies on oats, carried out in Finland, have included a five-year follow-up, and used biopsies to show that there was no damage to the intestinal lining among healthy adult celiacs eating oats. (What the study did not investigate was the question of cancer risk. It is known that celiacs who do not follow a strict gluten-free diet have a greater risk of certain cancers, unlike those who stick religiously to their gluten-free regime.)

Oats are certainly not safe for severe celiacs—those who are extremely sensitive to gluten. Some have an acute reaction to even the smallest amount of gluten, known as celiac shock. For such people, avoiding minute traces of gluten is essential, and this means being careful about medicines and vitamin supplements, for example (see page 457), as well as unexpected sources of gluten in food and drink (see pages 395–97). Ideally, such severely affected people should prepare their own food, because even products labeled "gluten free" may contain minute traces of gluten.

If regular ready-made foods are part of the diet, it is vital to check labels, even on foods that have been eaten before without problem—ingredients lists can change without warning. Be sure to understand the synonyms used on labels (see page 369). Restaurants have to be approached with caution, as in severe food allergy (see page 62). The Canadian Celiac Association (see page 454) produces useful information cards, aimed at chefs and waitstaff, including foreign-language versions for use when traveling.

Most celiacs do not need to avoid skin contact with wheat products (some even work as bakers), but those with dermatitis herpetiformis should do so.

The treatment for dermatitis herpetiformis is a gluten-free diet, to reverse the damage to the small intestine and so avoid nutritional deficiencies, plus drug treatment with dapsone, which promptly clears the rash. Once the diet has been followed for some time, the drug can be discontinued.

A few patients do not get better, even though they are very careful to avoid gluten. This may be because their gut lining is badly damaged and needs time to repair itself. Zinc deficiency can contribute to this problem, and a zinc supplement (see page 449) may be useful. Continuing symptoms can also be due to lactase deficiency (see pages 259–60), a consequence of structural damage to the gut lining. Avoiding milk or using lactose tablets (see page 455) may help in such cases. Soy milk can be used instead, and yogurt or cheese made from cow's, sheep's, or goat's milk can be eaten, but not cottage cheese.

Alternatively, persistent symptoms may be due to some other problem, such as a tumor or a defective pancreas. More commonly, however, the patient turns out to have sensitivities to other foods besides wheat. The damage done to the gut lining by celiac disease makes it much leakier, so other food molecules get through into the bloodstream, paving the way for food sensitivity. Soy is a common culprit, perhaps because it is so widely used in gluten-free products. Milk, fish, rice, and chicken have also been known to cause this problem. They can perpetuate the damaging reactions in the gut lining long after gluten has been eliminated from the diet. In theory, any food might have this effect. An elimination diet should help to track down the offender, but this should only be tried under medical supervision.

It makes sense to investigate such possiblities before treating the condition with steroids, where the risk of side effects is high. If there is a true food allergy involved, skin-prick tests or RAST may identify the culprit. More frequently, however, the problem is food intolerance, so such tests will be negative.

Mothers who may be at risk of having celiac children can reduce the risk by breast feeding for as long as possible, and weaning gradually rather than abruptly. Unfortunately, there is no specific advice at present on when to introduce gluten. Starting with small amounts is probably wise.

Immune Reactions Involved in Atopic Eczema

Research into the causes of atopic eczema over the past decade have revealed a complicated immune reaction to food—where food is a cause of atopic eczema—that cuts across the traditional categories of hypersensitivity reaction described on page 95. While IgE antibodies to the food are often involved, as in normal type I hypersensitivity, mast cells do not seem to play a central role. The IgE molecules are attached to special skin cells called Langerhans cells and dendritic cells, which have the role of presenting antigen to food-specific T cells in the skin. In cahoots with IgE, these cells become supercharged and excite the T cells to a far more powerful inflammatory reaction. This aspect of the reaction is more like a type IV hypersensitivity.

What does this mean, from a practical point of view, to the eczema sufferer? Since IgE is part of the reaction, skin-prick tests and RASTs (blood tests) can be positive in cases where food plays a part, but they are just as likely to be negative. Researchers in Finland have found that 52 percent of babies with atopic eczema give a negative skin-prick test despite having a genuine reaction to the food tested. This is called a *false negative*. (Older children and adults with atopic eczema are much less likely to give false negative skin-prick tests.) To make life difficult, false positives are also possible in babies—a positive skin-prick test but no reaction to the food. The Finnish researchers found that a different type of test, in which food is applied to intact skin and left there for two days (a form of patch test) is slightly more accurate, in that it only gives false negatives in 39 percent of babies. The surest way to pick up food sensitivities, in their opinion, is to use both tests, and take note of a positive reaction to either. This picks up 80 to 90 percent of eczema-causing food reactions in infants. Most doctors are not yet using patch tests for atopic eczema (although they are used for another type of skin condition, called contact dermatitis), because no standardized method has yet been devised. You may find a specialist who has developed a personal method for patch tests.

The response to the different tests seems to reflect a basic difference in the response to food as shown by an elimination diet. Babies with a positive patch test but negative skin-prick test tend to have a delayed reaction, usually with eczema symptoms only, when foods are tested after a period of avoidance. Those with a positive skin-prick test are more likely to have an immediate reaction with symptoms such as itching, hives, and a rash, sometimes vomiting and diarrhea, and occasionally wheezing or sneezing.

False Food Allergy

False food allergy, as used in this book, means unusual reactions to food that are caused by the foods triggering mast cells directly. In other words, these reactions involve mast cells, but they do not depend on IgE antibodies being formed to the food in question. Because the reaction is produced by mast cells releasing mediators, the symptoms are indistinguishable from true IgE-mediated food allergy. (But a modified RAST can distinguish between the two [see page 111].)

When Food Bites Back

Food, as we have already seen in chapter 1, is not necessarily the nice, passive, innocuous stuff that we have traditionally believed it to be: neither plants nor animals want to be eaten, and they have ways of fighting back. In plants particularly, there are many chemical weapons to deter would-be diners, and some of these chemicals persist even in modern crop plants. That we are not made ill by them more often is a tribute to our own abilities in breaking down such chemicals—abilities that have been acquired in the course of evolution.

One particularly cunning type of chemical weapon turns the body's most potent defensive force on itself: it fools the mast cells into degranulating. There are dozens of different substances found in food that can perform this trick. Some bind to IgE molecules, effectively bridging two adjacent molecules, in much the same way as an antigen might bridge them. This mimics the signal for the mast cell to degranulate, releasing damaging mediators such as histamine. Other substances may produce the same effect simply by binding to the mast-cell membrane and changing its structure so that it becomes more permeable.

One group of compounds that can have this effect on mast cells is the lectins. They are produced in particularly high concentrations by peanuts, beans, peas, and lentils, all of which are members of the legume family of plants. Lectins are also found in edible snails and wheat.

The main characteristic of lectins is that they bind to carbohydrate molecules carried on the surface of all cells. As a result they make red blood cells clump together, and this is how they are recognized in the laboratory. The deadly poison ricin used in the KGB's infamous umbrella-tip murder of Georgi Markov is a type of lectin. Fortunately, not all lectins are as potent as this, but many can cause more subtle damage. Apart from triggering mast cells, they can also bind to the lining of the gut wall and make it leakier, so that more undigested food molecules get into the bloodstream. These molecules can act as allergens, causing further damage as they travel around the body in the blood. There is also some evidence that, in atopic individuals, certain lectins can stimulate the body to produce IgE in preference to other antibodies. All these different effects could contribute to adverse reactions to food, but the major factor in false food allergy is the direct effect of lectins on mast cells.

Many lectins are inactivated by cooking, but they need to be heated for a long time and at fairly high temperatures to destroy all their activity. The powerful lectin found in kidney beans or haricot beans *(Phaseolus vulgaris)* can cause serious diarrhea and abdominal pain if the beans are not soaked and cooked properly. Using low-temperature slow cookers to prepare casseroles containing beans has caused many outbreaks of such illness.

Whereas the lectin found in raw or badly cooked kidney beans is damaging to almost everyone, other lectins are more selective—indeed, the word *lectin* comes from a Latin word meaning "choosing." Each of us is slightly different in our chemical makeup, and one important way in which people vary is in the short carbohydrate molecules that sit on the surface of our body cells. It is mainly these carbohydrates to which the lectins bind, and they are highly specific for the individual sugars that make up the carbohydrate. Each type of lectin is specific for a particular sugar. (There is also a short carbohydrate chain in every antibody molecule, and it may well be that lectins trigger mast cells by binding to the carbohydrate component of IgE.)

It seems likely that individual differences in the carbohydrate chains (either on the cell surface, or in IgE molecules) could make some people susceptible to a particular lectin that has no adverse effect on the majority of the population.

But if susceptibility to particular lectins causes false food allergy, why is this problem so rare? The answer must be that natural selection has weeded it out, because it would have been a serious disadvantage among our distant ancestors if an important ingredient in the common diet could not be eaten. Any individual who suffered such an affliction probably would have died early without leaving any offspring. In this way, the genes that could make a person susceptible to false food allergy would have remained very rare. But even such damaging genes can survive if they are capable of being masked by other "healthy" genes. This means that some people can carry the gene without suffering any ill effects and pass it on to their children.

The Radioallergosorbent Test (RAST)

The **radioallergosorbent test,** or **RAST,** measures the level of IgE antibodies that a person has to a specific substance, such as a food protein or a pollen. There are four stages to the test:

1. An extract of the food (or other potential allergen) is applied to beads made of a substance called sepharose. This is an inert substance that simply acts as a surface on which reactions between the allergen and the antibody can take place. The food molecules remain attached to the sepharose beads throughout the test.
2. A sample of the patient's serum (the liquid part of the blood) is allowed to flow over the beads. If the blood contains IgE antibodies to that food, these will bind to the food antigens on the beads. The beads are later rinsed to remove everything that is not bound—only the IgE molecules should remain.
3. Another liquid is poured over the beads. This contains a special type of antibody called anti-IgE, which binds specifically to the stem of IgE molecules. If there is IgE stuck to the beads, these anti-IgE antibodies will bind to it. If no IgE is present, then all the anti-IgE will be washed away.
4. The anti-IgE has been previously marked with a radioactive or colored marker. This means that the amount of IgE present can be worked out by measuring the radioactivity or color given off by the beads. The amount of anti-IgE present is a measure of how much IgE (specific for that food) there is in the patient's blood.

Of course, the test will also give a positive result if the food contains something that specifically binds to IgE (as long as there is some IgE in the blood). This does indeed happen in some patients with false food allergy, and is discussed on pages 112–13.

Should new drugs become available that specifically counteract IgE, these would not work for false food allergy. Similarly, vaccines designed to reduce production of IgE would be ineffective.

Other Foods That Can Trigger Mast Cells

Although lectins are probably the best-studied, they are certainly not the only food components that can trigger mast cells directly. Several foods contain **peptides** (small proteinlike molecules), which also bind to mast cells and make them degranulate. Among the foods known to contain such peptides are egg white, strawberries, crustacean shellfish (prawns, shrimps, crabs, lobsters), tomatoes, fish, pork, alcohol, and chocolate.

Pineapple and papaya both contain very powerful **proteolytic** (protein-breaking) **enzymes** that can attack the membranes of any body cell, including mast cells. This again may cause the mast cells to degranulate. It is not certain whether some individuals are more susceptible than others, but it is not advisable for anyone to eat raw pineapple or papaya on an empty stomach, because of the damage done to the stomach lining by these enzymes. Canned pineapple is safe, because the heat used in canning inactivates the enzyme.

Yet another group of foods contains substances that appear to trigger mast cells but whose chemical identity is unknown. The foods in question are buckwheat, sunflower seeds, mango, and mustard. The offending ingredient—which is assumed to be a peptide or protein—binds to the IgE of susceptible individuals.

Diagnosing False Food Allergy

Sorting out false food allergy from the real thing is far from easy. A skin-prick test (see page 34) will not distinguish someone with false food allergy from someone who has true IgE-mediated food allergy—both can produce a positive result. The radioallergosorbent test or RAST (see page 111) is usually positive as well, because the lectins or other offending food components bind IgE—in a true case of allergy, the IgE will bind the food antigen, but the results of the test look just the same. A simple modification of the RAST reveals the truth, however; if extra food extract is added to the mixture, false food allergy will still give a positive test, but true food allergy will not.

Distinguishing between these two distinct types of food reaction is important to researchers seeking to understand food allergy and establish its prevalence. As far as the patient is concerned, the distinction is less important, because the consequences and treatment are much the same. In most cases avoidance will be necessary. At present, if drugs are used, they will be ones that prevent mast cells from or counteract the effect of the mediators—in either case, it does not matter how the mast cells are being triggered.

It is possible that those with false food allergy have some underlying deficiency that may make them more susceptible. It has been found that 50 percent of patients with false food allergy are deficient in the element magnesium. A shortage of magnesium is known to affect histamine release and increase sensitivity to histamine. A nutritional assessment (see page 332) might be advisable for anyone known to have false food allergy.

Surprisingly enough, it is possible to grow out of false food allergy. Children who have such a reaction to a particular food sometimes lose it, usually by the time they are eight years old. Exactly why this should happen is far from clear. There could be a change in the structure of the tissues that surround the mast cells in the gut, making them less accessible to food molecules.

Histamine in Foods

Some foods contain large amounts of histamine, and this can cause unpleasant symptoms when they are eaten. The histamine has a druglike (pharmacological) effect on the body. Although this is not false food allergy (according to the definition we are using), it is appropriate to discuss it here—since histamine is also the main mediator produced by mast cells, the effects are similar.

Histamine is formed in foods by the action of certain bacteria. These are not disease-causing bacteria and their presence is normally harmless, but if they are too numerous, the histamine they generate can cause problems. The principal foods concerned are well-ripened cheeses and salami-like sausages, especially those that are kept for a long time. Some types of fish, principally mackerel and tuna, may cause similar problems if they are not kept at low temperatures before being eaten or canned. Bacteria in the fish produce a cocktail of toxins that includes generous quantities of histamine. Fish affected in this way have a sharp, peppery, or metallic taste and may be darker in color. Canned fish of any kind, sauerkraut, and many alcoholic drinks can also be rich in histamine.

Histamine levels are extremely high in some red wines, quite high in champagnes, but moderate in beer and white wine. People who are intolerant of wine may well have a diminished ability to break down histamine.

For those not affected in this way who simply eat or drink an unusually large amount of histamine at one meal, the symptoms of histamine poisoning are nausea, diarrhea, skin rashes, flushing, and headaches. The liver is well equipped to detoxify histamine, and these unpleasant symptoms are relatively short lived, usually clearing up within twelve hours. However, the drug isoniazid, used for the treatment of tuberculosis, reduces the liver's ability to break down histamine, and anyone taking this drug should avoid histamine-rich foods. Viral hepatitis and cirrhosis of the liver also make the body less able to detoxify histamine. Some people with chronic urticaria seem to be unusually susceptible to histamine and should avoid it for a while to see if the urticaria clears up.

Any increase in the leakiness of the gut wall increases susceptibility to histamine in foods, simply because more histamine gets through. It seems likely that greater permeability of the gut is a common feature of both food allergy and food intolerance, so avoiding histamine-rich cheeses and sausages may be generally advisable.

Treatment of Chronic Urticaria (Hives)

If you have had chronic urticaria for less than six months, take heart, because it clears up spontaneously in about 50 percent of cases. Those who have been suffering for more than six months have a much smaller chance of recovering unaided (only 6 percent), so treatment is advisable.

In the first edition of this book, we noted that only about 20 or 30 percent of people with this distressing problem are likely to discover the underlying cause. We are pleased to say that this figure has now been pushed up to 77 percent by some research teams who are studying chronic urticaria intensively. Indeed, one recent paper from doctors at the University of Munich in Germany states "there are probably few truly 'idiopathic' cases of urticaria." The word *idiopathic* will not need explaining to anyone who has been hunting for an explanation for their chronic urticaria for years—it's the label doctors apply when they cannot find a cause for the disease.)

The Munich researchers, and many others, believe that it's almost always possible to find a cause for so-called idiopathic urticaria if you just keep trying. Contrast this with the gloomy pronouncements of some United States allergists that 90 percent of the time your physician will not be able to find the cause of your hives or the cause cannot be determined in up to 85 percent of cases. These allergists generally test for the physical urticarias with an ice cube, heat, etc. (see page 51), check out the possibility of an inherited defect or a more serious underlying disease by taking skin biopsies and blood tests, and then stop.

Assuming you've had chronic urticaria for more than six months and have never been through this basic set of tests, start by seeing a conventional allergist or dermatologist who will take you through them. Should a cause for your symptoms, such as cold or exercise, be found by these tests, you will probably be advised simply to avoid these. This is good advice, as far as it goes, but many people with a physical urticaria have multiple causes for their symptoms, and dealing with other causes may mean that cold, exercise, or whatever is no longer a trigger (see the case history on page 117).

Assuming the standard tests find no explanation for your chronic urticaria, then look at the list of possible causes on page 51 and consider whether there is anything (such as ointments, creams, latex rubber, or pets) that you are in contact with regularly that could explain your symptom pattern. Do you have symptoms that come on mainly during the pollen season, but are not explained by heat or sunlight? None of these are common causes of chronic urticaria, but they are ones you could, in theory, track down for yourself. The problem, of course, is that chronic urticaria comes and goes all the time and can be affected by the temperature, by emotional stress, and by a host of other factors. You will need to keep a clear head when puzzling all this out, and you may need medical help to finally pinpoint the culprit.

The next logical step is to try an additive-free diet. You should eat at home and make all your own food from fresh produce (no shortcuts—even things like cooked chicken and ready-to-eat salad can contain additives). At the same time, cut out alcohol, spices, and all aspirin and related drugs (see page 79). Don't use toothpase unless its guaranteed additive-free (baking soda can be used instead) and drink mineral water or filtered water. Medicinal drugs can contain colorings and other additives, so you should try to get additive-free versions of all your medications. You may need to use a specialist pharmacy for this (see pages 457–458). Continue with this regime for at least six weeks before concluding that there is no improvement. If your urticaria does clear up, you can undertake cautious testing with small amounts of tap water, spices, and alcohol, but you will probably need medical help to work out which additives are at fault. It is difficult to organize these tests at home, because most foods contain such a mixture of additives. There is also the possibility of quite severe reactions on testing, so medical supervision is desirable. In particular, you should not test aspirin or aspirinlike drugs at home, as life-threatening reactions are common in sensitive individuals—avoidance can heighten your reaction.

Other dietary investigations that you can try for yourself are a low-histamine diet, and a low-carbohydrate diet. Research has shown that many patients with chronic urticaria cannot break histamine down as well as they should, and histamine absorbed from food could be causing their illness. The foods to avoid are given on page 113.

Histamine is also produced by the bacteria of the gut, and the amount can be excessive if a lot of starchy foods, or a lot of fruit and vegetables, are eaten. If someone suffers from chronic urticaria and it gets worse shortly after every meal, bacterially generated histamine is a possibility that should be considered. Reducing starch intake, fruit and vegetable intake, or both may help. Eating live yogurt may also be useful in improving the balance of different kinds of bacteria in the gut.

Should you have gas, bloating, or an itchy anus, yeast overgrowth in the gut is a possibility. For this you need a no-yeast, no-sugar diet (see page 244) and a course of antifungal drugs from your doctor.

After this, if you are still looking for a cause, you could also try an elimination diet, to look for food intolerance. However, this is a relatively unusual cause of chronic urticaria and quite a big undertaking, so you may want to explore other possibilities first. Note that food ingredients in medication—such as antihistamines—could interfere with the results of the elimination diet if you are very sensitive to a food such as corn. Food-free medicines are available (see pages 457–458).

Those with chronic urticaria should test foods in very small portions at first—just a mouthful. If there is no reaction whatever after four hours, test a normal portion.

A note of caution here—the elimination diet is for chronic urticaria only, not acute urticaria. Those who have prompt reactions to food, symptoms in the lips and mouth, or positive skin-prick tests should never undertake food testing at home. Should you ever have suffered any swelling (angioedema) of the throat from any food, do not test foods except under medical supervision.

Long-term unrecognized infection elsewhere in the body is an important cause of chronic urticaria. Possibilities include infected teeth, sinusitis, throat infections, tonsillitis, middle-ear infections, inflammation of the gallbladder, kidneys, ovaries or uterus, intestinal parasites, athlete's foot or related infections (intertrigo, onychomycosis, tinea), prostatitis, Epstein-Barr virus, and cytomegalovirus. If you have diarrhea and inflamed joints as well, Yersinia infection is a possibility. Ask your family doctor to help with investigation of these or find another board-certified doctor who will assist you.

Elizabeth

As a schoolgirl Elizabeth suffered from a rather odd type of hives that only came on when she was cold. It made her very miserable in winter, with an unbearably itchy rash on any exposed part of her body. She found this difficult to live with because she was very enthusiastic about sports and could not play hockey or other outdoor games in winter. Cold-induced urticaria, as her problem is known, can indicate more serious underlying problems, but medical tests showed that this was not the cause of the symptoms in her case. The standard test for cold-induced urticaria is to place an ice cube on the patient's arm for three minutes. When the doctor tried this on Elizabeth, she reacted with hives on the arm. Purely as an experiment, the doctor decided to try Elizabeth on an elimination diet. After five days of excluding all commonly eaten foods, she did not react to the ice cube test. But when she reintroduced milk, and later eggs, she reacted in the same way as before. By avoiding these foods in winter, or eating them only occasionally, she is free of hives. This has allowed her to do something she never thought possible before—go on a skiing vacation!

Some researchers believe that *Helicobacter pylori* in the stomach, a common infection that can be a cause of recurring stomach ulcers, may also be a source of chronic urticaria. The research is conflicting on this point, but if all other inquiries have proved fruitless, and you have an active *Helicobacter* infection (shown by a breath test for urea and a stomach biopsy) then it is worth trying eradication treatment. You must take three antibiotics simultaneously for one to two weeks. This is not always successful the first time around, so a second stomach biopsy is essential, followed by a second round of antibiotic treatment if the bacteria are still found.

Very occasionally, chronic urticaria is an early symptom of adult-onset celiac disease.

These investigations could take some time, and it is important to control symptoms in the meantime. Medical opinion at present favors a nonsedating antihistamine, as used for hay fever, plus a type of drug that is usually used for those with stomach ulcers, called an H-2 receptor antagonist. This blocks a different kind of receptor for histamine. The two drugs together block both kinds of histamine receptor (H-1 and H-2) and many doctors believe that the combination achieves better control of chronic urticaria. If you are sensitive to colorings, other additives, or to any foods, you should obtain special formulations of these drugs that are guaranteed free from such extras (see pages 457–458).

Antihistamines can become ineffective if taken continuously for years. Switching to another kind of antihistamine may help.

Leukotriene antagonists, new drugs currently prescribed only for asthma, may also be useful for chronic urticaria, according to preliminary trials.

SIX

The Great Controversy

No one writing about food intolerance can claim to be reflecting majority opinion, because there are such widely differing views on the subject. By looking at those differences in opinion first, before considering food intolerance in detail, we hope to give you a better understanding of our own viewpoint on the subject.

Why is there so much disagreement over food intolerance? And why do so many doctors regard it as a "media illness," the outcome of ill-informed publicity? There is no simple answer to this question, but it is an important one nonetheless. The disagreement is not over whether food intolerance exists—few doctors would dispute that it does. What is at issue is the prevalence of the problem, and the sort of symptoms it can cause.

The question of prevalence is problematic because there are no reliable data available. Estimates of how many people suffer from food intolerance range from a very conservative 0.3 percent to a rather implausible 90 percent. A more realistic figure is probably somewhere between 10 and 25 percent.

Controversy over the sort of symptoms caused by food intolerance is equally fierce. The orthodox view is that foods are unlikely to cause symptoms such as rheumatoid arthritis or Crohn's disease (a severe inflammation of the bowel), and that only certain sorts of foods might trigger migraines. The idea of foods causing mental problems, such as depression, anxiety, hyperactivity, or even psychosis is considered quite outrageous by most orthodox doctors and psychiatrists. The list of complaints attributed to food intolerance, given in chapter 7, contains many other controversial items.

A related issue is the type of symptoms caused by food allergy. Although most allergists have now come around to the idea that allergic reactions to foods may cause asthma and eczema, not all have. And few are willing to accept that other problems, such as hyperactivity in children, might be linked to food allergy. For historical reasons, these debates are linked to those over food intolerance (see page 10), so they, too, form part of this chapter.

In the course of this chapter we will look at these bones of contention in some detail, assess the scientific evidence, and try to discover why the question of food sensitivity generates so much heated debate.

Cause-and-Effect Thinking

In the eighteenth and early nineteenth centuries, doctors tried to explain why they saw certain patterns of diseases. Epidemics broke out in the crowded urban slums created by the Industrial Revolution due to a lack of sanitation and clean water supplies. Knowing nothing of bacteria and viruses, doctors constructed the theory of "miasmas" to explain them.

Miasmas were elusive, unidentified atmospheric conditions that could somehow cause disease. To explain the great variety of diseases that appeared in the same crowded areas, the miasmas were assumed to be nonspecific—they might cause cholera in some people, yellow fever in others, and so on. As an extension of this idea, other factors in the environment were assumed to cause disease. Cold was an obvious one, and it too was seen as being nonspecific—different people suffered different symptoms when they lived in cold houses or breathed cold air.

In the 1860s and 1870s, a revolution occurred in medical thinking. Dr. Robert Koch in Germany and Louis Pasteur in France discovered that microorganisms caused a great many diseases. More important, they found that specific bacteria caused specific illnesses. This is a fact that we now take for granted, but in its time it was a remarkable and novel idea. The **germ theory,** as it was known, quickly replaced the old idea that a miasma or other environmental factor could cause a great variety of different ills.

The change in medical thinking brought about by the germ theory was a radical one. In a reaction to the vagueness of the old ways of thought, a dogmatic insistence on cause-and-effect thinking took over. From then on, each disease had to have a specific set of symptoms and a specific cause. This way of thinking, with its obvious scientific merits, has dominated medical education for the past century.

Food intolerance, as it is presently understood, is anathema to this way of thinking. The range of symptoms claimed for it is vast. No two patients are alike, and there is no single symptom that is common to all. Different foods are at fault in different patients—and they cause different symptoms. Some patients are apparently sensitive to other things as well, such as house dust mites or synthetic chemicals. There are no tests for food intolerance and no obvious physical signs—indeed, the patients often look well. To cap it all, there is no obvious mechanism.

As Dr. William Bynum, a medical historian at the Wellcome Institute, observes:

> There is a general reluctance among the medical establishment to accept things that are nonspecific and don't always cause the same symptoms. It smacks too much of the old ideas of causation in medicine—cold weather was supposed to cause head colds in some people and rheumatism in other people and so on. Causal thinking before the germ theory was extremely loose and it did not satisfy the usual canons of scientific explanation about cause and effect. There has been a strong reaction to that, and the problem with so-called food intolerance is that it goes against the grain of present-day thinking.

Two other factors help make food intolerance seem dubious. Many of the symptoms that are claimed for it are symptoms of a general type that can be caused in all sorts of different ways. Headache, for example, can be due to a bump on the head, anxiety, overwork, a brain tumor, or a wild party the night before. What is more, many of the symptoms are those that can be produced by psychosomatic illness, in which emotional or mental distress evokes physical symptoms in the body (see pages 195–98). Both these factors make the phenomenon of food intolerance seem even less credible.

Doctors come to food intolerance with a set of preconceived ideas that automatically prejudice them against the whole concept. And unlike the general public, they are not readily swayed by stories of miracle cures, however numerous those stories might be. This sort of evidence is referred to in medical science as "anecdotal," and is quite rightly treated with great caution. The human body and mind interact in mysterious ways, and a person may recover from an illness spontaneously or in response to an entirely ineffective treatment. The latter is known as the **placebo effect,** and is described on pages 199–201. These and other factors make individual case histories a doubtful item of evidence. Even if diets are helpful in clearing up the symptoms, it may be for some other reason entirely—perhaps the person's previous diet was unsound nutritionally, or contained an unhealthy amount of caffeine or some other druglike substance that was causing the symptoms.

The history of medicine is littered with bogus miracle cures that apparently worked wonders in their day. Hydropathy, popular in the nineteenth century, was said to be a cure for all sorts of nervous complaints and long-term illnesses. The treatments consisted of alternate hot and cold baths, wrapping the patients in wet blankets, and requiring them to drink huge quantities of water. These measures were supposed to "strengthen the fibers" of the body and rid it of poisons. Direct Faradism (named after Faraday, who helped discover electricity) involved giving mild electric shocks to the arms and legs. It was recommended to anyone who was tired or run down, or had other nervous afflictions. The electric shocks supposedly stimulated the constitution. Both these therapies were highly regarded in their day, and thousands felt they had benefited from them. Mass enthusiasm is a strange thing—simply feeling caught up in some wonderful new discovery may be a powerful form of treatment.

There are various other preconceived ideas that work against food intolerance—the belief that food is essentially passive and innocuous, for example (see pages 17–18); the notion that what we have eaten for thousands of years must be good for us (see pages 22–23); and the simplistic model of digestion that assumes no complex molecules reach the bloodstream (see pages 23–24). These mistaken ideas all contribute to the understandable skepticism of the medical world.

Seeing the Light

A combination of factors such as these makes it very difficult for doctors, however open minded they may be, to accept many of the effects now being claimed for food sensitivity. Dr. Doris Rapp describes in her book *Allergies and the Hyperactive Child* how she became a convert to the idea that foods and inhalants could cause hyperkinetic syndrome:

> I am ashamed to admit that from 1960 to 1975 while in practice as a pedriatric allergist, I seldom recognized or

diagnosed this problem. Then, as often happens in medicine, my patients taught me.

One of the patients involved was a five-year-old girl who had nose, eye, and chest allergies, for which Dr. Rapp was consulted. The parents mentioned that she was also irritable, overactive, depressed, and weepy, and suffered from stomachaches, headaches, and diarrhea. Dr. Rapp suspected brain damage as the cause of the behavioral problems, which of course would be incurable. Her main concerns were the allergies, and these she attempted to treat with an elimination diet, plus suggestions for the removal of major allergens from the home:

> In three days, her mother called to say she was extremely pleased. I assumed Paula's hay fever and asthma had improved, but her mother said no, Paula's disposition and her activity were better. I was amazed and perplexed. The mother said Paula's teacher had called to find out which "drug" the child was taking. . . .

A succession of similar experiences were enough to change Dr. Rapp's outlook. "How could I have missed it for so long?" she goes on to ask. "The answer is that a doctor often sees what he wants to see and is trained to see. If parents noticed their child had a better disposition, stopped wetting the bed, or seemed less tired or less overactive after a diet, I always believed that it was because the nose and chest allergies were better. . . ."

Many other doctors who work in the field of food sensitivity have similar tales to tell. Some have come to the idea because they themselves, or members of their families, were plagued by mysterious illnesses. In desperation they tried an elimination diet and found that symptoms that had troubled them for years cleared up within a week or two. This encouraged them to look again at some of their long-term patients with unidentified illnesses, and when they began to try elimination diets on such patients they found that many of them responded very well.

Belief and Disbelief

So far we have only looked at attitudes to food intolerance in terms of beliefs and preconceived ideas, which will undoubtedly seem odd to anyone with a scientific turn of mind. In theory medical beliefs should be secondary to the scientific evidence, for or against, although in reality they rarely are. Dr. David Atherton of the Institute of Child Health in London, who specializes in treating eczema, writes:

> I am often asked by skeptical colleagues whether I "believe in all this food business." It is a sad reflection on current medical practice that such an important question as the relationship between a patient's diet and their disease should be relegated to one of belief or disbelief.

In the next section we will consider the scientific evidence, but as we do so the importance of prejudice will again become evident. Even in the most scientific studies of this subject, it seems that the beliefs of the experimenters can influence the outcome. In general, those who believe in food intolerance tend to get positive results, while the disbelievers usually get negative results. The conclusions you draw from this will, of course, be influenced by what you believe! But as we hope to show, there are simple explanations for these apparently contradictory findings.

The Scientific Evidence

Safety in Numbers

Medical science is never exact, for a variety of reasons. For a start, people are different, both in the genes that make them what they are and in the environmental conditions that shape them from birth. Those environmental conditions include childhood and adult illnesses, standard of nutrition, type of work, nature of relationships with other people, past medical treatments, and present living conditions. A collection of patients also differs in age and sex, two very important factors in health and illness. Their response to treatment is bound to differ for these reasons alone.

A second major factor is the imprecise nature of diagnosis. Names may be given to diseases—*rheumatoid arthritis*, for example, or *migraine*—but this does not mean that they are single, clearly defined conditions in the way that infectious diseases such as measles or cholera are. Doctors suspect that although the symptoms look similar, there are a multitude of different disorders sheltering under such umbrella terms. One of the ways in which medicine advances is by recognizing different subgroups within such diseases, and giving new names to the symptoms shown by those subgroups—*classical migraine* and *common migraine,* for example. But in many diseases there are no obvious subgroups, even though it is clear that the patients are not all the same. This is particularly true in food intolerance.

To overcome these problems in medical trials, it is important to study as large a group of patients as possible. Because the patients suffering from a disease can be so diverse, a new treatment may only be effective for, say, 10 percent of them. A study that includes only twenty patients should, in a perfect world, include two patients who will respond. But when numbers are this small, the laws of chance dictate that there could easily be no patients of this type in the group. So a group of one hundred patients may be needed to give a convincing result—but such large-scale trials are costly and difficult to organize.

Different Doctors, Different Patients

A third factor that influences medical trials is the type of patients a particular doctor sees. To take one example, a consultant gastroenterologist working in a large hospital will see a wide range of patients with persistent diarrhea who have been referred by their family doctors. These patients will vary in all sorts of ways, including their own ideas about their illness. Some may think that particular foods cause their symptoms, but most will have no clue at all why they are ill. An allergist, on the other hand, will not see many patients with diarrhea, but those he does see will probably have been referred by their family doctor because the patients believe their symptoms are caused by allergies to food. Experience shows that such patients have often tried some form of self-diagnosis, or alternative therapy, without success.

A proportion of the allergist's patients may be people with psychosomatic problems who have latched on to diet as an explanation for their symptoms because they find the label *psychosomatic* unacceptable (see page 203). Despite their lack of success in identifying dietary triggers for their symptoms, they are unwilling to give up. Of course, the first group of patients—those seen by the gastroenterologist—may well include some with psychosomatic problems, but they are probably fewer than in the group seen by the allergist.

When referring patients, family doctors take account of the consultant's views, and, it must be said, their own personal preferences. A difficult patient whose diarrhea is accompanied by a patently neurotic personality is likely to be referred to a doctor whose main interest lies in psychosomatic causes. Another patient with much the same bowel symptoms but whom the family doctor believes to be mentally well balanced will probably be referred to a doctor who is more interested in physical causes. This again biases the sample of patients that a particular doctor sees and tends to reinforce medical prejudices.

Neither of these two groups of patients is a representative sample of everyone in the country with persistent diarrhea. A survey indicating that a third of apparently healthy people suffered some form of bowel disorder (see page 153) also discovered that the majority had not sought medical treatment. So the statistics produced by any medical study are not necessarily applicable to the population at large.

Studies of Food Intolerance

In the face of all these difficulties it is reasonable to ask why anyone bothers with such studies. But they do, in the interests of establishing scientifically valid forms of diagnosis and treatment. Attempts to do this in relation to food intolerance are many and varied, and we will not try to cover them all. What matters in such studies is the care with which they are designed and the details of how they are carried out. To assess a trial properly the details must be carefully considered, and we will therefore concentrate on five trials—two dealing with rheumatoid arthritis, two with irritable bowel syndrome, and one with migraine. These trials are the main ones carried out within the past twenty years, and they are among the most scientific attempts to evaluate the food-intolerance concept.

Trials Dealing with Rheumatoid Arthritis

Rheumatoid arthritis is a disease in which the joints become painful, swollen, and warm due to internal inflammation. There are characteristic changes in the level of certain factors in the blood that help confirm the diagnosis. Contradictory results from different trials are often due to a failure to diagnose rheumatoid arthritis properly. This disease should not be confused with other forms of joint pain, which are milder, more transient, and do not produce the same sort of changes in the blood or damage to the joint—it is well known that joint pains of this type can be due to allergic reactions to food. What is at issue is whether foods can ever be a factor in true rheumatoid arthritis. In the two studies described here, all the patients involved were diagnosed as cases of rheumatoid arthritis by a standard set of tests.

Dr. Gail Darlington, a rheumatologist, carried out one such trial with the help of Dr. John Mansfield, a private practitioner with many years' experience of elimination diets.

This was a reasonably large-scale study with fifty-three rheumatoid arthritis patients involved, and forty-four actually completing the trial. They all underwent a two-week "washout" period during which the medicines they had been taking were withdrawn; instead they all received acetaminophen, plus a dummy tablet that they were told was a new drug. This sort of treatment is known as a placebo. Placebos play an important part in scientific trials, as explained on page 199.

After two weeks the patients were split into two groups, one of which began an elimination diet. For the first week, this diet consisted of five rarely eaten foods. All milk products, eggs, cereals, beverages, and additives were excluded, along with most meats and all commonly eaten fruits and vegetables.

After the first week these excluded foods were reintroduced, one at a time. Any foods that caused a flare-up of symptoms were not eaten again. The assessment of the patients continued for six weeks—long enough for them to have tested most foods and established a workable diet that excluded all incriminated foods.

While the first group of patients was undergoing the elimination diet, the other group kept on taking their dummy tablets. After six weeks they were told that a different form of treatment would be tried—and they were then put on the elimination diet. The objective here was to use the second group to assess the placebo effect—the improvement that is produced by any new form of treatment. Their response during the first six weeks on the dummy tablets was a measure of the placebo response that might be expected in the other group during the elimination diet.

The joint symptoms of all the patients were assessed using various standard measurements of pain and stiffness, plus routine blood tests that help evaluate the severity of rheumatoid arthritis. The assessor was unaware of which patients belonged to which group and was therefore unbiased. The patients who received the dummy tablets first did show some improvement—so there *was* a placebo effect—but the group that undertook the elimination diet did far better. When the placebo group later went on the diet its members, too, showed a much more striking improvement.

Notice that these measurements are a rather crude assessment of improvement in the group as a whole: when considered individually, some showed little change, while others seemed to respond dramatically to the treatment. (The reasons for assessing patients as a "job lot," rather than individually, will become clear when we look at the next trial.) At the end of the diet three-quarters of the patients claimed to feel better or much better than at the outset.

Elimination diets often act as weight-reducing diets, and on average, Dr. Darlington's patients lost about ten pounds during the trial. Being overweight has a bad effect on diseased joints, especially those in the knees and ankles. So it could be argued that the loss of weight might have contributed significantly to the improvement seen. To check this, Dr. Darlington compared weight losses in those who had responded well and in those who had responded poorly. There was no difference, so this seemed unlikely to have been an important factor.

Despite these striking results, Gail Darlington is in no way a propagandist for the food-intolerance idea:

> I'm a very routine, orthodox physician and rheumatologist. If I spend the next ten years of my life helping to prove that the whole thing is a nonsense, or a placebo effect, or a nonspecific manipulation of the immune system, I won't be at all concerned—I simply feel it's an area that needs to be investigated in just as scientific a way as we look at Drug A versus Drug B. Before 1981 most people in the United Kingdom thought that food intolerance was rubbish in a rheumatological context, as indeed I did at that time—one is fairly definitely trained to believe it's rubbish. But I was impressed by the results I saw in my patients who had gone to other people to have their diets manipulated. After seven years working in this field, I've gradually come to believe that it is relevant to some patients. To take one example, I have a patient of thirty-three who has changed from being a limping acute arthritic to being a perfectly fit, normal young man—and that is an improvement he has maintained for two and a half years.

Rheumatologists tend to attribute such results to natural remissions, because rheumatoid arthritis is a disease that comes and goes for no apparent reason. It is also notoriously susceptible to placebo effects. Gail

Darlington understands these doubts, but feels they are misplaced:

> Yes, obviously, it could be purely coincidental, but I do
> have quite a few patients in this bracket now, and it does
> seem unlikely that they all just happened to go into natu-
> ral remission at the moment they began their diet. As for
> placebo effect, our trial was carefully designed to measure
> this in the control group. We showed that there was a
> placebo effect, but that it certainly couldn't account for all
> the improvement seen in the patients on the diet. What is
> more, when the control group were later put on elimina-
> tion diets, they responded just as well as the first group—
> far better than they had done on the placebo.

If Dr. Darlington is right, then why did a similar trial, carried out
three years earlier, produce such different results? This trial was conducted at a different hospital by Dr. Michael Denman, Dr. Bruce
Mitchell, and Dr. Barbara Ansell. They studied eighteen patients with
rheumatoid arthritis, putting them on diets that excluded various foods
for periods up to six months. In their opinion the effects of eliminating
foods cannot be assessed over shorter time intervals, because rheumatoid arthritis is such a variable disease. (Dr. Darlington's study overcame
this problem by using a large group of patients and measuring their symptoms as a whole—in this way, the week-to-week variations in individual
patients should cancel each other out.)

Only three of Dr. Denman's patients stuck to the course for the full
six months. Thirteen dropped out before two months, and the report
does not say how long they were on the diet. None of the patients showed
any improvement.

One problem with this study was that the diet did not eliminate
wheat, which other studies of food intolerance have identified as one of
the most common offending foods. The diet also allowed chicken, tea,
coffee, and all kinds of vegetables—including commonly eaten ones such
as potatoes that are often incriminated by elimination diets. This failure
to exclude several suspect foods, combined with the small number of
patients involved, could well explain the poor results.

Despite its obvious drawbacks and serious limitations, this trial is
quoted remarkably often as showing that elimination diets don't work
for rheumatoid arthritis. Fortunately there are now several other trials

that demonstrate the usefulness of elimination diets for a proportion of patients—about 30 to 40 percent of the total—with rheumatoid arthritis. One Norwegian study used a diet that was both an elimination diet and a vegetarian diet (in that meat was never reintroduced). In this study 44 percent of patients improved a great deal, and many of them were able to identify culprit foods. Straightforward vegetarian and vegan diets have been studied by several other research groups and are of no value in rheumatoid arthritis, so it is clear that it was the elimination diet that helped these Norwegian patients, not the avoidance of meat.

Other researchers, in India and in the Netherlands, have also produced evidence for the importance of food intolerance among some patients with rheumatoid arthritis. Again, they found that 30 to 40 percent of patients tested did very well. Only one study found that none of their rheumatoid arthritis patients responded well to the diet. This was a study carried out at Addenbrooke's Hospital in Cambridge, England, and the reasons for the anomalous result remain unclear. But while there were no "good responders" in this study, many patients did find that their symptoms improved a little during the exclusion phase of the diet, and that they worsened when testing foods. (What is particularly interesting is that a quarter of the patients felt they had reacted badly to tap water. The researchers tested their reactions double blind—giving them coded bottles of water to drink, so that neither the researchers nor the patients knew whether tap water or bottled mineral water was being tested at any one time. The double-blind tests showed that the reactions to tap water were all genuine.)

Trials Involving IBS

Irritable bowel syndrome or IBS is a disorder characterized by chronic diarrhea or constipation, or a mixture of the two. (*Chronic* in medical parlance means "long term.") In most patients there is also abdominal pain. A major trial of IBS patients was carried out at Addenbrooke's Hospital in Cambridge by Dr. John Hunter and Dr. Virginia Alun-Jones. Twenty-one patients were involved, and they were placed on a diet of nothing but lamb, pears, and water for the first week. Other foods were then reintroduced one at a time. Fourteen of the patients—66 percent—improved considerably on the diet and were then able to identify culprit foods. Eleven of these patients were later tested double-blind to check that the effects were not purely psychological. Normal-sized portions of the food were eaten, disguised in a strong-tasting lentil puree that effectively concealed the identity of the food. All the patients responded in much the same way as they had when they could taste the food being tested.

One obvious criticism of this trial is that the numbers involved were small. However, Dr. Hunter and Dr. Alun-Jones followed it up with another trial involving 122 patients. The percentage who responded to the diet was slightly higher—about 70 percent. When a follow-up questionnaire was sent out, two to three years later, 86 percent of patients replied, and 87 percent of those who replied were still following the diet and benefiting from it.

In another trial of IBS, although there was a response to an elimination diet, the percentage who benefited was much smaller. This study was carried out by Dr. David Pearson and Dr. Stephen Bentley of the University Hospital of South Manchester, England, and Dr. Keith Rix, a psychiatrist at the University of Manchester. The patients had all been referred to an allergy clinic at the hospital because they suspected that their bowel symptoms were caused by food.

Nineteen patients completed the diet, and fourteen of these showed an improvement in their symptoms. When tested with foods, ten produced consistent reactions to foods, while four did not.

At this stage two patients with consistent reactions dropped out of the study, so only eight were left. They were tested double-blind with food in capsules, and five of them failed to react to foods that they had previously identified as causing problems when they could taste the food. This left just three whose bowel symptoms could definitely be related to food—only 15 percent of the number who took part. Some of the patients were diagnosed as having mild psychiatric disorders, and this led the doctors involved to conclude that psychosomatic problems were an important factor in causing the symptoms for the remaining 85 percent. (This aspect of the study is discussed on page 204).

Unfortunately, there are several major drawbacks to this study. First, the number of patients involved was very small, and they were probably what doctors call a "highly selected group": that is to say, they were not representative of IBS patients as a whole, for reasons that have already been discussed (see pages 124–26). Second, 59 percent of the patients studied refused to undertake a full elimination diet, and according to the authors, "Wheat was not excluded in all these patients." Third, the methods used for double-blind testing were highly questionable. Some patients were given the food disguised in soy milk, which will inevitably give false results if patients are sensitive to soy. (Reactions to soy are increasingly common.) Other patients were given the food in powder form, contained in a gelatin capsule. The amount contained in the capsules was much too small to identify food intolerance (rather than allergy), as was pointed out in a joint report by the Royal College of Physicians and the Nutrition Foundation entitled *Food Intolerance and Food Aversion*. It is widely accepted, by orthodox and unorthodox doctors alike, that food-intolerance reactions do not occur with such small amounts of food. Food-allergy reactions can, of course, and the test procedure was probably designed with these sorts of reactions in mind. It is significant that the three patients who showed consistent positive reactions also had a range of atopic symptoms—asthma, eczema, hives, or hay fever. In other words, the double-blind test was probably detecting those with IgE-mediated allergic reactions to food and missing others with food intolerance. As the authors themselves admit, "Even patients with clear evidence of immunologically mediated sensitivity may not react every time they are exposed, particularly if the dose is limited."

Another trial of IBS patients, carried out two years later by a different group of doctors, produced similar results. In this study, only three out of forty-nine patients were found to be food intolerant. Unfortunately, this study followed a similar procedure to that of the Manchester group—wheat and citrus fruits were not excluded, and capsules were used for double-blind testing.

Trials Involving Migraine

Migraine is generally defined as "a severe headache, usually one sided, that may be accompanied by nausea, vomiting, and visual or perceptual changes." The symptoms vary greatly from one person to another, and there is considerable disagreement among doctors about what should or should not be described as a migraine. This makes the design and interpretation of trials involving migraines especially difficult.

The most comprehensive and frequently quoted trial of migraine patients was carried out at England's Great Ormond Street Hospital for Sick Children in 1982–83. It involved eighty-eight children with severe and frequent migraine, most of whom had other symptoms as well. More than two-thirds suffered from abdominal pain, diarrhea, and flatulence, and almost half showed disturbed behavior, the majority being hyperkinetic (see pages 264–70). Aching limbs and runny or congested noses were also common, and some children also suffered epileptic fits, recurrent mouth ulcers, vaginal discharge, asthma, or eczema. A few showed signs of permanent damage to the nervous system.

The majority of children with migraine do not show such a huge range of other symptoms, and in this sense the children studied were a highly selected group. Because Great Ormond Street is the major specialist center for children's diseases, its patients tend to be the most severely affected. This is the major criticism made of this study—that it is not generally applicable. Even so, it is of great interest because of the high degree of response obtained.

The children were initially placed on a low-risk diet consisting of one meat, one fruit, one vegetable, and either rice or potatoes. Vitamin and calcium supplements were taken to compensate for any deficiencies in this diet. The children stayed on this diet for three to four weeks, and those who showed an improvement then began reintroducing other foods, one per week. Those who did not improve after four weeks were put on another very simple diet, with a different selection of foods, to check whether they were sensitive to one of the components of the first diet.

If foods caused symptoms when they were reintroduced, they were withdrawn again, and the children continued until they had tested all commonly eaten foods. They were then tested again with one of the foods that seemed to cause a bad reaction, but this time the tests were done double-blind—neither the child, the parents, nor the experimenter knew which foods were being eaten. Toward this end, the foods were disguised in a strongly flavored puree and supplied in cans to be given to the children at home. The cans were identified by a code number, and it was only when the code was broken at the end of the experiment that it became clear which can contained the suspect food and which the placebo—unadulterated puree that should have caused no symptoms.

For various reasons, some children could not be tested double-blind, but forty were tested in this way.

The results of this trial were a surprise to many doctors, not least to those involved. Of the eighty-eight children who completed the diet, seventy-eight recovered completely on one or another of the simple diets that were tried during the first stage of the experiment. Another four children "improved greatly," and only six showed no improvement whatever. The response, in other words, was 93 percent, a staggeringly high figure by any standards. Of the children who improved, eight remained well even when foods were reintroduced, and they continued to be healthy on a normal diet. That left seventy-four children for whom particular foods could be identified as a cause of migraine in open trial. Of the forty who were then retested double-blind, thirty-five were made ill by the can containing the suspect food, but not by the placebo can. Three reacted to neither can, and two were made ill by the placebo. Given the vagaries of food reactions generally, thirty-five out of forty is an impressive response. The results would have been more convincing if the children could have been tested for all the foods to which they reacted on open trial, and if they could have been tested more than once, but the practical difficulties of doing this in such a large-scale trial are obvious.

One of the most unexpected features of this trial was the extent to which other symptoms cleared up during the diet. These symptoms—such as epileptic fits, hyperactivity, and aching limbs—were generally assumed to be unconnected with the migraine. Yet in the majority of children they disappeared during the initial stages of the diet, and reappeared when incriminated foods were eaten. So, too, did symptoms such as abdominal pain, diarrhea, flatulence, mouth ulcers, and vaginal discharge. The atopic symptoms—rhinitis (runny nose), asthma, and eczema—cleared up in only about half the children, suggesting that unidentified airborne allergens were playing a part. The only major symptoms not to clear up in any of the children were those due to permanent nervous-system damage.

One interesting feature of this trial is that four of the five researchers involved were highly skeptical about the importance of food at the outset. The exception was Professor John Soothill, who wished to set up the trial and persuaded the others to assist him. Their report of the experiment records that they "embarked on this study believing that any favorable response, such as that claimed to substantiate the dietary hypothesis, could be explained as a placebo reponse. The positive double-blind controlled trial . . . provides clear evidence that a placebo response was not the explanation."

Two American research teams have carried out similar studies with adult migraine sufferers. Professor Lyndon Mansfield of the University of Texas looked at forty-three migraine patients. The patients were given skin-prick tests for allergy, and if the tests were positive these foods were eliminated from the diet. Patients with no positive skin tests were put on a diet eliminating wheat, corn, milk, and eggs. There are several problems with this approach. Skin-prick tests rarely pinpoint problem foods in migraine, as Professor Mansfield now acknowledges. And the elimination diet used for the other patients was not really strict enough.

Despite these defects, the research team still found that 30 percent of the patients had far fewer migraines. Of those tested with double-blind challenges, 70 percent responded to the food that had already been incriminated by "open" challenges (those where the patient knew what food was being eaten).

Another study, by Dr. T. Ray Vaughan of Fitzsimons Army Medical Center in Colorado, looked at 104 patients, asking them to eliminate wheat, corn, milk, and eggs, as well as any food that gave a positive skin-prick test and any foods suspected of causing migraine. This approach produced an improvement in 66 percent of the patients, and 38 percent had less than half as many migraines. Not all patients could identify a food that caused migraine when they tested them openly, but 75 percent could. More than half of these identified the same food on double-blind challenges.

In both these studies the double-blind challenge was carried out with capsules, and these contained only about a third of an ounce of freeze-dried food. This was taken three times a day for each challenge, so an ounce was eaten in all, but it is still a very small quantity. This capsule test probably failed to identify some genuine reactions simply because so little food was given.

Other tests in adult migraine sufferers, using a full elimination diet, have produced a very good response (total or almost total relief from migraines) in 60 to 70 percent of sufferers. (Unfortunately, these trials did not use double-blind challenges to check the subsequent food reaction.) If the trials by Vaughan and Mansfield had used a more extensive elimination diet, they would almost certainly have gotten a higher recovery rate among their patients. As it is they found that about a third of patients were significantly better, and up to 10 percent lost their migraines altogether. Their studies are useful because of the double-blind challenges, which showed convincingly that common foods, such as wheat, milk, eggs, and corn, can cause migraine.

Migraine—The Arguments Against

With rheumatoid arthritis and irritable bowel syndrome, we were able to present another scientific trial that failed to find any response to an elimination diet. As far as we know, there has been no such trial with migraine. Paradoxically, the fact that foodstuffs already have an accepted role in the orthodox view of migraine is partly reponsible for this. Certain foods, such as chocolate, cheese, red wine, and citrus fruits, are well-known migraine triggers. They are thought to spark migraine attacks because they contain chemicals known as vasoactive amines that can have a druglike effect on the blood vessels. For more about these amines, see page 170.

A great many migraine sufferers have benefited by avoiding these trigger foods, but few find that their migraines clear up altogether when they avoid them. Other trigger factors, such as bright lights, television screens, or emotional upsets, still have to be avoided, and some migraines are experienced regardless of all these precautions. This is an important difference between the chocolate/cheese/red wine type of food response and the intolerance of commonly eaten foods, such as wheat and milk, diagnosed by elimination diet. When foods are identified by elimination diet and then avoided, it is common for migraines to disappear altogether—nonspecific triggers, such as bright lights, no longer seem to be a problem. This was noticed in the Great Ormond Street study, and is commonly reported by other doctors treating migraine with elimination diets.

In the orthodox approach to migraine, getting patients to avoid high-risk foods such as chocolate and then record any reduction in their attacks is a standard part of treatment. Unfortunately, as ideas about intolerance of everyday foods have filtered through, this same method has been extended to those foods. So patients who inquire if commonly eaten foods might cause their symptoms are told to omit wheat for a couple of weeks, then milk for a couple of weeks, and so on. The collective experience of all those treating food intolerance is that this approach simply does not work. The majority of people, if they are sensitive to any foods, are sensitive to more than one, and it is only if all are withdrawn at the same time that any improvement is noticed. This is why a proper elimination diet is necessary to detect this sort of food sensitivity. Yet the majority of migraine specialists dismiss the idea of food intolerance as a major, fundamental cause of migraine—and they do so on the basis of having asked patients to exclude foods from their diet one at a time.

Assessing the Evidence

Skeptics might suggest that we have deliberately chosen to describe trials that support our case—ignoring trials with negative results unless they had some obvious flaw, for example. In fact, the studies described here are not a carefully chosen selection—they represent the major scientific trials of food intolerance carried out during the past twenty years.

We believe the studies that produced no evidence for food intolerance in rheumatoid arthritis and irritable bowel syndrome were both seriously flawed. The doctors carrying out these studies are skeptical of the whole idea, and this has led them to disregard some important aspects of food intolerance—that it is vital to exclude all the likely foods at once, that wheat and citrus fruits are common culprits, and that normal-sized portions are usually needed to provoke a reaction during testing. The number of patients studied in these trials was small, and in the case of the IBS trial, they may not have been representative.

No medical trial is ever perfect, and various criticisms can be made of the three trials that showed a good response to an elimination diet. But they are all fairly minor criticisms, and they do not invalidate the overall findings. The doctors who carried out these trials were well aware of the controversial nature of their approach, and all took special care to design their trials very carefully. Moreover, some of the doctors who planned these trials believed that they would not see any response, or that it would be a placebo effect if they did. *Their own results changed their minds.*

Food and the Medical Fringe

Thus far it might seem that the controversy over food intolerance is a two-cornered fight: orthodox medical opinion on the one hand, various unconventional doctors (often called clinical ecologists in the United States) on the other. Life would be a great deal easier if this were true, but it is not.

To complicate matters, a great many unqualified practitioners have moved into the food-intolerance field.

Many people turn to alternative therapies, such as acupuncture or homeopathy, for treatment of migraines, irritable bowel syndrome, and other long-term illnesses. Some such treatments may have some benefits, perhaps through their effects on the autonomic nervous system (see page 196), and most do no harm. But the more recent involvement of alternative therapists in dietary treatments is far more worrying. Many of these therapists have little understanding of nutrition—or of food sensitivity, for that matter. Some have endangered the health of their patients by putting them on such restricted diets that they are short of essential vitamins, minerals, or protein. A case of scurvy (a serious deficiency of vitamin C) has been reported. Young patients are especially vulnerable, since children need food to fuel their growth and development. Over the past few years pediatricians have begun to see children with severe malnutrition as a result of ill-advised diets.

This has caused great concern among the medical profession and led some doctors to mount what can only be described as a crusade against the whole idea of food intolerance as a commonplace illness. Qualified and reputable private practitioners working in this area have found themselves as much under attack as the unqualified practitioners—everyone has been tarred with the same brush. These vociferous critics have been very influential, and the air of controversy and doubt that surrounds food intolerance owes a lot to their activities.

While their anger at cases of malnutrition is entirely understandable, in a sense these doctors are helping to perpetuate the very situation they deplore. The reluctance of most family doctors and specialists to take food intolerance seriously undoubtedly springs from its disreputable image, rather than from a careful weighing of the scientific evidence. Unable to get help from their doctors, patients who think that food might be at the root of their problems turn to alternative practitioners, and so the situation is perpetuated.

Of course doctors should not go along with every fashionable therapy simply because there is a demand for it from their patients. And of course there are some ailments that really are incurable, and for which "you'll just have to learn to live with it" is the best advice. But we believe that the scientific evidence is now strong enough to merit a major medical rethink on food intolerance. That same evidence suggests that common illnesses such as migraine, irritable bowel syndrome, and rheumatoid arthritis should not be regarded as incurable in all patients. For a significant number of people, eliminating certain foods can bring relief from such symptoms.

Dubious Tests for Food Allergy and Intolerance

An elimination diet is not an easy method of diagnosis, and unless the patient fully understands the procedure, it may not work at all. Doctors have been searching for a simpler method of diagnosing food intolerance for many years, but so far without success.

As alternative practitioners have moved into this field, they have found the elimination diet too difficult and time consuming, and have sought easier diagnostic tests. Some, such as the pulse test and the cytotoxic test, are based on methods that were originally devised by conventional doctors but found to be too inaccurate. Others are frankly unscientific. All have helped their practitioners to earn a very comfortable living, without necessarily doing the patients a great deal of good. We will only consider the most common tests.

The Cytotoxic Test

This involves taking a blood sample, extracting the white blood cells (immune cells), and then exposing them to food extracts. The theory behind the test is that if a patient is sensitive to a particular food it will affect the white blood cells, causing changes that are visible under a microscope. In severe reactions, the white blood cells are said to swell up and break open.

Scientific appraisals of the cytotoxic test show that food extracts do sometimes affect the white blood cells in this way, and a recent study under carefully controlled conditions produced 70 to 80 percent accuracy. If this could be achieved consistently—and, perhaps, improved upon—the test might be of some value, but the commercial tests presently available give so many wrong answers that they are of very little value. Tests sometimes show a reaction to foods that the patient can eat without getting any symptoms (a **false positive**) or they may fail to pick up a known food sensitivity (a **false negative**). In several investigations commercial laboratories offering cytotoxic tests have been sent duplicate samples of the same blood. Unaware that these were from the same person, the laboratories invariably give a different list of food sensitivity reactions for each sample.

There may well be some value in the cytotoxic test, but not as currently practiced. Scientific attempts to improve it are going on at present—in particular, the assessment of the reaction by the blood cells needs to be automated rather than assessed by someone looking down a microscope. Such assessment is highly subjective, and the results are known to vary from one observer to another. A more accurate version of the test may be available in a few years, but at present it is not worth the money.

Hair Analysis

Hair is mainly made up of a protein called keratin. Analyzing it involves breaking it down to determine the mineral content of the hair, which can be useful in showing if the body is deficient in certain minerals. This is the main use of hair analysis.

It is very difficult to see how the composition of hair could possibly indicate anything about the body's response to foods, but hair analysis is advertised as a method of diagnosing food intolerance. Objective trials have shown that the test has no value in the context of food sensitivity.

Pulse Rate Changes
This is a diagnostic method that was devised by an American allergist, Dr. Arthur Coca, in the 1940s. According to Coca, the pulse would increase markedly after a food-sensitive patient ate an offending food, and this could be used in diagnosis. Most doctors who have tried it say that although there is sometimes a rise, it is not dependable enough to be of diagnostic value—there are plenty of false negatives. The pulse can also quicken for many other reasons, so that there are also many false positives.

Other Diagnostic Tests
The other diagnostic tests available include those that use pendulums or dowsing rods to test patients; others use radionic boxes, "energy boxes," Vegatest electrical devices, or other instruments. There are also tests derived from applied kinesiology, which mostly measure muscle strength. Most of these tests are based on ideas about energy fields or energy flows in the human body that are said to be disturbed by illness. There is no reliable evidence to show that these tests actually work.

The implausible nature of the reasoning behind these tests becomes evident if you look more closely at what some practitioners actually do. Some claim that they do not need to have the patient present at all to perform the diagnosis—they can get to the root of the problem by swinging a pendulum over a list of foods while thinking about the patient. And it does not matter if the practitioner and patient have never met, apparently.

No amount of logic will dissuade those who firmly believe in this type of medicine, of course. But there are a great many others who turn to such therapists simply because they are ill, and desperate to find out the source of their illness. Such methods can seem attractive shortcuts to a cure, but in reality they are highly unlikely to work, and none has been evaluated scientifically. All those who think they may have food sensitivity would be much better advised to put their time and energy into an elimination diet—it is far more likely to help, and it will be a great deal cheaper.

"But It Worked for My Friend"

The therapists practicing these techniques would not stay in business if they had no successes, of course, and you may well meet people who claim to have been cured by such methods. This proves very little, however. Given that the most common sources of food intolerance are wheat and milk, such therapists can achieve a reasonable success rate by diagnosing sensitivity to these two foods in all their patients. If eggs, oranges, chocolate, tea, and coffee are added to the list, they may well achieve success with 50 percent or more, and some patients will benefit from the placebo effect alone (see pages 199–201). But there will be other patients who are not helped at all, or who are only partially better because the therapist's list does not include culprit foods.

Even those who are better are not getting a very good deal—they are almost certainly avoiding some foods unnecessarily. Quite apart from the inconvenience and social disruption that this causes, such people may not be eating an adequate diet. Indeed, anyone who cuts out certain foods without medical advice runs this risk, which is why we urge you to consult your doctor before embarking on an elimination diet, and to check with him or her subsequently to ensure that the diet you are eating is adequate.

SEVEN

Food Intolerance

There is a disease that is well known to doctors, although it does not feature much in medical textbooks. It is called "thick note syndrome." Those who suffer from it are waiting room regulars, and they have been referred to innumerable specialists for further examination—which is why their medical notes are so voluminous. Their symptoms are usually minor ones, but very varied and affecting many different parts of the body—the patients may have headaches, indigestion, diarrhea, aches and pains, rashes, and a host of other problems. In most cases, no physical disorder can be found to explain them.

It is generally assumed that patients with "thick note syndrome" are suffering from psychosomatic illness (which is discussed in the next chapter). But as food intolerance has become more widely recognized, doctors have begun to realize that many of these people may be sensitive to food. Multiple symptoms, affecting any and every body system, are a key feature of this disorder.

The second part of this chapter looks at each of those symptoms in turn, while the first considers the general features of food intolerance. Because so little scientific research has been done on food intolerance, much of what follows is based upon general impressions gained by many different doctors treating large numbers of people. This is not hard evidence, from a scientific point of view, but it is all we have to go on at present.

Given the controversial nature of food intolerance, many of the statements in this chapter might be disputed by some doctors. Ideally, we should qualify each contentious statement, but this would make the chapter very long and ponderous. We have therefore summarized the arguments over food intolerance in the previous chapter. On the basis of the evidence presented there, we believe that the case for food intolerance is very strong, and the present chapter is written from that viewpoint.

General Features of Food Intolerance

Everyday Foods

In food intolerance, it is almost always commonly eaten foods that are the source of the problem. In the United States, this means wheat, milk, and corn, which are usually consumed several times a day. Corn may often be eaten unwittingly—it finds its way into many prepared foods in the form of cornmeal, cornstarch, and corn syrup. As eating habits change, so, too, do sensitivities. Now that soybeans and soy flour are more widely used in processed foods, more cases of intolerance to soy are being seen. Where wheat and milk are not staple foods, other sensitivities prevail— a doctor practicing in Taiwan found that the most common culprit foods there were rice and soybeans.

The impression gained from patients' case histories is that a large intake of one food, regardless of what it is, can trigger intolerance of that food. For the breast-feeding mother, large amounts of a food can have a sensitizing effect on her baby.

Any food can produce intolerance, but it does seem that some foods are more likely to be a problem than others. Oranges, for example, are regularly identified as culprit foods, whereas apples are incriminated much less frequently. Yet apples and oranges are probably eaten in roughly equivalent quantities. Similarly, wheat appears to be a more potent cause of intolerance than other cereals. However, the idea that some foods are completely safe and can never produce food intolerance is wrong—this claim is sometimes made by alternative therapists, particularly those "dietary therapists" who emphasize the supposedly magical qualities of rice.

The general pattern of food intolerance seems to be as follows. Patients begin with sensitivity to milk, wheat, corn, eggs, or some other commonly eaten food. At this stage they probably have just one or two minor symptoms. As time goes by new sensitivities appear, to foods that are eaten less often. With new sensitivities come new symptoms, and the patients' health deteriorates. In those who have had food intolerance for many years, a large number of foods may be at fault—sometimes as many as twenty or thirty. Such people tend to be quite severely affected by their symptoms, to the extent that they cannot lead a normal life. However, these cases are a minority. Most people who need treatment for food intolerance are sensitive to between one and five foods, and they are able to function quite well despite their illness.

The amount of food needed to provoke symptoms is generally much larger in intolerance than in allergy. Someone with true food allergy may react to a single drop of milk or a trace of food left in a cooking utensil. One young man who was allergic to fish even fell victim to his girlfriend's kiss—she had eaten fish half an hour beforehand. Food-intolerant individuals never show this sort of exquisite sensitivity. They usually need normal-sized portions to provoke a reaction, although some will react to just a few mouthfuls of the food.

Slow Reactions

Unlike food allergy, where the reaction to a food can happen within minutes, food intolerance generally produces very slow responses to food. The symptoms may appear several hours after the food is eaten, or the following day, or even forty-eight hours later in the case of bowel symptoms. Because the food (or foods) in question are being eaten so frequently, there is no obvious link between the food and the symptoms. This effect was referred to as masking by the early clinical ecologists, and the name *masked food allergy* is still sometimes used for food intolerance.

For many of those with food intolerance, it is difficult to pinpoint a moment when the illness started. The symptoms can begin with mild problems that most of us take for granted, such as headaches or excessive tiredness or frequent bouts of indigestion. Over the years there is a slow decline into ill health, but it is often so gradual that the person does not really notice how bad things are getting. For some patients, however, food intolerance has a more definite beginning. It may follow a bad bout of influenza or other viral infection. Or it may stem from a course of antibiotics, such as those given before some operations, including hysterectomies. Where people have been exposed to toxic amounts of pesticides or other synthetic chemicals, food intolerance sometimes sets in immediately afterward.

Most people with food intolerance have symptoms that fluctuate from day to day, and there may be periods when they are worse for a while, or better. Changeable factors, such as stress, probably play a part in these fluctuations, by making patients more or less susceptible to the foods they are eating.

Following an elimination diet during which the offending foods are withdrawn for a week or more, the reaction time may speed up considerably. If a culprit food is eaten again after this period of avoidance, the reaction is likely to be both more prompt and more severe. In some people there is an almost immediate reaction, such as vomiting, flushing, itching, or a sudden flow of mucus from the nose. (However, sudden severe swelling of the lips and tongue—the characteristic symptom of immediate reactions in food allergy—is not seen.)

More puzzling still, the symptoms that appear upon testing are not necessarily the same ones that the patient had before. To orthodox doctors this is a very dubious aspect of food intolerance, and one that puts the whole phenomenon in doubt—it is a fundamental part of the scientific approach to medicine that the same cause should always produce the same effect. However, the common observation with food-intolerant patients is that the symptoms really do vary in some people, especially after abstinence from the food. How this might be explained is not known at present. But given the fact that food intolerance is probably a result of many interacting factors (see chapter 12), then changing symptoms may not be so implausible as they seem at first sight. If changes occur following exclusion of the food, it may be because one cause of sensitivity is more easily cured by avoidance than another. Not eating the food could also alter the balance of causative factors, and thus produce a different type of symptom.

Getting Over Food Intolerance

Food allergy, especially the immediate-reaction type, is usually lifelong. Food intolerance, on the other hand, tends to diminish if the food is avoided for a while. After a period of months or sometimes a year, the same food can be eaten without ill effects. But the potential for a reaction remains: if the food is eaten on a daily basis again, the intolerance is likely to reappear within a month or so. A viral infection can also spark food intolerance again.

Sometimes intolerance reactions disappear very quickly after avoidance of the food, and do not reappear even though the patients return to their previous diet. This seems to happen more often in children than in adults.

In general, the longer offending foods are avoided, the better patients become (as long as other foods are not eaten too regularly or in too great a quantity). With improving health, the people are better able to cope with both their diets and other environmental factors—airborne allergens, for example, or synthetic chemicals. Just as there was a gradual decline into ill health, so there is now a steady recovery, with the body becoming stronger and less sensitive at each step.

Food Addiction

Craving the culprit food is the most bizarre aspect of food intolerance— it affects about 50 percent of patients, at a very rough estimate. These patients tend to crave the particular food or foods that cause their problems. They may be aware of the craving and just regard it as a personal quirk, or they may be unaware of it but unconsciously select foods containing their culprit food. With wheat and milk, it is quite easy to do this unawares—the person who has to have cookies and a milky drink before bed, eats wheat cereal and milk for breakfast, and always has a cheese sandwich for lunch may well be a food addict of this sort.

If the food is avoided for a while, the cravings eventually disappear. But unfortunately, they reappear all too easily. Eating the same food (or a related food—see page 324) on a regular basis again can quickly reestablish the addiction, and the downward spiral is particularly difficult to combat. Because eating the food initially gives great satisfaction and well-being to a person in this addicted state, self-control is all the more difficult.

We do not want to take the analogy with drug addiction too far, but "food junkies" seem to suffer withdrawal symptoms when they give up their favorite food just as heroin addicts and alcoholics do when they try to kick their habit. One of the problems of following an elimination diet is that the first few days are often very unpleasant due to these withdrawal symptoms.

Although this aspect of food intolerance sounds peculiar and unlikely to anyone new to the subject, none of the doctors working in this area is in any doubt about it—they have all seen too many people with this same curious pattern of eating behavior. There is now a tentative explanation for this strange phenomenon (see pages 294–96).

The Symptoms of Food Intolerance

Every illness dealt with here can be caused in some other way as well, and it is important to remember this when thinking about your own problems. What makes food intolerance likely is if you have two, three, or more of these symptoms, especially if your doctor has been unable to find any cause for them.

No one with food intolerance will have all these symptoms—most patients have two or three major symptoms and several minor ones, but some people have just one symptom. No two patients with food intolerance are the same, and each one has a different collection of symptoms, acquired in a different order, and at a different time of life. Food intolerance can begin at any age, and it may disappear in a child as it grows up, only to reappear later, often in a different form.

The Digestive System

This is the front line as far as food is concerned, and it is hardly surprising that many of the symptoms of food intolerance occur here. Most patients show some disturbances of the digestive system, although they may be quite minor—but not all patients are affected in this way.

Mouth Ulcers

An ulcer is an area where the top surface of the mouth lining is lost, producing a small crater. Mouth ulcers are painful, especially when acidic fruits or spicy foods are eaten. There are two main types of ulcer—those caused by injury, and those caused in other ways. The first type is larger and can be caused by a rough edge on a tooth, badly fitting dentures, or careless brushing of the teeth. Those of the second type are smaller, about $1/16$ to $1/8$ inch across. Most people suffer from mouth ulcers of this type from time to time. They are only unusual if you have large crops of ulcers that recur frequently—roughly one person in ten is affected in this way.

Viral infections, the most common cause of mouth ulcers generally, are *not* found in cases of recurrent mouth ulcers. No one knows exactly what causes this problem, but it is thought to be some sort of infectious agent that induces the body to make antibodies against its own mouth cells. The infectious agent itself has not been tracked down yet, because it is not present in large numbers. According to this theory, the ulcers are produced by the body's immune system attacking the lining of the mouth. Heredity seems to play a part—recurrent mouth ulcers often run in the family.

Some vitamin and mineral deficiencies can also produce this symptom (see page 330), and those with Crohn's disease (see page 158),

---

John

For the past fifteen years John had suffered from regular bouts of mouth ulcers. Sometimes these were so painful that he could not eat for several days. Eventually the ulcers would clear up, only to come back again a few weeks later. During a long vacation in Southeast Asia, John's mouth ulcers were much less of a problem, and this made him wonder if food might be the culprit, because he was eating a very different diet while he was on vacation. Soon after his return, the mouth ulcers began to trouble him again. His doctor suggested that being on vacation and free of stress could have effected the cure, but John pointed out that they had never gotten better on vacations before. The foods he had eaten very little of in Southeast Asia were bread, milk, butter, and cheese, so he decided to try cutting these foods out for a while. There was no improvement, so the doctor suggested that John should also cut out foods containing wheat, such as cookies, pastry, and pasta. When he did so John's mouth ulcers improved considerably but did not disappear. The doctor then advised a gluten-free diet, cutting out oats, barley, and rye as well as wheat. On this diet, John has not suffered from mouth ulcers for over two years.

---

ulcerative colitis (see pages 181–84), and celiac disease (see page 104) also tend to suffer from persistent mouth ulcers.

In general, food intolerance is a relatively unlikely cause of recurrent mouth ulcers—but there are certainly some cases where such ulcers clear up during an elimination diet. Those with classical allergic symptoms, such as hay fever or asthma (atopics), are more likely to fall into this group than others. In most of those whose recurrent ulcers are due to food, there are other food-related symptoms as well, but sometimes recurrent mouth ulcers are the sole symptom of food sensitivity.

How foods might produce mouth ulcers is not known, although in atopic patients mast cells probably play an important part. Any food can be responsible (as in all forms of food intolerance), but there is some evidence that **gluten**—the mixture of proteins found in wheat, rye, barley, and oats—is a common offender here. Those who have mouth ulcers as their main symptom, or sole symptom, could try a gluten-free diet before embarking on the main elimination diet.

Burning Mouth

A burning sensation in the mouth is often mistakenly attributed to food sensitivity. Recent research has shown that an allergic reaction to the materials used to make dentures is quite often the problem, or a sensitivity to metals used in fillings, particularly gold (in the form of gold chloride).

Nausea and Indigestion

Everyone gets indigestion at some time or another. By far the most common cause is unwise eating habits—eating too much, eating too quickly, trying to eat when you are anxious, excited, angry, upset, or tense, eating standing up, rushing about after a meal, eating late at night, or having too much rich food. Smoking makes matters worse, as does too much alcohol, very acid food, spicy food, or too much oil and fat. The fashion for drinking large quantities of fruit juice is likely to produce indigestion

---

Maggie

Like many mothers with young children, Maggie found it difficult to make time for a proper breakfast or lunch. She made up for this by eating a large evening meal with her husband, after which she usually suffered indigestion. By sucking antacid tablets she could settle her stomach in time for bed, but then the pattern would be repeated the next day. Eventually the pain in her stomach became quite severe, and she began to feel generally unwell. Once the children were old enough to go to school this improved, but she still suffered indigestion most days. She now had a job as receptionist at a doctor's office, and the doctor noticed Maggie constantly sucking antacids. He discovered that Maggie had never consulted a doctor about her problem, which had now been going on for almost eight years, and suggested that she should do so. After examining her carefully, her own doctor decided that there was nothing seriously wrong, and suggested that she try to relax and eat more slowly. She also recommended a bland diet, so Maggie began to eat more cottage cheese and drink warm milk instead of tea. Within two weeks her indigestion was a great deal worse, which provided a clue to the cause of the problem. As an experiment, Maggie switched to a diet containing no milk at all, and her indigestion cleared up completely a few days later.

in some people: when fruit is eaten, the stomach has time to adjust to the influx of acid, but drinking a large glass of orange juice all at once is a different matter. For some people there are specific foods that cause indigestion, and these should simply be avoided. In some cases nausea and indigestion are purely psychosomatic (see page 195).

More seriously, a peptic ulcer (stomach ulcer or duodenal ulcer) can be at the root of nausea and indigestion. Other possibilities include gallstones, a hiatal hernia, and, very rarely, cancer of the stomach. If your indigestion becomes more severe or very frequent, or if you lose your appetite, lose weight, or begin vomiting regularly, then there may be something seriously amiss, and these possibilities should be investigated by your doctor.

Food intolerance can cause nausea and indigestion, although these are rarely the sole symptoms. It seems that if the food affects the stomach in this way, then it affects the digestive system as a whole. So there is usually diarrhea or other bowel symptoms as well. In babies the equivalent of indigestion appears to be colic (see page 255).

Heartburn

This is usually caused by the contents of the stomach, which are acidic, welling up into the esophagus (the tube that leads from the mouth to the stomach). The correct medical term for this is gastroesophageal reflux. There is a narrow opening between the esophagus and the stomach that should prevent the stomach contents moving back into the esophagus—this is called the esophageal sphincter. Several foods are known to widen the esophageal sphincter and so contribute to the problem of heartburn. These include peppermint and spearmint, alchohol, coffee, and chocolate. Fatty meals also increase the amount of reflux from the stomach. Avoiding all these foods may help substantially with heartburn.

You could also eliminate foods that stimulate the stomach lining to produce acid and so make the stomach contents more acidic. These include tea and milk (ironically enough—its usefulness in heartburn is something of a myth, as it neutralizes the acidity only temporarily, then stimulates a surge in acid production). Coffee, chocolate, and alcohol also stimulate acid production, but these should be avoided anyway (see above). Finally, foods that directly irritate the esophagus on their way down to the stomach (notably chile and other hot spices; orange, lemon, and grapefruit juices; and concentrated tomato products) should be avoided if symptoms persist. Not eating too late in the evening may also be helpful.

Heartburn can make asthma much worse or even produce symptoms that mimic asthma if droplets of stomach acid are inhaled during the night. One asthma drug, theophylline, can aggravate heartburn. If you think this could be your problem, consult your doctor. *Do not stop taking this drug without medical edvice.*

Stomach (Gastric) Ulcers

A stomach ulcer, like a mouth ulcer, is a craterlike area where the upper layer of the stomach lining is missing. But it is much larger than a mouth ulcer and a far more serious problem. The main symptom is a burning pain that extends across the chest and upper abdomen. The pain lasts for between half an hour and three hours, and episodes of pain tend to come and go.

No one is sure what causes stomach ulcers, but the acid that the stomach produces to help in digestion may be a factor—if there is an eroded or inflamed area in the stomach lining, then the acid could begin to break it down. A tendency to suffer from stomach ulcers runs in some families. Smoking, drinking too much alcohol, and taking aspirin and similar painkillers (see pages 443–444) can all contribute to the development of a stomach ulcer. So can stress, particularly if this means hurried, irregular, or unrelaxed mealtimes. Investigations for a bacterium called *Helicobacter pylori* should always be carried out with stomach ulcers, especially recurrent ones. A blood test is needed to look for antibodies, followed by a breath test for urea, then endoscopy (looking into the stomach), a biopsy (taking a sample of stomach lining for examination), or both.

Whether food intolerance can ever produce stomach ulcers is a controversial issue. Certainly, there are case histories of patients with persistent or recurring stomach ulcers who have recovered remarkably well on an elimination diet. However, these people are probably a minority of all patients with this problem. What might arouse suspicion is if the symptoms get substantially worse during the conventional treatment. Such treatment relies heavily on milk as a safe, bland food. For anyone who is sensitive to milk, this sort of diet will make matters worse.

The presence of allergic symptoms, such as asthma, hay fever, or urticaria, makes it more likely that a stomach ulcer is due to food sensitivity. Some patients of this type (atopics) who also have stomach or duodenal ulcers turn out to have high IgE levels for certain foods. Objective evidence that foods are causing their ulcers comes from direct observation of the stomach lining in contact with a few drops of food extract. This can be achieved by lowering an observation tube into the stomach, a method developed by Polish allergist Dr. Bogdan Romanski. Dr. Romanski reports that inflammation occurs rapidly in the stomach lining where the food extract touches it—the action of stomach acid on such inflamed areas is the likely cause of ulceration. A drug that prevents mast cells from reacting, cromolyn sodium (see pages 431–33), is an effective treatment for these people. All this points to the ulcers being produced by IgE antibodies and mast cells—in other words, being truly allergic. At present, however, stomach and duodenal ulcers are not generally accepted as a possible symptom of food allergy, which is why they are dealt with here, rather than in chapter 3.

There is little doubt that psychosomatic factors (see page 196) play a part in stomach ulcers, even where there is some other underlying cause. Research has shown that by learning to relax, patients can reduce the likelihood of their ulcer recurring after treatment.

Duodenal Ulcers

These are very similar to stomach ulcers but occur in the first part of the small intestine—the duodenum. The main symptom is pain several hours after eating. This pain is usually felt in the upper abdomen, although sometimes it appears to be in the back.

Most duodenal ulcers result from excessive acid production in the stomach. All the causative factors described above for stomach ulcers are also operative in duodenal ulcers, particularly anxiety, tension, smoking, and drinking too much alcohol. Wine and spirits are the main offenders. Duodenal ulcers also seem to be linked with eating a lot of pickled food and eating refined carbohydrates—sugar and white flour. Duodenal ulcers tend to heal themselves, provided the original causes are removed.

Again, a small minority of patients with duodenal ulcers may be suffering from food allergy or food intolerance—but there is little hard evidence to support this belief, only individual case histories.

Diarrhea

Bowel function varies a great deal from one person to another, making it difficult to say exactly what diarrhea is. For most people, one bowel movement a day seems to be the norm, but some people only go once every three or four days, while others go twice a day or more. An important question here is whether "average" is the same thing as "normal and

---

Jenny

Jenny had been in excellent health until she went on vacation to Morocco and picked up a very unpleasant stomach infection. This resulted in severe diarrhea that lasted for more than a week. Although she recovered from this illness, her bowels never really got back to normal, and she continued to have mild diarrhea most of the time. When this had gone on for a couple of years Jenny consulted her doctor, who suggested she try a whole-food diet with plenty of brown bread and vegetables. She did so for two months, but had to report that she was no better—in fact, she was worse than before. This prompted her doctor to try Jenny on an elimination diet, cutting out wheat, milk, and eggs. Avoiding these foods proved very effective, and, when she reintroduced each of them in turn, it was clear that wheat was the source of her problems. After avoiding wheat for a year, Jenny is now able to eat the occasional slice of bread without ill effects.

---

healthy." One survey of 301 apparently healthy adults found that almost a third of them reported bowel symptoms of some sort (diarrhea, constipation, and so on), although most had not consulted a doctor for their problem. This study can be interpreted in two ways. It either shows that everyone's bowel function is different and there is no such thing as a normal pattern—or it shows that a large percentage of the population is suffering from minor bowel complaints. We would lean toward the latter view and suggest that some of those people, at least, are sensitive to the food they eat.

In general, a healthy bowel pattern *feels* healthy, whether you go three times a day or twice a week. There is a regularity to the pattern—it is not erratic. The stools are fairly firm and well formed and there is no particular urgency, nor any great difficulty in going. There is no sense of malaise or pain, either before or afterward, and the movement feels complete—not as if you still have some feces left to pass. In diarrhea soft, loose, or semiliquid stools are passed several times a day; there is generally a sense of urgency and, usually, some feeling of malaise.

Diarrhea is basically a means of ridding the body of toxins, harmful bacteria, or other unwanted substances—it is a healthy reaction to infection and should only be considered a problem when it serves no useful purpose. However, acute diarrhea can lead to dehydration because so much water is lost, and this can be dangerous (see page 264).

Diarrhea can be caused in many different ways. Infections are the most common cause—they tend to bring on an acute attack of diarrhea that clears up of its own accord within a few days, as long as no further food is taken. Sometimes a temporary deficiency in the enzyme lactase (see page 259) follows the infection, and this can perpetuate the diarrhea if milk is consumed. One form of infection that often goes unrecognized is infestation with the parasite *Giardia* (see pages 249–50). Disturbance of the gut flora can also produce diarrhea, usually with other symptoms as well (see page 241).

Celiac disease numbers diarrhea among its symptoms, and in mild cases there may be few other signs (see page 104). A permanent lactase deficiency is another possibility—this will produce persistent diarrhea, usually with gas and some abdominal pain, if milk is consumed. Both problems can affect adults as well as children, but because they usually come to light in infancy they are dealt with in chapter 11. One estimate suggests that lactose intolerance afflicts about 80 percent of African Americans.

Recent studies by the National Institutes of Health suggest that the average time between first symptoms and correct diagnosis for celiacs in the United States is about ten years. The incorrect diagnoses offered in the meantime can include anemia, irritable bowel syndrome, "nerves," chronic fatigue sydrome, infection, ulcers, gallbladder disease, colitis, and lactose intolerance. It is vital that anyone with celiac disease is diagnosed properly (preferably with a biopsy) before altering their diet. If a wheat-free or gluten-free diet has already begun then accurate diagnosis can be very difficult. Such diagnosis is important because of the potential complications of celiac disease. So if you suspect celiac disease— if you are tired and pale as well as having diarrhea, for example, if your muscles feel weak, or if you have relatives with celiac disease—ask your physician for a test.

Crohn's disease (see pages 158–62) and ulcerative colitis (see pages 181–184) also result in diarrhea, but they are serious conditions that produce other symptoms as well. Psychosomatic illness can result in diarrhea (see page 197), and intense stress can produce diarrhea directly, by stimulating the sympathetic nervous system (see page 197). Finally, cancer of the colon can cause diarrhea, although this is the least likely of all the causes listed here.

One potential cause of recurrent diarrhea that is often overlooked is poor food hygiene. People vary greatly in their ability to resist foodborne infections. Some have a cast-iron constitution and remain well however filthy the kitchen, while others need far more stringent hygiene. Judging hygiene standards by the way other people live is not necessarily a good policy.

Many people are unaware that food that has been kept for a long time is not always rendered safe by thorough cooking—some bacteria produce toxins that are not destroyed by heat, even though the bacteria themselves are killed. These toxins can produce a short-lived bout of diarrhea. So anyone in the habit of keeping food or leftovers for long periods of time may be regularly exposed to this sort of "food poisoning." Food should be eaten as fresh as possible, and other basic hygiene measures adopted. These include washing the hands with soap after visiting the lavatory and before preparing food—water alone does not remove bacteria. Kitchen work surfaces should also be kept clean, knives and chopping boards should be washed in hot soapy water after cutting up meat, and raw meat should never be stored alongside or above cooked meat. Pets should be kept off surfaces used for food preparation. Any leftovers should be heated for twenty minutes or more to kill bacteria.

Cooked rice is particularly liable to cause food poisoning. A bacterium called *Bacillus cereus* is found on the grain and is not killed by cooking, but instead forms hard-coated spores. These come to life about one to five hours after the cooking process, and they multiply fast. Even if kept in a refrigerator, rice should not be eaten more than a day after it was cooked, and should not be fed to babies more than twelve hours after cooking.

Another potential cause of diarrhea is the natural laxative effect of some fruits (see page 18). Prunes, rhubarb, and figs are well known for such properties, but other fruits can have similar, if milder, effects, and so can avocados. Eating too much of foods such as these may produce diarrhea in the susceptible person. Eating beans, lentils, chickpeas, or other legumes can also cause problems, especially if they have not been properly cooked (see page 110). Shellfish are another common cause of diarrhea— they quite often contain toxins that are not destroyed by cooking.

These are common reactions to food or food contaminants that anyone might have. In food intolerance there is a more specific reaction to one or more foods that do not produce diarrhea in most people. The sort of diarrhea caused by food intolerance is likely to be fairly mild, although with occasional more acute attacks, perhaps in reponse to a change in diet or stress. There might also be periods when the bowel reverts to normal function for a while, or brief episodes of constipation. Opinions vary, but some doctors would classify this sort of chronic diarrhea, without any pain, as a form of irritable bowel syndrome. It is therefore dealt with below, under that heading. For diarrhea in children, see pages 263–64.

Diarrhea is not necessarily caused by food—there can be other causes. For example, marathon runners and other long-distance competition runners are frequently afflicted by diarrhea while training, and sometimes while competing. In one survey almost half the runners questioned were so affected, and 12 percent had suffered fecal incontinence while running. Some had severe abdominal cramps after races, and had noticed blood in their stools. No one knows how these symptoms are caused, but they seem to be a direct outcome of the running itself and nothing to do with food. Some runners did observe that high-fiber diets, milk, and fruit seemed to make the problem worse, but the basic problem persisted even if these foods were avoided.

Constipation

The difficulty of deciding what is normal or healthy in terms of bowel function is just as much a problem here as for diarrhea (see above). In general, it is not so much a question of how infrequently the bowels are opened as it is of the accompanying symptoms. If there is a feeling of bloating and discomfort, of wanting to go and not being able to, of straining or incomplete evacuation, then this really is constipation.

Overuse of laxatives makes the bowel dependent on them, and this is one possible cause of chronic constipation. Other medicines may have a similar effect, notably cough mixtures. Lack of fiber in the diet is another common cause—but the answer is not to eat mountains of bran (see page 328). Hemorrhoids can cause constipation, and so can various psychological problems. In rare cases constipation is the main symptom of celiac disease.

Whether food intolerance can ever be a cause of constipation, as some doctors believe, is still debated. There may be some individuals who do respond in this way (see page 266 for an example), and occasionally constipation might be the sole symptom. Quite often, patients taking large quantities of bran for constipation improve markedly when this, and all other forms of wheat, are eliminated.

Irritable Bowel Syndrome

Irritable bowel syndrome or IBS (also called irritable colon or spastic colon) is a diagnosis that means different things to different doctors. However, it usually denotes abnormal bowel function—either constipation or diarrhea—without any sign of infection or other physical cause (such as bowel cancer), and without any structural damage to the wall of the bowel. Within this group there is plenty of scope for variation—some patients suffer diarrhea most of the time, others are usually constipated, while for some these symptoms alternate. Most patients suffer pain that is relieved by defecation, but not all do. In effect, *IBS* is little more than an umbrella term for various minor bowel disturbances of unknown origin. In some cases there may be a more serious underlying problem, or a very simple problem that is easily cured (see above, under Diarrhea and Constipation).

Since there is no damage to the gut in IBS, there is usually no blood in the stools. Neither is there any weight loss or nighttime diarrhea—either of these symptoms indicates more serious conditions such as Crohn's disease or ulcerative colitis. IBS is a fairly "minor" problem in the sense that it does not affect general health, does not usually get any worse as the years go by, and does not predispose the sufferer to any other illnesses. (However, the experience of having IBS can be far from minor. Those who suffer chronically from it find it extremely disruptive, painful, and exhausting.)

There appear to be two distinct subgroups within IBS patients. The first group suffers from mild diarrhea most of the time, often with pain, and sometimes with brief episodes of constipation. The second group suffers from constipation for some or most of the time, with bloating and occasional bouts of mild diarrhea. They may also suffer pain. For people in this second group, food sensitivity is unlikely to be at the root of their symptoms. For those with chronic diarrhea—the first group—food sensitivity is worth investigating, especially if they have bloating and gas as well. Some studies have shown that as many as 70 percent of IBS sufferers may be food intolerant (see page 130).

Alternative explanations for IBS are few in number. The most widely accepted theory is that the complaint is usually psychosomatic, an idea discussed further on pages 204–7. Another theory suggests that lack of fiber in the diet is responsible. Although this idea is now largely discredited, extra bran and other bulk-forming agents are still prescribed for IBS, regardless of whether diarrhea or constipation is the main symptom.

The latter might be helped by this strategy, but not the former. Indeed, there is evidence that some people with IBS are made worse by eating bran, suggesting a sensitivity to wheat or other grains.

Exactly what goes wrong in IBS is far from clear. In many cases it may be that the muscles of the gut are contracting too much, or too little, or are simply unsynchronized. The muscles that control the bowel are smooth muscles, like those in the bladder and the bronchi (the tubes leading to the lungs). Some patients with IBS have to urinate frequently, and this can be a sign that smooth-muscle spasms are at the root of the symptoms, although frequent urination can also be a straightforward psychological problem.

What causes these spasms? It could be an effect of the sympathetic nerves, if IBS really is psychosomatic. Or it could be mediators released by mast cells (see page 30), if there is a true allergic reaction. The term *asthma of the gut* is sometimes used to describe this sort of reaction—in just the same way as there are spasms of the bronchial muscles, producing asthma, there could be spasmodic contractions of the smooth muscles of the gut, producing diarrhea.

Another important causative factor in IBS may be the **gut flora**— the menagerie of bacteria and yeasts that live in our intestines and are harmless or beneficial in most people. Research done by Dr. John Hunter at Addenbrooke's Hospital in Cambridge, England, suggests that many IBS sufferers have a disturbed gut flora. Some bacteria or yeasts are over-represented while others are lacking (see chapter 10). How a disturbed gut flora might be treated is discussed on pages 250–51.

There are various other ways in which adverse reactions to foods might bring on diarrhea and pain, but at present there is too little evidence to choose among them. In the end it may turn out that several different factors are at work.

Crohn's Disease

This is a serious bowel disorder that produces patches of inflammation in the intestines, mostly in the second part of the small intestine (the **ileum**) or the large intestine (the **colon**). These patches have a characteristic appearance under the microscope. They may heal themselves in time, and some patients recover after just one or two attacks of Crohn's disease. Others suffer recurring attacks throughout their lives. As they heal, the inflamed areas may develop scar tissue that narrows the intestine, making passage of food difficult. In terms of actual symptoms,

Crohn's disease produces diarrhea and cramps or more generalized pain in the abdomen, especially after eating. There is usually a general feeling of malaise and, sometimes, a slight fever. If left untreated, weight loss and deteriorating health will occur, because nutrients are not absorbed properly. Other symptoms, such as joint pains and mouth ulcers, often accompany Crohn's disease.

Despite intensive study, doctors still have no clear idea what produces Crohn's disease. The damaged areas of intestine, when studied under the microscope, contain a great many immune cells—it is these that produce the inflammation. The obvious explanation is that some infectious agent attracts them there—but there is no evidence that Crohn's disease is infectious, and the fact that the disease mostly affects people in their twenties makes an infection unlikely. However, some researchers believe that they may now have found an infectious agent—a slow-growing bacterium related to the one that causes tuberculosis. Attempts to show that this bacterium really does produce Crohn's disease are now in progress.

Another line of research has pinned the blame for Crohn's disease on substances produced by bacteria that are a normal part of the gut flora. These substances are peptide molecules (see page 295) that happen to act as attractants for certain cells of the immune system. It is believed that most people have bacteria that generate these peptides, but that they can neutralize them by means of a special enzyme (see page 21) that breaks them down. What goes wrong in Crohn's disease, according to this theory, is that the patient lacks the enzymes to break down these peptides. It has been shown that the peptides attract the immune cells known as phagocytes ("eating cells"), and that these come pouring through the gut wall into the intestine. Once there, they can set up an inflammation reaction.

Although interesting, all this research has not resulted in any new form of treatment for Crohn's disease as yet. The conventional treatment is to use drugs such as corticosteroids (see pages 439–42) to suppress the inflammation. Surgery may also be used if parts of the bowel are so badly scarred that they are causing congestion.

Recent research in the United States, however, has led to a form of treatment—and a highly unusual one. Guessing that Crohn's disease might be linked to the eradication of parasitic worms in the West, these researchers tried infecting patients with worms—(a kind that could not establish a permanent infestation, you'll be pleased to hear). This apparently produced a dramatic clearance of symptoms for most patients. (It is interesting that the epidemic rise of allergic diseases in the West has also been linked, by some researchers, with a reduction in parasitic worm infections.) However, this was only a very small experimental trial, and much more research would be required to confirm the finding.

So what about the role of food? In the first edition of this book we wrote that the proposed link between food intolerance and Crohn's disease was "highly controversial." We are pleased to report that, in the eleven years since then, the idea has become respectable, thanks to the excellent scientific work of Dr. John Hunter at Addenbrooke's Hospital in Cambridge. With his own Crohn's disease patients, Dr. Hunter found that over 80 percent recovered on an elimination diet, and then reacted to specific foods when they were reintroduced. By cutting out the incriminated foods, these patients can remain well. Some relapse later—as is common with Crohn's disease—but after two years 80 percent of those still on their diet remained well.

The latest trial, instigated by Dr. Hunter but carried out at nine different hospitals under the supervision of several different doctors, has vindicated the original results. The long-term recovery rate, at 50 percent, was not as good, but still much better than a comparable treatment using steroid drugs. The doctors assessing the patients were totally impartial in that they did not know whether their patients were receiving the dietary treatment or the drug treatment.

Because patients with Crohn's disease are often very ill, carrying out an elimination diet is not all that easy, and other doctors have been reluctant to try this new approach. The technique that Dr. Hunter uses is to feed his patients an elemental diet (see page 321) during the first part of the elimination diet, or to feed them in some other way—using an intravenous drip, which puts nutrients straight into the bloodstream, for example. Other doctors who are skeptical about food intolerance suggest that the Crohn's disease symptoms clear up simply because the patient's gut is being given a rest from digesting real food, or because the patient's nutritional status is improved. But if this were the case, you would not expect the patients to remain well afterward on a normal diet that just excluded certain food items. And in the latest trial this possibility was investigated, by giving the elemental diet to all the patients involved. Of those who recovered on the elemental diet, half were then told to return to their normal diet, but given corticosteroid drugs. The other half tested foods on a one-by-one basis, noted which ones they reacted to, and then avoided those. They were not given any drugs, yet twice as many in this group were still well two years later.

How specific foods might cause Crohn's disease is not clear. Dr. Hunter believes that an abnormal population of bacteria in the gut might be the problem, as in IBS (see page 158). The discovery that bacterial peptides attract immune cells into the gut (described above) could fit in quite well with this explanation, and Dr. Hunter suspects that enzyme deficiencies might play a part. It certainly looks as if several different factors could be at work in producing this puzzling disease.

Given that corticosteroids have some side effects, including making the patient more susceptible to infections, an alternative nondrug treatment with a good success rate should seem very attractive. At present, however, elimination diets are not widely used for Crohn's disease, and the serious nature of this illness makes it unsuitable for self-help treatment. *If you have Crohn's disease, you should not consider trying an elimination diet without full medical supervision.* If your doctor is willing to help, he or she can prescribe an elemental diet for you. When testing foods, very small amounts should be tried initially because there is a risk of experiencing strong reactions with lasting ill effects.

Some recent research has suggested that certain substances produced by yeasts might have a special role to play in triggering Crohn's disease, because patients have very high levels of antibodies to these substances. In view of these results, it might be worth trying a yeast-free, sugar-free diet (see pages 244–48), which is relatively easy and without risk. See page 412 for full details of the foods that contain yeast.

A separate line of research has looked at the eating habits of people in the five years before they develop Crohn's disease. This study, carried out in Sweden, has shown that eating fast foods twice a week or more increased the risk of contracting Crohn's disease dramatically— numbers of cases were 3.4 times higher in the fast-food eaters. Of course, this does not necessarily mean that cutting out fast foods will cure or dramatically improve Crohn's disease; the disease process that is triggered or partially triggered by the fast food, once begun, may be difficult to reverse. Nevertheless, cutting out fast foods is clearly worth a try for such a serious and debilitating disease. High sugar and low fiber consumption also increased the risk of Crohn's disease, so an increased intake of fruits and vegetables (not bran—see page 328) and a reduction in soft drinks and sweet snacks might also help.

Bloating and Flatulence (Gas)

Bloating of the abdomen after meals is usually caused by overgrowth of certain bacteria or yeasts in the gut. These feed on food residues, producing gas in the process. Certain foods are notorious for producing this effect, notably kidney beans (haricot beans, baked beans, and the like) and Jerusalem artichokes. Jerusalem artichokes contain an unusual type of sugar that human beings cannot digest and which therefore passes through to nourish bacteria in the hind part of the gut. Other foods that tend to produce gas in a wide range of people include lettuce, apples, cabbage, brussels sprouts, and malt extract.

Where belching is the main problem, it may be due to swallowing air when eating. Gas can also indicate more serious problems, such as gallstones, hiatal hernia, or malabsorption of food, but there will usually be other symptoms as well. A possible cause of flatulence and bloating that is not widely recognized is an imbalance in the gut flora (see page 236). Infection with *Giardia* can also have this effect (see page 250). Alternatively, food intolerance may be the cause of the problem, although there will usually be other symptoms as well, such as diarrhea, abdominal pain, nausea, or indigestion.

The Skin

Itchiness

Itchy skin is usually accompanied by a rash of some sort, as in eczema (see page 52) and urticaria (see page 50). Itchiness, without any spots or rash, can be caused by all sorts of things. The most likely sources of trouble are clothing, toiletries, and cosmetics. Woolens and synthetics are the most common offenders, while cotton or silk clothes are the least irritating. Changing to unscented brands of soap and using a minimum of cosmetics may relieve the itching. Adding a few drops of baby oil or lavender essential oil to the bathwater can also help. Chlorinated water can be the culprit, and reducing the number of baths or showers taken and avoiding swimming pools can produce a dramatic improvement. Some people are sensitive to traces of detergent or fabric conditioner left on clothes, and simply rinsing clothing more thoroughly may be the answer. If the itching is mainly on your hands, then cleaning agents may be the culprit. Wear rubber gloves for housework, preferably with cotton gloves inside them, or wear cotton-lined PVC gloves.

Various parasites cause itching, including scabies, threadworms, lice, and ringworms. Generalized itchiness is also one of the symptoms that may clear up on a no-sugar, no-yeast diet (see chapter 10). Itchiness of the vulva or vagina is likely to indicate a *Candida* overgrowth, and an itchy anus may also be due to *Candida*. However, anal itching could be due to some other problem with the gut flora, food intolerance, or even hemorrhoids. In general, itchiness in other parts of the body does not seem to be a common symptom of food intolerance, but it is reported in a few cases.

The Joints and Muscles

Muscular Aches (Myalgia)

It is unusual to experience aches in the muscles that are not the result of overusing the muscles, or of a viral infection such as influenza. However, they are a feature of postviral syndrome (see page 294) or, if severe, they may indicate a disease known as polymyalgia rheumatica, which requires drug treatment. Tension can produce muscle aches, especially in the neck, shoulders, and face. Misaligned vertebrae can also produce aches and pains in the back, shoulders, and neck, and these may respond to treatment by an osteopath.

More generalized, but mild, muscle aches may also be a symptom of food intolerance, although this is unusual. One group of food-intolerant patients who regularly include muscle aches among their symptoms are hyperactive children (see page 265).

Aching Joints (Arthralgia)

The joints are a very vulnerable part of the body, and misuse or overuse can easily produce pains. Too much kneeling can produce bursitis, for example, commonly known as housemaid's knee or parson's knee. Sports enthusiasts may also suffer joint pains in certain susceptible joints.

Generalized joint pain can accompany some illnesses, such as rheumatic fever, or it may follow on from influenza, *Salmonella* poisoning, and other infections. *Giardia* (see page 249) and a gut flora imbalance (see page 235) may also produce joint pain among their symptoms. Diseases that make the gut wall more permeable to food molecules can produce aching joints as well—these include Crohn's disease, celiac disease, and ulcerative colitis. If the underlying disease is sorted out, the joints tend to get better. In children, vaccination sometimes results in an attack of joint pain. Rarely, generalized joint pain may be an indication of a serious autoimmune disease called systemic lupus erythematosus or SLE (see page 97).

In many of these disorders, the pain is produced by immune complexes (see page 96) forming in the blood, and then becoming deposited in the joint. These immune complexes consist of masses of antigens and antibodies. In the examples mentioned above, the antigens are either bacteria (in an infection), the vaccine (in vaccination), food molecules (in Crohn's disease and celiac disease), or the body's own proteins (in autoimmune diseases such as SLE). Because so many immune complexes are formed at once, the system that normally mops them up cannot cope.

Food intolerance can apparently cause aching joints in some people. It is likely to be the most heavily used joints, such as the knees, that are afflicted first, but it may later spread to other joints. Assuming that all the disorders mentioned above have been ruled out, then food intolerance is a very likely cause for joint pain, especially in patients with a variety of other minor symptoms as well. Studies have found that between 50 and 85 percent of patients respond to an elimination diet.

Since immune complexes are known to produce joint pain in several other diseases, they are a logical suspect in food intolerance as well. In this case, the immune complexes might well consist of food molecules (absorbed intact into the blood from the gut) and antibodies to the food. At present there is no evidence to show whether this idea is right or not, and it is possible that food produces joint pain by some completely different mechanism.

An acute, immediate *allergic* reaction to a food, with characteristic symptoms such as swelling of the lips, can also include transitory pain and swelling in the joints, especially those of the hand and wrist. Other atopic (allergic) patients experience more long-lasting joint pain, which may be due to food. Whether this is food allergy or intolerance is a debatable point, but mast cells do seem to be involved in some of these patients.

Rheumatoid Arthritis

Rheumatoid arthritis is characterized by painful, swollen joints that feel warm to the touch and are often stiff. The stiffness and pain are usually worse in the morning. Various blood tests are used to confirm the diagnosis—they look for certain factors in the blood that are characteristic of rheumatoid arthritis.

Inflammation is the cause of the problem, and the part to be affected first is the **synovial membrane**. This membrane has an important role to

George

George was in his midforties when his joints began to feel painful and stiff. The affected joints were red and swollen, and he also felt feverish at times. After running some blood tests, his doctor diagnosed rheumatoid arthritis. George was a landscape gardener who had always done a lot of the hard physical work himself, and the gradual loss of mobility affected his business badly. Although the drugs he was given helped a little, the disease gradually got worse. By the time he was fifty simply getting out of bed in the morning was difficult. His shoulders were so stiff that he could not comb his hair or put on a tie, and gripping a mug was difficult because of the stiffness in his hands. At this stage his doctor suggested that George might try an elimination diet, which was said to help some people with rheumatoid arthritis. She told him to cut out grains, dairy, eggs, citrus fruit, and other common foods. His symptoms got slightly worse in the first few days, but he stayed on the diet anyway. By the end of the second week he began to feel better and some of his joints were less swollen and painful. Over the next week things improved noticeably every day, and after three weeks he was almost back to his former good health. When he tried reintroducing foods, George found that milk, potatoes, and yeast triggered his joint symptoms again. By avoiding these he has remained fairly well, although he still has a few aches in his joints and his shoulders are a little stiff. He suspects that some of the foods he is still eating may be at the root of this, but rather than restrict his diet further he relies on low doses of an antirheumatoid drug to reduce the inflammation. His gardening business is expanding again, and he feels better than he has for years.

play in the joint, because it produces the fluid that lubricates the joint. The **synovium,** which surrounds the joint, is filled with this fluid. In rheumatoid arthritis the synovial membrane is invaded by large numbers of immune cells, which cause the inflammation.

The presence of all these immune cells suggests that there is an infection in the membrane, and early theories about rheumatoid arthritis invoked some bacterium or virus. But despite many years of searching, no infectious agent has been found. An alternative theory suggests that the body is mounting an immune reaction against its own proteins—

in other words, that rheumatoid arthritis is an autoimmune disease. Recent discoveries do not tend to support this idea—there is an autoimmune element that appears later in advanced rheumatoid arthritis, but autoimmunity does not play a part in the initial causes of the disease. A third theory suggests that there is an overgrowth of cells in the synovial membrane that attracts the attention of the immune system. This idea is currently being tested.

The standard treatment for rheumatoid arthritis at present is to use drugs that suppress inflammation, such as aspirin, ibuprofen, methotrexate, and penicillamine (see pages 443–45). Unfortunately, these can all have various side effects, and they do little more than suppress—or partially suppress—the symptoms. Corticosteroids, the most effective anti-inflammatory drugs, are used only in severe attacks.

The idea that food intolerance can play a part in causing rheumatoid arthritis is not widely accepted among rheumatologists. However, some specialists in this field report excellent results when they try their patients on an elimination diet. One of these is Dr. Gail Darlington, whose work is described on pages 127–29. According to Dr. Darlington, about three-quarters of patients show some improvement when they identify culprit foods and eliminate them from their diet. Some of these patients lose their symptoms entirely—a dramatic improvement that drug treatment rarely achieves.

How food intolerance might trigger the inflammation in the joint is still an open question. The idea that immune complexes (consisting of food molecules and their antigens) are deposited in the joint is tempting, but there is no evidence for this at present.

Other Forms of Arthritis

Some other forms of arthritis may respond to an elimination diet, notably palindromic rheumatism or episodic arthritis. This disease produces bouts of joint pain and swelling, which clear up spontaneously, without any treatment, only to recur months or years later. Food intolerance is very often at the root of these attacks. Often sufferers can relate their bouts of arthritis to the consumption of some rarely eaten food. It may be sufficient just to keep a note of foods eaten and see how this compares with the onset of attacks. You should test the food or foods that come under suspicion, especially if it is a food that is difficult to avoid normally, such as milk or wheat. Follow the testing procedure given in chapter 14.

If a food diary does not produce any answers, then an elimination diet may be worth trying. The diet should begin during an episode of arthritis, so if your attacks are normally short lived, read through chapter 14 in advance and be prepared to start as soon as possible when your next bout of joint pain begins. If the exclusion phase of the diet is going to produce an improvement, this will happen within seven days or, more rarely, within ten days. You need to be aware how long your attacks normally last, so as not to confuse the spontaneous recovery that occurs at the end of the attack with any improvement resulting from the diet.

Inflammatory polyarthropathy is another form of arthritis that might benefit from an elimination diet. Get your doctor's approval before trying such a diet.

Very occasionally, food sensitivity plays a part in juvenile chronic arthritis. However, food does not seem to be the source of trouble for many children with arthritis, and in this it differs from adult rheumatoid arthritis. Because of the risks of malnutrition and stunted growth when children are put on strict diets, most doctors are reluctant to prescribe elimination diets for their young patients. If you are particularly anxious to try such a diet, discuss the matter with your family doctor or rheumatologist. The Stage 2 elimination diet (see page 342) is adequate, and there is no point in progressing to the Stage 3 diet.

Finally, a rare form of arthritis known as Behçet's syndrome may be related to food sensitivity. In one American study, walnuts often seemed to be the culprit food (and one of the patients who deteriorated considerably upon eating walnuts dated the start of his problems to a time when he was milling a lot of walnut timber and inhaling the dust). Whether these observations are relevant to other groups of patients, particularly those in other countries, is unknown. Note that if walnuts are the culprit, then related nuts—pecans and hickory nuts—could also cause problems. Some patients with Behçet's syndrome report that they also react to chocolate, to other kinds of nuts, and to a variety of other foods such as tomatoes, oranges, and lemons. Clearly, an elimination diet would be worth trying for Behçet's syndrome, as long as your doctor approves.

Backache
Most backache is a result of injury or misuse of the back. Very occasionally, however, long-term back pain has abated as a result of an elimination diet. In all these cases there are other symptoms as well, such as joint pain, aching muscles, or irritable bowel syndrome.

The Heart and Blood Vessels

Irregular Heartbeat

There may be many causes for an irregular heartbeat (sometimes called palpitations), and since any condition affecting the heart can be serious, it is wise to seek medical advice without delay. If there is no serious underlying problem, then overconsumption of caffeine (see page 213) or hyperventilation (see page 210) should be considered. Some doctors have reported that sensitivity to foods or to chemicals (see chapter 9) may cause irregularities in the heartbeat, and these factors may be worth investigating if other possible causes have been ruled out.

Chest Pain

Chest pain is reported as a symptom of food intolerance by some doctors, but this is certainly not common. There are a great many other possible causes, some of which may be serious and require immediate attention. If the doctor can find no underlying cause for the chest pain, then the possibility of hyperventilation (see page 210) is worth considering.

The Head

Headaches

The brain itself has no pain receptors. But the blood vessels supplying the brain, and the membranes that surround it (the **meninges**) do feel pain. It is these that produce a headache.

Most people experience headaches from time to time, and they are usually nothing to worry about. The possible causes are too numerous to list, but tension, anxiety, overwork, irregular meals, eyestrain, and alcohol are the most common ones. Regular headaches are a sign that something is amiss, and simply suppressing this warning sign with a painkiller and ignoring the underlying cause is a mistake. Mild or moderate headache that is continuous is generally regarded as psychosomatic (see page 196). A sudden attack of severe recurrent headaches, or daily headaches, may be a sign of some serious underlying illness, such as meningitis or brain tumor—medical help should be sought without any delay.

Recurrent headaches are often reported as a feature of food intolerance, and in some people they may be the sole symptom, although there will usually be some other problems as well. Hyperventilation (see page 210) and abnormalities of the gut flora may also cause headache, among other symptoms.

Migraine

Defining *migraine* is no easy task. It is generally described as a severe, throbbing headache that is usually restricted to one side of the head and is often accompanied by nausea and a dislike of loud noises and bright lights—or any light (photophobia). Some people also experience split vision, half vision, flashing lights, or other visual disturbances—the term for this sort of migraine is *classical migraine*. Where there are no visual phenomena, the term *common migraine* is used. In both types of migraine, there may be indications that an attack is imminent—visual effects or just mood changes.

Doctors differ in their interpretation of these criteria. Some will tell you that it is not migraine unless you feel nauseous and your head throbs. Others maintain that the pain has to be incapacitating for it to qualify—if you are walking about, it's not a migraine. In reality, migraine refuses to fit into these rigid definitions. Many patients with migraine experience varying symptoms. Sometimes their attacks are incapacitating or make them vomit violently; at other times the attacks are fairly mild but have that same essential "migrainey" quality. Whereas a headache is just a pain in the head, a migraine seems to disrupt the mental functioning and perception of the world—even if the visual disturbances of classical migraine are lacking. There is a spaced-out, cut-off-from-things, groggy, disoriented quality to a migraine that sets it apart from a headache, even when the pain is mild and there is no throbbing or nausea.

One characteristic feature of migraine is that patients recognize certain things that tend to trigger attacks. For some people it is alcohol, or certain foods. For others it is bright lights, flashing lights, television, very hot baths, strong winds or changes in climate, loud noises, strong smells, excitement, anxiety, shock, or sleeping too long. Although this might seem like a very miscellaneous list, it is striking how often migraine patients report the same sorts of triggers—especially bright lights and oversleeping. When stress is a factor, the migraine attack often develops after the pressure is off—weekend migraines, or those that spoil the first few days of any vacation, are commonly reported.

Migraine attacks usually begin between the ages of twenty and thirty, but there are a few unfortunate people who develop them in childhood. Sometimes children suffer more in their stomachs than in their heads, with vomiting as the main feature of an attack. They may have these bouts of vomiting without any head pain at first, only developing a one-sided headache as they grow older.

As a result of extensive research into migraine, doctors have a fairly clear idea of what happens during an attack. They know that there are two distinct phases. During the first, the blood vessels throughout the body—including those in the brain—become constricted. In the second phase there is a backlash reaction, and the blood vessels open (or **dilate**) more than is normal. It is the expansion of blood vessels in the brain during the second phase that causes the pain. The premonitions of migraine that some sufferers feel occur during the first phase, and may be caused by a reduced blood flow to certain parts of the brain as the blood vessels narrow.

Playing a central part in this reaction are tiny "cells" in the blood known as platelets. These are very numerous—there are fifteen million of them in a single drop of blood—and their main function is to help the blood clot around a wound. During clotting the platelets clump together and release a substance called **serotonin** or **5HT** that makes the blood vessels constrict. This reduces blood flow so that less blood is lost from the wound.

What happens in a migraine attack is that the platelets clump together and release serotonin when it is not needed. During the first phase of a migraine attack something makes the platelets in the blood clump together—they do not actually form clots, of course, but they do release large amounts of serotonin. The serotonin makes the blood vessels constrict and thus reduces the blood flow to the brain. The body has control mechanisms that counteract the effect of the serotonin, but when these come into play they cause a violent swing in the opposite direction: the blood vessels in the brain open out too much, bringing on the throbbing pain that is a feature of the second phase of the attack. Pressure on certain parts of the brain might produce the feelings of nausea.

But what makes the platelets clump together in the first place? The answer to this question may be two **vasoactive amines,** known as **tyramine** and **phenylethylamine,** that are found in certain foods. These substances are usually broken down by the platelets, which produce various enzymes for the purpose. Doctors suspect that some people with migraine do not produce enough of these enzymes, or produce defective versions of them. So if they eat foods rich in these substances, they cannot break them down fast enough—and platelet clumping follows. The foods that are rich in these amines are well known as migraine triggers—principally chocolate, cheese, and red wine.

However, studies of the enzymes involved in breaking down tyramine

Tom

Tom was in his late thirties when he first started to get migraines. With a demanding job as a social worker in a hostel for alcoholics and three young children to raise, he chalked up his symptoms to stress. Over the next ten years the problem gradually got worse, until he rarely had a day without some sort of head pain. He was also very tired and lacked the energy to join in with family activities or help look after the children on weekends. This inevitably led to friction, and his marriage was in danger of breaking up.

In the hope of improving his health and keeping the family together, Tom and his wife decided to move to the country. He gave up social work for a job in a garden center that did not pay as well, but was much less taxing. The move also involved finding a different doctor. At an initial checkup, Tom's new physician asked him what he thought the cause of his headaches and tiredness might be. "Stress," Tom replied, without hesitation. "That's why we've moved out here." The doctor suggested that he come back and see him after a year, when he had had time to settle in and judge the effects of a slower pace of life.

Tom did so and had to report that, while there'd been some improvement, it was not nearly as much as he had hoped; he was still very tired and experiencing migraines several times a week. The doctor then suggested that he try changing his diet for an experimental period, telling him to eat nothing but meat and vegetables, and drink only springwater, for ten days. Tom felt very ill on this diet at first, with stomach pains and a severe migraine. But after a week he noticed a remarkable improvement: his energy was restored and his head free of pain. The doctor then explained to Tom that he should test foods individually, which he did. To test wheat, he ate some spaghetti. Within an hour of eating the pasta he was his old self again, and with a vengeance—exhausted, depressed, nauseated, and with a throbbing pain on one side of his head. Cow's milk, oranges, and rye had similar effects. After avoiding these foods for a year, he finds he can now eat them occasionally without ill effects. His children are amazed and delighted with the transformation in their father, who now plays football with them, takes them swimming, and is a lot more fun to be with. The family have decided they like country life, but Tom is planning to go back into social work as soon as he can get a job locally.

and phenylethylamine have produced rather puzzling results. Many migraine patients *are* defective for one of the enzymes involved, called a monoamine oxidase. But those who are sensitive to triggers such as chocolate or cheese are no more defective than other migraine patients. If tyramine and phenylethylamine are involved in migraine (and it is by no means certain that they are), then the underlying enzyme deficiencies are obviously not simple ones. For more on enzyme deficiencies in migraine, see page 301.

There must be other factors that can make the platelets clump together, because it is only a minority of patients whose migraines are triggered by these foods. The hormone adrenaline is known to have similar effects on platelets, and other substances produced by the body may act in this way. Presumably the migraine sufferer produces too much of these substances or lacks the control mechanisms that normally keep them in check.

Although the blood vessels play an important part in migraines, many doctors believe that they are not the whole story. Some things are difficult to explain on the basis of blood vessels alone—why the pain is usually on one side of the head, for example, or why bright lights should trigger a migraine. These facts suggest that the nervous system is involved as well, but exactly how is not known.

The conventional view of migraine is that it cannot be cured, except in rare instances where a misaligned vertebra, usually in the neck, is at the root of the problem—and this may not be true migraine anyway. For such patients, treatment by an osteopath may be effective. (How a misaligned vertebra might cause migraine in the first place is something of a puzzle, but one that we will return to at the end of this section.) Given that there is no cure, the main form of conventional treatment is drug therapy, using drugs that can stop an attack, or at least alleviate it (see pages 447–48). Patients are also advised to identify their particular triggers and avoid them.

The relevance of food intolerance to migraine is hotly debated. The conventional wisdom is that certain foods (chocolate, cheese, citrus fruits, and red wine) can act as triggers but that commonly eaten foods, such as wheat and milk, are unlikely to play a part in migraine. However, several carefully conducted scientific trials using elimination diets to treat migraine sufferers have produced good results. One of these studies, involving children with severe migraine, is described on pages 132–34. Studies with adults have shown that about 70 percent of patients recover very well when treated in this way. Doctors working in this field in fact achieve a better success rate than this because patients who do not respond to a simple elimination diet often turn out to have chemical sensitivities, or they respond to a no-sugar, no-yeast diet (see chapter 10). When this much broader approach is taken, then the success rate rises to 80 or 90 percent.

The foods identified by an elimination diet seem to be acting in a different way from the accepted food triggers. When they are eliminated from the diet, the migraines usually clear up completely—whereas excluding trigger foods only makes the migraines less frequent. Following an elimination diet and the avoidance of culprit foods, patients often find that they can once more tolerate their triggers—both food and non-food. It looks as if the milk, wheat, or whatever was creating some serious underlying problem that made the body vulnerable to any external change. Thus bright lights, stress, the flickering of a television screen, or the druglike substances in chocolate could upset the delicate balance and tip the whole system into a migraine attack. Once the underlying food intolerance has been sorted out, the system is far more stable and can better cope with external circumstances.

How food intolerance might create this underlying instability is not known. One study suggests that migraine patients, although not apparently atopic, have a mild IgE/mast-cell reaction to the food when it comes into contact with the lining of the gut. This may set up inflammation locally, make the gut wall leakier, and thus allow more food molecules through. These might then provoke an immune response in the blood, although it is not clear how this could make the person susceptible to migraines.

Another possibility is that certain naturally occurring chemicals in the foods, which require detoxification by enzymes, are to blame. If the patient has a deficit in certain detoxification enzymes, this could be made much worse by overloading them with particular foodstuffs. There might then be less spare enzyme capacity to deal with triggers such as tyramine. At present this is just speculation, and much more research is needed.

Although elimination diets do seem to be useful for many people with migraine, they are probably not worth trying for those who only get migraines occasionally—once a month or less. In such circumstances it would be difficult to tell if excluding foods had had any effect, unless there were other symptoms as well. Testing might also be rather inconclusive. But for anyone who has migraines at particular times—

during menstruation, for example—then it might be worth carrying out an elimination diet timed to start about a week before the moment when migraines usually occur.

There is one final puzzle in relation to migraine. Within the past few years several dentists have apparently discovered a "miracle cure" for it. As dentists, they did not set out to treat migraines, of course. What they were doing was treating people who habitually ground their teeth together in their sleep. This habit, which is usually due to stress and tension, tends to leave telltale marks on the teeth—a polished area where they rub together. Anyone whose teeth has these marks is usually offered a dental plate to wear in bed, which is designed to prevent the grinding action. Surprisingly, some patients who had previously suffered migraines, reported that these had cleared up after they began using the dental plate.

Further research was carried out involving patients with classical migraine, all of whom experienced migraines upon waking up—the theory was that such migraines are far more likely to be due to nocturnal tooth grinding. Some of these patients showed signs of grinding on their teeth, but not all did—it seems that only the most enthusiastic grinders actually manage to wear the teeth down. The effect on the patients of using dental plates at night was remarkable: almost all of them suffered far fewer attacks.

How can this discovery be reconciled with the finding that food intolerance is at the root of most migraines? One possibility is that the subgroup of patients being studied by the dentists are uncharacteristic of migraine patients as a whole—that they are part of the 10 or 20 percent of patients who cannot be helped by an elimination diet, chemical avoidance, or by a no-sugar, no-yeast diet. Another possibility, and a more likely one, is that tooth grinding is a trigger, just like bright lights and chocolate. The underlying tendency to get migraines is already there, and probably remains there after the dental treatment.

Dr. Phillip Lamey, of Glasgow University, who carried out this research on dental plates, suggests a way in which tooth grinding could produce a migraine. The continuous tensing of the jaw muscles during sleep might well produce toxins—overworked muscles do this. These toxins might then affect the blood vessels in the vicinity, precipitating a migraine attack. A misaligned vertebra can also cause migraines, as mentioned earlier—again, excess muscle tension, due to the skeleton being awry, could spark the migraine.

Generalized muscle tension due to psychological stresses also contributes to migraine, probably because the tension tends to focus on the muscles of the shoulders and neck. Learning to relax can be very beneficial for migraine sufferers, even if food intolerance is the root cause of the problem. Mental factors can also play a part in migraine by means of adrenaline production, which affects the blood vessels as described above. Feeling angry or afraid, or being under constant stress, boosts adrenaline production and can trigger migraines. An elimination diet may work wonders, but for many migraine sufferers it is only part of the solution. They also need to adopt a calmer approach to life to attain real physical health, and to protect them from other stress-induced illnesses.

Mental Symptoms
The question of whether food intolerance can cause mental symptoms is discussed fully in chapter 8. In general, mental disorders are much more likely to be caused by emotional or social problems than by foods. Where they are a result of food intolerance, there will usually be physical symptoms as well, although a few patients have mental symptoms only.

The mental symptoms most often mentioned in connection with food intolerance are anxiety and depression—often accompanied by excessive fatigue (see page 178). Other minor symptoms that are reported include dizziness, confusion, tension, nervousness, insomnia, emotional instability, mental exhaustion, sleepiness, lack of concentration, and memory lapses. In children there may be various mental and behavioral problems that are described as the hyperkinetic syndrome (see pages 264–66).

The possibility of hyperventilation should always be kept in mind when there are minor mental symptoms—see pages 210–12 for further details. Finally, abnormalities of the gut flora (see chapter 10) can cause lethargy and depression.

The Eyes, Nose, Throat, and Lungs

Red, Itchy, or Watery Eyes
Assuming there is no infection causing these symptoms, then the most likely explanation is sensitivity to airborne allergens—see page 42 and pages 85–87. Occasionally, however, food sensitivity can produce symptoms in the eye or along the margins of the eyelids.

Other Symptoms

Bed-Wetting and Other Forms of Incontinence

Most children wet the bed until they are three or four. Thereafter about 25 percent of children continue to wet the bed, and some may also wet themselves during the day. In some children this may continue until age ten or older. Sometimes a urinary infection causes bed-wetting, and so can diabetes. However, in the vast majority of cases the cause is probably psychological, with anxiety or insecurity at the root of the problem.

In many children with food sensitivity, bed-wetting has unexpectedly stopped when they were treated for other symptoms, and recurred, along with those other symptoms, when certain foods were reintroduced.

At first this was put down to coincidence, but most doctors now accept that food sensitivity (either allergy or intolerance) can cause bed-wetting. It probably does so by making smooth muscles throughout the body contract. As well as being found in the bronchi (where their spasms can cause asthma) and the bowels (where they can cause diarrhea), smooth muscles make up the wall of the bladder. If they contract excessively, the bladder empties much more frequently, and with less control.

Some adults with food sensitivity have to empty their bladder very frequently, and the mechanism is probably the same. Severe constipation can also lead to urinary incontinence, as described in the case history on page 266.

Water Retention (Edema)

The symptoms of edema are a sudden gain in weight and a general puffiness all over the body, most noticeably around the eyes, on the face generally, and around the ankles. The most common cause of edema is kidney disease, and it is important that anyone with these symptoms see their doctor without delay.

Edema sometimes occurs in food allergy (see pages 50 and 98–100). It is also reported in some patients with food intolerance.

Epileptic Fits

There are two types of epileptic fit. In **grand mal** epilepsy the sufferer falls to the ground unconscious, goes very stiff, and then jerks and twitches uncontrollably. In **petit mal** epilepsy the sufferer does not usually fall but simply stares blankly for a few seconds, and is unaware of external events. It is mostly children who suffer from petit mal epilepsy, and they usually grow out of it by their teens. Epilepsy is a disorder of the brain, in which one group of brain cells becomes overactive and sends out strong electrical signals that overwhelm other parts of the brain.

Children with severe migraine sometimes suffer from seizures, probably epileptic in nature. Studies at Great Ormond Street Hospital in London have shown that eliminating certain foods can help these children (see pages 132–34), and the seizures often clear up along with the migraine. So it is probably worth investigating the role of food in epileptic children, but only if they also have migraines or some well-recognized allergic condition, such as asthma, allergic rhinitis, or eczema. How foods might provoke a seizure is a mystery, but they may affect the blood vessels supplying the brain, as they are thought to do in migraine.

Flushing, Sweating, and Chilling

Flushing and sweating are natural reactions to being too hot—both help cool the body off. They also occur as a nervous reaction to various emotions—fear, embarrassment, anger, or excitement—and they are a symptom of menopause, which usually begins during the forties or fifties but can start earlier in some women. Flushing and sweating are

---

Anna

Anna had suffered from an allergy to house dust mites since she was a child. If she breathed in too much dust, she suffered with a streaming nose and watery eyes. By keeping her house scrupulously clean and dust-free she had remained well for many years. In her thirties, however, she began to be troubled by a new problem. When she ate certain foods, her face flushed scarlet and remained hot and itchy for an hour or two. This caused her a great deal of embarrassment if she had to eat out. She kept a record of the foods responsible, which included onions, wine, vinegar, and cheese. But even when she avoided these foods, she still had episodes of flushing that she could not explain. The doctor suggested that she try a very simple diet, avoiding all commonly eaten foods for a while. This seemed to help considerably, and Anna reported feeling much more energetic and cheerful as well. When she reintroduced foods, she found that wheat, milk, and corn caused her to flush and brought on a headache. By avoiding these foods, she is able to eat other things, including wine, vinegar, and onions, which no longer make her face flush.

only a cause for concern if they occur regularly for no obvious reason.

People with food intolerance sometimes report flushing or sweating, or both, among their symptoms. They often say that they also get chilled easily, or "feel the cold." A few patients seem to have a slight fever, either intermittently or for much of the time. The general impression given by these symptoms is that they have difficulty controlling their body temperature—or adapting to normal changes in air temperature. It is unlikely that this would be the sole symptom of food intolerance, and it is not obvious how food might produce such an effect.

Fatigue

Excessive tiredness that is not relieved by rest is usually a sign of some mental disorder, such as depression. It can also be caused by many infectious diseases, by anemia, or by an underactive thyroid gland. Sometimes fatigue persists following a viral infection; this is now known as postviral syndrome or chronic fatigue syndrome (see page 293).

Fatigue is very often reported as a symptom of food intolerance, especially in connection with migraine and irritable bowel syndrome. Early-morning tiredness is the most frequent problem. Looking back over case histories, it seems that fatigue may be an early warning sign as food intolerance develops. How food might produce fatigue is not known. Exorphins (see page 294) may play a part, or it may be a side effect of some generalized immune reaction, as is suspected in postviral syndrome.

No one should embark on an elimination diet without first consulting a doctor, but this point should be emphasized for anyone with severe fatigue. There can be several other causes for this problem, and some are serious diseases.

Hypoglycemia

What gasoline is to a car, **glucose** is to the body—an energy-rich fuel that keeps every part of the body alive and powers our muscles. Glucose is carried around the body in the blood, and cells that need glucose can absorb it from the blood. It is very important that the level of glucose in the blood is always kept at about the same level. The brain is the organ most sensitive to a change in glucose level—too little produces tiredness, confusion, irritability, aggression, and other symptoms, while too much may result in loss of consciousness.

The body keeps glucose at the right level with the help of several hormones, the main ones being glucagon and insulin. **Glucagon** releases glucose from the liver, where it is stored, when the blood sugar is low. Insulin comes into play when the blood sugar is too high—it takes glucose out of circulation and puts it into storage. The level of glucagon is kept fairly steady, whereas the level of insulin changes rapidly in reponse to changes in blood glucose. After a meal, especially one containing a lot of sugar or starch, large quantities of glucose pass into the blood. Insulin is therefore produced to keep the blood glucose down. In diabetics, too little insulin is produced. They must compensate with injected insulin and avoid foods that release a lot of glucose at once—mainly sugar and other sweet foods.

Hypoglycemia is the medical term for low blood sugar, and it is usually a result of too much insulin being produced (or too much injected, in the case of diabetics). Everyone suffers from this condition to some extent—especially when they eat meals containing a lot of sugar and starch. Drinking alcohol with the meal makes matters worse. Extra insulin is produced to cope with this onslaught of high-glucose food, and in an excess of zeal it reduces the blood sugar to a very low level, producing symptoms of tiredness, confusion, and hunger about two to five hours after the meal. If the blood sugar drops to a very low level, then epinephrine (see page 196) is produced to help the body cope with what is a major crisis. The effect of the epinephrine is to make the subject irritable and aggressive. He or she will also sweat more, tremble, and look pale; there may also be a change in the heart rhythm. Since this type of hypoglycemia is a response to too much sugar, it is known as **reactive hypoglycemia.**

In the past doctors often advised people with reactive hypoglycemia to drink a cup of sweet tea, or suck sweets or glucose tablets, whenever they felt symptoms coming on. This may relieve the symptoms temporarily, but in the long term it just perpetuates the problem. The influx of sugar will simply stimulate the body to produce more insulin, and so make matters worse.

People who are overweight and eat a lot of starchy or sugary food may suffer from reactive hypoglycemia on a daily basis. Because they have to cope with such a high glucose load, their body cells become more responsive to insulin and they easily become hypoglycemic, especially if they miss out on one of their usual sugary snacks. Simply changing their diet will help such people, although they may find it quite difficult to wean themselves from the high-sugar diet that their body has become accustomed to. They should eat more meat, fish, eggs, cheese, and vegetables, and cut out sugar and honey entirely. White flour and bread should be replaced by whole wheat, since this is digested more slowly and does not release a lot of glucose at once. Even so, the amount of bread, pastry, and potatoes should be restricted, and no cakes, cookies, candies, puddings, or jam must be eaten. If there is an improvement, then some sweet foods can be reintroduced to the diet later, once the body has regained its natural equilibrium.

Various things can make hypoglycemia more likely. Alcohol, tea, and coffee can all do so, especially in excess. Smoking increases the amount of both glucagon and insulin, producing a rise in blood sugar followed by a fall about an hour later. The thyroid hormone plays an important part in controlling glucose levels, and either too much or too little thyroid hormone can cause hypoglycemia. Some vitamin and mineral deficiencies make people more prone to hypoglycemia. Drugs can cause hypoglycemia, and stress makes it a great deal worse. Gut flora overgrowth or imbalance can also be at the root of hypoglycemia (see page 240). Finally, there are some people who simply produce too much insulin, regardless of their diet or other circumstances; these cases seem to be quite rare.

The relationship between hypoglycemia and food intolerance is a very tangled one. For one thing, the standard laboratory test for hypoglycemia uses glucose that is derived from corn (known as dextrose). This is fed to the patient, and the level of glucose in the blood is measured some time later. Those patients who are very sensitive to corn may well react badly to the traces of corn protein in the dextrose, which could mean that their blood glucose falls whether they are hypoglycemic or not. So there is a suspicion that the tests for hypoglycemia may sometimes be measuring food intolerance, without anyone being aware of this. Patients may be told that they are hypoglycemic when in fact they are intolerant of corn.

More important, some doctors claim that hypoglycemia can sometimes be a symptom of food intolerance. The basis for this is that many patients previously diagnosed as hypoglycemic have found that such problems disappear following an elimination diet—although in most cases they were undertaking the diet for other symptoms and did not expect any improvement in their hypoglycemia. In children there seems to be a link between hyperkinetic syndrome and hypoglycemia: a great many hyperactive children handle glucose abnormally. If the proposed link between food and hyperkinesis is a reality (see page 267), then it may be that food sensitivity is causing the hypoglycemia in such children. Some of the children's symptoms, such as poor concentration and irritability, could be due to low blood sugar. The craving for sugary junk food that is common in these children may also be a result of hypoglycemia. Some doctors believe that a high proportion of hypoglycemia cases might be caused by food intolerance, but at present there is no hard evidence to support this. How foods might cause hypoglycemia is an open question, but a small group of doctors in the United States is investigating the idea that food sensitivity can make the insulin-producing cells in the pancreas overactive.

Premenstrual Syndrome

Some doctors report that a proportion of patients with severe premenstrual problems improve considerably following an elimination diet. These patients usually embark on the diet because they have some other symptoms, such as migraine or irritable bowel syndrome. Upon avoiding the foods that bring on these symptoms, they find that their premenstrual problems also disappear or become much less troublesome.

Symptoms That Have Been Reported in Food Intolerance

Many other symptoms have been attributed to food intolerance over the years. Those discussed below are mentioned fairly regularly in connection with food.

Ulcerative Colitis

Ulcerative colitis is an inflammatory disease that affects the large intestine (also called the **colon**—hence **colitis,** inflammation of the colon). It causes bouts of abdominal pain and diarrhea, often with blood and mucus in the stools. There were reports in the 1960s and 1970s that ulcerative colitis patients recovered on a milk-free diet, and this was attributed to food intolerance. But subsequent experience has not borne this out.

Dr. John Hunter, who pioneered the study of food intolerance in Crohn's disease, has had little success in treating ulcerative colitis by the same methods. When all food is withdrawn and elemental diets (see page 321) or intravenous feeding used instead, the ulcerative colitis patients do not make a sustained recovery. Perhaps the milk-free diets in the original studies seemed to be effective because the patients were short of lactase, the enzyme that breaks down milk sugar (see page 259).

Diarrhea often makes the gut deficient in lactase temporarily, and by drinking milk the patients may have been perpetuating their attacks of colitis. Despite these negative results, efforts to treat ulcerative colitis with elimination diet continue sporadically, and successes are sometimes reported. It is important to have full medical supervision for such a diet and to proceed cautiously when testing foods, using very small portions initially, because there can be a violent reaction.

Taking a different approach to the problem, one study carried out in Japan looked at what ulcerative colitis patients actually ate in the five years before contracting the disease, and compared this with the diets of healthy people. They discovered that sufferers had a far higher consumption of bread and margarine than healthy people, who tended to eat more of the traditional Japanese foods. Whether this study is relevant to non-Japanese is unknown. A study in Sweden has shown that eating fast foods twice a week or more increased the risk of contracting ulcerative colitis dramatically—numbers of cases were four times higher in the fast-food eaters.

One form of ulcerative colitis, known as **proctitis,** produces inflammation mainly in the lower part of the large intestine, near where it opens at the anus. It is possible that food allergy plays a part in this disorder, as a great many IgE antibodies have been found in the vicinity. So far, however, there has been little investigation of this possibility.

There is one type of colitis that is commonly due to food, and that is **infant colitis,** especially when it affects children under a year old. This rare condition is regarded as a form of ulcerative colitis by some doctors, but not by others. The main symptom is diarrhea containing blood and mucus. A sample is taken and examined under the microscope (a biopsy) to assess the degree of inflammation in the gut. Dr. Peter Milla, of the Institute of Child Health in London, has made a special study of infant colitis; he has found that the symptoms are caused by food in about 75 percent of cases. There are clear signs of immune-system involvement, so this is in fact food allergy. In some babies IgE and mast cells are involved; in others it is a different type of immune reaction.

This condition is known as **food-allergic colitis** or **FAC,** and most of the babies suffering from it are are bottle fed. However, some are breast-fed infants responding to foods that the mother is eating (see page 278). For bottle-fed infants, switching to a hydrolysate feed (see page 275) is the usual treatment. For those being breast fed, it is usually enough for the mother to eliminate certain foods from her diet—the most common culprits being milk, eggs, soy, and wheat. When this alone does not work, the mother can also be treated with the drug cromolyn sodium (see pages 431–33) to reduce absorption of intact food molecules by suppressing her own allergic reactions to them. Some babies are best treated by taking them off the breast and giving a hydrolysate feed instead.

A few babies with colitis have a type of autoimmune disease—they are making antibodies to their own cells. These antibodies start to attack various body cells, including those in the large intestine, and this sets off the inflammation that causes the bleeding and diarrhea. By looking for

---

Kate

"I had lots of headaches, particularly migraines and sinus pains, and I just felt tired all the time. I always woke up feeling sick, had stomachaches after eating, asthma, diarrhea, and lots of menstrual problems. My doctor was quite sympathetic at first, but every time I went it was a different diagnosis, and eventually he began to get fairly irritable with me.

"At one point he thought I might have myalgic encephalitis, then hyperventilation, and then he said perhaps it was the early stages of multiple sclerosis, because I kept going numb in one leg, and had trouble moving about and kept falling over. I used to have quite bad bouts of this, then it would go away. I had joint pains, too, but I didn't even tell the doctor about those—there were too many other things.

"I tried various alternative treatments, such as acupuncture, but they didn't really make any difference. In the end I came across something about diet and thought I would try cutting out certain things. I stopped eating wheat, dairy products, chocolate, and sugar, and cut out all alcoholic drinks. The effect was pretty astonishing. Almost all the symptoms went, even my asthma, which I'd had for years. I've never had another bout of numbness or falling over since then, either. I think I was just lucky in guessing what foods might be a problem.

"It's only since coming off these foods that I've really recognized how ill I felt before. When I felt better I dashed around and cleaned the whole house and just ran about outside in the garden for joy—it was really amazing to feel so well."

auto-antibodies in the blood, doctors can tell if colitis is being caused in this way. Interestingly enough, Dr. Milla has found that changing to a hydrolysate feed or chicken-based feed helps these babies considerably. Some still need immunosuppressant drugs to control the inflammation, but others do not. It would seem that immune reactions to foods are aggravating the autoimmune reaction in such cases. Some babies with food-allergic colitis grow out of it, but others are still sensitive to the same foods five or more years later. For other causes of diarrhea in babies and children, see page 263.

Multiple Sclerosis

Multiple sclerosis is a degenerative disease affecting the nerves and brain. The cause is not known. Several doctors have tried investigating MS patients for food intolerance. They claim that by treating them for supposed "candidiasis" (see chapter 10) and eliminating suspect foods, the patients' symptoms can sometimes be greatly alleviated.

Some patients treated in this way have recovered sufficiently to be able to walk again, when previously they had been confined to a wheelchair. However, it is very difficult to know if these improvements have anything to do with the treatment, because MS is characterized by natural periods of remission anyway. As yet there is no hard evidence that these measures make any difference in MS.

One new theory is that chocolate plays a part in developing MS. Clearly it does not produce MS in everyone, but there may be a small number of people who are unusually susceptible to something in chocolate. The limited evidence available suggests that the reaction is a slow one, perhaps taking as long as a week, so it may not be obvious that eating chocolate (or an especially large amount of chocolate) has triggered a deterioration in the condition of an MS patient.

Some MS patients have halted the progress of their disease by cutting out chocolate. While the existing damage to the nerves does not disappear, no further decline occurs. Since chocolate is not an essential part of anyone's diet, nutritionally speaking, there can be no harm in trying this out. Some doctors also advise cutting out coffee, cola, and strong tea at the same time, as they contain some of the same druglike chemicals that are found in chocolate.

Because of the natural cycle of remissions described above, it may be necessary to live without chocolate for some time to assess the effects realistically.

Diabetes

Diabetes is a shortage of the hormone insulin that controls the level of glucose in the blood (see page 179). There are two types of diabetes. One form (type 1 diabetes) comes on in childhood and is due to the body forming antibodies against its own cells. In this case the cells under attack are the islet cells of the pancreas, which produce the insulin. The other form (type 2) of diabetes comes on in adults, usually those who are overweight, and is probably due to exhaustion of the islet cells through overconsumption of sugar and starch.

It has been suggested that diabetes might be due to an immune reaction to cow's milk. Some researchers claim that children who are susceptible to diabetes due to their genetic makeup are at risk if they take cow's milk in early infancy, or drink a lot of cow's milk (three glasses or more a day) later in childhood. Such children can first develop antibodies against a particular protein in cow's milk. Then, because the milk protein is similar to proteins in the pancreas, these antibodies turn against the pancreas, gradually destroying it. No one is claiming that this is the sole cause of type 1 diabetes, and many other researchers dispute the whole milk-diabetes connection. It is a subect of heated debate.

Our advice, to any parents with type 1 diabetes in the family, particularly if one child already suffers from it, is to exclusively breast-feed a new baby for at least the first four months, and delay introducing cow's milk for as long as possible after that. Prolonged breast feeding is good for the prevention of many diseases, so you cannot really lose by doing this. Once the child is weaned, keep cow's milk consumption to two glasses a day or less.

Alcoholism

This is a very controversial area. The putative link between food intolerance and alcoholism is based on case histories of recovering alcoholics, many of whom were seeking treatment for other symptoms. Regardless of what these other symptoms were, most also complained of extreme tension, great fatigue, continuous headaches, or the like.

These symptoms had begun when the subjects gave up drinking but did not clear up despite many years on the wagon. Some sought treatment because these symptoms had become so unbearable that they felt they were about to hit the bottle again.

According to the doctors treating these cases, the stories show a common pattern. For many of these patients, the elimination diet was apparently very successful—it brought relief from the tension, fatigue, and other symptoms. More surprisingly, the craving for a drink, which is the bane of recovering alcoholics, also disappeared for the first time. When they began to reintroduce foods, they experienced unusual reactions to some of them: in some patients certain food items supposedly produced symptoms akin to drunkenness. It invariably turned out that the food concerned was a major ingredient of the drink the patient had formerly favored—potatoes for the vodka alcoholic, wheat, barley, or corn for the whiskey addict, grapes for the confirmed brandy drinker.

These discoveries were first made by Dr. Theron G. Randolph, one of the founders of the clinical ecology movement in the United States. Dr. Randolph interpreted the findings as follows:

The patients concerned were primarily intolerant of/addicted to a *food*. (Addictive eating is often a feature of food intolerance, as explained on page 146.) Small amounts of food protein remain in an alcoholic drink, and these can pass through the gut wall and into the blood much more readily than food proteins that are eaten in the ordinary way—simply because of the alcohol. Alcoholics are addicted both to the food and to the alcohol. When the potent combination of the two is withdrawn, the recovering alcoholic is still eating the culprit food. So the addiction is kept alive, and the craving for the favorite drink—the "jet-propelled" version of the addictive food, in Dr. Randolph's words—persists. If the culprit food can be identified and avoided for some time, this lingering addiction is broken.

The revolutionary implication of Dr. Randolph's theory is that recovering alcoholics can drink again, as long as they avoid the drinks that contain their culprit foods. Because this goes against the conventional wisdom on alcoholism—which forbids the recovering alcoholic to ever drink again—Dr. Randolph's work has been rejected out of hand by organizations such as Alcoholics Anonymous. There have been no scientific studies of his claims, although his basic findings have been confirmed by several other doctors working in this field.

Cancer

Claims that cancer is a result of "allergies" are now cropping up, and treatments are being offered by some practitioners. Like any life-threatening disease for which conventional medicine offers no certain cure, cancer attracts all kinds of implausible treatment claims. Extreme skepticism is advisable.

Other Reported symptoms

Some of the other symptoms attributed to food intolerance are excessive hunger or thirst, twitching muscles, muscle cramps, numbness, insomnia, sleeping too much, and sexual impotence. Experience suggests that none of these is a very likely indicator of food intolerance, although excessive hunger and thirst are often reported in hyperkinetic syndrome (see pages 264–68). Numbness is a common symptom of hyperventilation (see page 210).

EIGHT

Mind and Body

Can food allergy or intolerance cause mental symptoms? This is without a doubt the most controversial aspect of food sensitivity. Reports of mental disorders that were apparently caused by foods began with the work of the early clinical ecologists in America. Since then, many other doctors who treat food intolerance and chemical sensitivity have claimed that such sensitivity can produce a wide range of mental problems. The most common are anxiety and depression, but many more serious illnesses, including psychosis and schizophrenia, have also been attributed to food.

For the most part, objective evidence to support these claims, in the form of scientific trials, is still lacking. But this may simply reflect the tremendous difficulties involved in such trials. For doctors specializing in the treatment of food sensitivity, the many positive responses they have seen in their patients are sufficient evidence that food can cause mental symptoms. But the case has been greatly overstated in some popular publications, and genuine psychological problems have been wrongly attributed to food sensitivity, both by patients and by fringe practitioners.

This is just one of the mind-body controversies that beset the question of food sensitivity. Equally acrimonious are the disputes over the purely physical symptoms of food intolerance, which some regard as psychosomatic—conditions in which the mind produces genuine physical symptoms in the body. On the one hand are those who see most "food intolerance" as misdiagnosed psychosomatic illness; on the other hand are those who see most "psychosomatic illness" as unrecognized food intolerance.

The effects of the mind on the body, and the problems of disentangling physical and emotional causes in chronic health problems, are also considered in this chapter. The mind has the power to produce health as well as illness, and ways in which its healing powers can be harnessed are described here.

Psychological Problems in Food Allergy

Some doctors believe that true, IgE-mediated allergy can produce mental symptoms as well as physical ones, but others would dispute this. Certainly, some studies have shown that those with serious allergic disorders, such as severe, disabling asthma, tend to have more emotional and social problems. The difficulty lies in separating cause and effect. The disabling symptoms of the allergy and the restrictions incurred by having to avoid certain allergens are bound to cause mental suffering. Indeed, studies that have compared asthmatic children with children suffering from other physical handicaps find little difference in the level of psychological problems.

However, there are innumerable reports of children with allergic disorders, such as asthma or perennial rhinitis (runny or congested nose), who also show a cluster of symptoms that includes an inability to keep still, excitability, clumsiness, poor memory, and short attention span. These symptoms, often known collectively as hyperactivity or the hyperkinetic syndrome, are dealt with more fully in chapter 11. Some of these children show an interesting reaction when the allergenic foods are removed from the diet and other allergens avoided: their mental and behavioral symptoms clear up at the same time as their physical ones. Reintroducing those foods brings the bad behavior back, along with the wheezing or runny nose. Although the mental symptoms could be a result of the physical ones, this seems unlikely.

One study showed that some such children had high IgE levels for the particular foods that caused behavioral problems, so it seems that this could sometimes be a true allergic symptom. This is a controversial area, however, and conventional allergists do not seem eager to welcome behavioral disorders such as hyperactivity into their domain.

Less controversial is the notion that some allergic symptoms may affect the brain and cause mental problems, these being secondary to the allergic response itself. In people with severe asthma, for example, the reduction in oxygen reaching the brain can cause changes in mood and abnormal behavior. Lack of concentration, poor memory, "slowness," drowsiness, depression, anxiety, and irritability can all result from lack of oxygen.

Hay fever and nonseasonal rhinitis (constant runny nose) can also have secondary effects on the brain. The congestion in the nose may result in the normal breathing pattern stopping entirely during sleep (**sleep apnea**). This wakes the patient, and breathing starts again, but repeated attacks during the night can produce severe fatigue and drowsiness the following day.

Overall, the evidence suggests that IgE-mediated allergy probably *can* affect the brain, either directly or indirectly. But the mechanism of direct action is unknown, and the subject remains highly contentious. Nevertheless, there is considerable evidence that the immune system interacts with both the nervous system and the hormones. This evidence, which will be looked at in the next section, is an indication that a direct link between allergy and mental problems is not impossible.

Interlocking Systems

One of the newest and most exciting fields of biological research at present concerns the relationships among the immune system, the nervous system, and the hormones. The realization that these three systems can interact, and the identification of the mechanisms involved, has come only within the past few years. This new science has been given the rather daunting name of **psychoneuroimmunology**.

Among the discoveries made in psychoneuroimmunology is that stressful events can make the immune cells far less responsive to infection. Bereavement can have devastating effects on our defensive cells, but even something as minor as taking an exam can make us more vulnerable to infection. With long-term stress, it appears that a sense of being in control makes all the difference—feelings of helplessness and inability to improve matters are the most damaging. Controllable stress, on the other hand, can actually improve immune status. (However, expecting to have absolute control over external events is obviously unrealistic, and can eventually increase stress levels.) Another important factor in reducing stress is having the support of family, friends, and colleagues. Having little social contact, or not turning to others for comfort, sympathy, or advice when in difficult circumstances, tends to magnify stress.

The mechanisms behind the interactions of mind and immune system are still waiting to be unraveled, but there are indications that small messenger molecules may be important. These small messengers include the major chemical signals produced by the body (**hormones**), messenger substances released by the nerves for communication with adjacent nerves (**neurotransmitters**), and mediators released by immune cells that stimulate or suppress other immune cells (**lymphokines**). Some of the hormones known to affect the nervous system, such as the endorphins (see page 295), now appear to bind to immune cells as well, and probably influence their behavior. Conversely, mediators produced by immune cells can influence nerve cells—histamine and prostaglandins both have this effect. One lymphokine with marked effects on both body and mind is interferon (see page 292). The hormone norepinephrine also acts as a neurotransmitter for some nerves. In other words, these are three closely interconnected systems.

There are also direct links between the nerves and the immune system that do not rely on messenger substances. Detailed anatomical studies have revealed nervous connections that were not previously suspected. It turns out that several parts of the immune system—including the lymph nodes, the spleen, the thymus gland, and the bone marrow—are connected by nerve fibers to the central nervous system. Exactly what effect the nerves have on these organs is as yet unknown.

So far research into psychoneuroimmunology has done no more than scratch the surface of this potentially important topic. But it indicates that the idea of allergies affecting the mind—and vice versa—is not implausible.

Food Intolerance and Mental Symptoms

Many of the doctors now working on food intolerance trace their interest back to a book, published in 1976, with the intriguing title *Not All in the Mind*. Written by Dr. Richard Mackarness, a psychiatrist then at Britain's Basingstoke District Hospital, it described the good results of dietary change on a patient called "Joanna" whose severe mental disturbance had been variously diagnosed as schizophrenia, schizo-affective psychosis, presenile dementia, temporal lobe epilepsy, neurotic depression, and anxiety hysteria. During seven years of illness she had been admitted to the hospital thirteen times, often compulsorily during episodes of violent behavior when she was a danger both to her children and herself. She had made determined attempts at suicide by slashing her wrists several times.

The outlook for this patient was very poor. Although his fellow psychiatrists were thoroughly skeptical about the usefulness of an elimination diet—which Dr. Mackarness had learned about from clinical ecologists in America—they were desperate enough to try anything. During a five-day fast Joanna showed a "very marked improvement in her condition," and when subsequently challenged with individual foods, she responded sharply to some but not others. In follow-up tests, the same foods were given by a tube leading straight into the stomach (thus avoiding the taste buds) to check whether she would still respond in the same way. By using the stomach tube and portions of liquefied food identified only by a code number, the test could be carried out without either the patient or the nurse giving the test food knowing its identity. (This sort of test—known as a **double-blind test**—is a must if the observations are to be verified objectively. Even if the patient does not know the identity of the food—as in a **single-blind test**—the expectations of the experimenter can still influence the outcome.) In Joanna's case the double-blind test confirmed the severe mental reactions to culprit foods already identified in open testing.

This is how one of the more skeptical psychiatrists involved later described the patient's case:

> I must admit that such a remarkable response has been a surprise to me. However, it has been so dramatic that I think it would be difficult for us to say that it was due to anything but the dietary changes, especially in view of the double-blind trial.

These and other well-documented case histories lend support to the idea that food sensitivity can sometimes be at the root of serious mental illness. But it seems unlikely that it is often so, and it would be a mistake to extrapolate to other cases of mental illness that have been given the same diagnostic labels. There is little doubt that a variety of different diseases are concealed under umbrella terms such as *psychosis* and *schizophrenia*. No one is suggesting that the mental hospitals are full of food-sensitive individuals who simply need an elimination diet to set them free from their illness. Nor is it possible to say what percentage of cases might be attributable to food, because nobody has even attempted to find out. It is extremely difficult to set up a large-scale trial of dietary treatment among patients who are seriously disturbed.

Rosemary

Rosemary was sixty-seven and lived alone. From time to time she suffered from bouts of depression, as she had for many years. At one stage, in her early fifties, the depression had been so bad that she had been admitted to the hospital. But this was not her reason for seeking medical help now. She suffered from diarrhea with pain and bloating, which had been diagnosed as irritable bowel syndrome. Her doctor had told her that there was nothing he could do for this problem, so she decided to consult a physician whom a friend had recommended. He put her on an elimination diet, and within two weeks her bowels were functioning normally for the first time in many years. She also reported feeling much more cheerful, alert, and confident than before, and the doctor assumed that this was an effect of losing her unpleasant bowel symptoms. What surprised them both was Rosemary's reaction upon retesting food. Milk taken at breakfasttime produced itchy skin by lunchtime, and severe bloating and diarrhea in the afternoon. A profound depression set in at the same time, despite the fact that she knew her bowel symptoms could now be controlled quite easily. The depression took two days to clear, but afterward Rosemary felt as well as before, both mentally and physically. Two years later she is still very healthy on a milk-free diet, and no longer suffers from depression.

Less serious forms of mental illness, such as depression and anxiety, are commonly reported among those with food intolerance, usually accompanied by some physical symptoms. Doctors who treat food intolerance have observed the mental problems to clear up at the same time as the physical symptoms during an elimination diet, and to reappear when the patient tests particular foods. In many cases it was the physical symptoms alone that were the target of the treatment, and both doctor and patient were pleasantly surprised at the change in mood that occurred simultaneously. It is possible, of course, that the depression or anxiety is felt in response to the physical symptoms—rather than being directly caused by the food itself—or that people experience certain mental responses to certain foods simply because they expect to do so. But the pattern of response that is observed is not easily explained in this way: with most patients there is a strong impression that the food itself is directly responsible for the symptoms.

Proving this is not easy, however. It involves administering food in such a way that the patients cannot taste it, and somehow assessing their mental symptoms objectively. As well as being disguised, the food must also be given in sufficient quantity, a task that has taxed the ingenuity of many a researcher (see page 130 and page 133). For the present, mental responses to food must be regarded as unproven, but with considerable circumstantial evidence in their favor.

Apart from depression and anxiety, the following mental symptoms are reported in cases of food intolerance: fatigue, mental exhaustion and confusion, inability to concentrate, poor memory, insomnia, tension, dizziness, disorientation, overexcitement, nervousness, irritability, violent mood swings, and aggressive behavior. In children hyperactivity is frequently reported (see pages 264–265), while in adults the most common symptom is excessive fatigue that is not relieved by rest. Children may also show great lethargy and drowsiness. Some doctors interpret both fatigue and hyperactivity as part of a common set of reactions that they describe as the tension-fatigue syndrome, in which the patient may be profoundly tired, or tense and irritable, or both. For many, the fatigue is worst in the morning; they have difficulty waking up and feel terrible upon getting out of bed. As the day progresses, the fatigue begins to clear.

Schizophrenia

One mental disorder, schizophrenia, deserves special mention here, because it has been strongly linked with food sensitivity by some doctors. The idea originated with the observation that schizophrenia was more common among those with celiac disease than among the population at large. (Celiac disease is an extreme sensitivity to wheat that causes damage to the structure of the small intestine; see pages 104–7.) Because of the damage to the gut wall, there is often a greater absorption of intact food molecules, which creates the potential for further food sensitivities.

The earliest studies designed to test this idea gave promising results. A gluten-free, milk-free diet produced fewer symptoms in some schizophrenics, while feeding extra gluten made the symptoms worse. Later studies failed to find any response, for the most part, although one found that two out of sixteen schizophrenics responded. It may be that gluten is important, but only in a fairly small proportion of schizophrenia cases.

Autism

There are a lot of claims being made at present for the role of "allergies" in autism. Three main strands of thought are emerging here. One is that autistic children are slow to break down the opioid-like peptides (see page 295) that are normally formed from foods such as wheat and milk. The levels of these build up in their blood and cause the mental dysfunction. A second idea is that imbalances of the gut flora are to blame. A third suggests that autistic children have difficulty breaking down natural toxins (see pages 297–98). There is little sound evidence to back up any of these theories, but they are certainly worth further investigation.

Treatments for autistic children, based on these tentative theories, are now available from some practitioners. It is worth pointing out that any serious disease for which conventional medicine offers no cures is likely to attract such treatment claims, and skepticism is advisable. On the other hand, if the treatment has no risks attached, there is probably no harm in trying it, provided your specialist agrees.

One treatment program that seems to meet with success is a course of the antifungal drug nystatin, taken by mouth for about three months, plus a strict wheat-free, milk-free diet. This regime has never been tested scientifically, but there have been many cases of striking improvement that are difficult to explain away.

Not every autistic child benefits from this treatment. However, those who were normal for the first twelve to eighteen months of life and then developed autism may improve, particularly if they have obvious digestive problems, or have taken many courses of antibiotics. It is important to begin the treatment early, before the child is five years old. Ideally, for those children who improve, wheat and milk should be tested to see if they do bring the autistic symptoms back. In reality, most parents are unwilling to carry out such tests, because the child may take several weeks to recover from the effects of the test.

Psychosomatic Illness and Hypochondria

A large proportion of those with food intolerance are diagnosed as having psychosomatic illness by their family doctors, or by specialists to whom they are referred. Although this is distressing and frustrating for the patient, the confusion is understandable because the two disorders do present a very similar picture in terms of symptoms.

Psychosomatic illness, like *hypochondria,* is a term that is frequently misused by the public and the medical profession alike.

The term *psychosomatic* is derived from the Greek words *psyche,* meaning "soul," and *soma* meaning "body." It denotes an illness in which the action of the mind creates a damaging reaction in the body, with physical symptoms that can be observed or measured. There is *no* sense in which the symptoms are imaginary or all in the mind, as is often implied in both medical and casual use. Nor is it possible for the sufferer to "snap out of it," as is often suggested with varying degrees of tact.

There are several ways in which psychosomatic symptoms can be generated. One major route is via the **autonomic nervous system,** which regulates the bodily functions that are not under conscious control, such as digestion, circulation of the blood, breathing, and sweating. The autonomic system consists of two parts, the parasympathetic and the sympathetic, which have largely opposing effects. The **parasympathetic** is responsible for the day-to-day running of the body—for keeping things ticking nicely. The **sympathetic** system comes into play when there is an emergency to deal with. It increases the heart rate and blood pressure while mobilizing glucose, the body's energy source. It diverts blood from the gut and increases the flow to the muscles, preparing the body for action. The sympathetic system can also cause bowel movement so that the contents of the gut are voided promptly, making the body lighter and therefore faster moving. The benefit of these reactions have to be understood in terms of life in the wild, where fighting off predators, or fleeing from them, may literally be a matter of life or death. The reactions produced are often summed up as the **flight-or-fight response.**

The sympathetic nerves achieve their effects by releasing the hormone **norepinephrine** from the nerve tips, which are located close to the organs that they influence. A very similar hormone, **epinephrine,** can also be generated by a pair of glands known as the adrenals that sit above the kidneys. The sympathetic nerves control the adrenals' activity, so they are really part of the same system. The inner part of the gland, the adrenal medulla, produces epinephrine, while the outer part of the gland, known as the adrenal cortex, is responsible for producing **corticosteroids** (steroids derived from the cortex). As the bloodstream carries these hormones around the body, the adrenaline produces the flight-or-fight

TABLE 1 SOME COMMON SYMPTOMS OF PSYCHOSOMATIC ILLNESS

Body system affected

Digestive system	Dry mouth or excessive saliva production. Spasm of the esophagus (the tube leading from the throat to the stomach). Nausea and vomiting, stomach ulcers, frequent indigestion, loss of appetite. Diarrhea or constipation.
Nervous system	Headache, fatigue, insomnia, tremors, nervousness, dizziness, and loss of balance.
Circulatory system	Abnormal heart rhythms, pain in chest.
Respiratory system	Runny or congested nose, constant sore throat, catarrh or postnasal drip, difficulty in breathing, hyperventilation.
Skin	Excessive sweating, skin irritation.

reaction already described, while the corticosteroids have a great variety of effects. They, too, are capable of mobilizing glucose, but they also suppress inflammation (see page 440) and inhibit some immune functions. Their main function in emergencies is to release glucose and thus perpetuate the flight-or-fight reaction initiated by epinephrine and norepinephrine—they have a longer-lasting effect on the body.

Overstimulation of the sympathetic nervous system can produce psychosomatic symptoms such as diarrhea, nervousness, tremors, high blood pressure, and abnormal heart rhythms. To make matters worse, epinephrine production is encouraged by smoking and by too much sugar, alcohol, or coffee.

Overactivity by the parasympathetic can also result in bowel disturbances; contraction of the bronchi producing asthma; or oversecretion of acid by the stomach, eventually leading to stomach ulcers.

A third way in which symptoms can be produced is through mental tension being translated into muscle tension, especially in the muscles of the neck, jaw, and head. Prolonged tightening of these muscles can produce headache, and possibly migraine (for more on this, see pages 174–75).

The full range of symptoms attributed to psychosomatic mechanisms are shown in table 1. In addition there are conditions in which the psychological component is only a small part of the story—it can make the symptoms worse, but not initiate the illness. This is true of eczema, psoriasis, and most cases of asthma. Exactly how the mind affects such symptoms is not known.

Diagnosing Psychosomatic Illness

A diagnosis of psychosomatic illness should not be made lightly. First, the possibility of any organic illness must be ruled out. (*Organic* in this sense means "of the body," and organic illness includes infections, autoimmune disorders, allergies, and other problems with an identifiable cause.) Even if all organic diseases have been ruled out, there are still other criteria to satisfy. The patient should have the right sort of symptoms and should have been subject to some stressful emotional experience before the onset of the illness. A typical pattern in psychosomatic illness is for the disease to fluctuate, with periods when the symptoms disappear, only to return again at a later date. If this pattern is present, and if other members of the family have had psychosomatic complaints, then the diagnosis is strengthened.

Unfortunately, a diagnosis of psychosomatic illness is often arrived at by a much shorter and less strenuous route than this, particularly with female patients, who tend to be perceived as more "nervy." All too often doctors use "psychosomatic" as a diagnosis of convenience, to cover any illness with no obvious cause. What is more, little is offered in the way of treatment. This is paradoxical, because physical illness is taken seriously and given adequate treatment, and mental illness with mainly mental symptoms is taken seriously and treated (if not always very effectively or humanely). Yet for some reason, mental illness that produces physical symptoms is relegated to the status of an imaginary disease.

Hypochondria

Hypochondria is an anxious preoccupation with the body or a part of the body. The patient characteristically believes that the part is diseased or not fully functional. He or she generally reports pain and other bizarre sensations of bodily disturbance and internal movement. There are few physical symptoms that can be observed, apart from vomiting, fainting, and sweating in some cases. Hypochondria is thought to be a result of repressed emotions and secret fears, and it is far more likely to develop in families where there is a preoccupation with illness, or in people who had a great deal of contact with invalids as children.

In earlier centuries hypochondria was recognized as a real illness, with a distinctive set of characteristics. And it was considered to be worthy of treatment. The dismissal of hypochondria by most doctors is a relatively new attitude, and one that is lamented by those that have studied this disorder. Robert Meister, in his book *Hypochondria*, writes:

> Those physicians who shrug off a suffering patient because they regard his condition as psychosomatic or hypochondriacal are not acting as professional healers. . . . The cultural and social norms that affect considerations of health and illness have established what might be called an unspoken "Acceptability Index" of various forms of illness. On such an index, bacterial pneumonia, which is regarded as a "real" illness, would indubitably outrank peptic ulcers, which are viewed suspiciously as being of "psychosomatic" origin, and all illnesses known to man would outrank hypochondria. . . . The prevailing negative attitudes towards hypochondria are largely unexplained, unjustified, and certainly unjust to victims of the condition.

The best type of treatment for both psychosomatic complaints and hypochondria is some form of psychotherapy, cognitive therapy, or hypnotherapy (see pages 207–8), which should make it possible for the sufferer to identify the underlying emotions that are responsible for the symptoms. Once aware of the source of the problem, the patient can come to terms with these emotions; the physical symptoms should then diminish.

In some cases, however, the symptoms are a vital element in the way the patient deals with the world and with his or her own conflicts about life and relationships. For such people the symptoms are indispensable, and the best hope is to keep the condition within limits so that it causes the least possible disruption to the patient and his family.

The Placebo Effect

One intriguing aspect of illness is that it can often be cured—at least temporarily—by *any* form of medical attention. A medical investigation or injection can work wonders, and a course of tablets is almost as good.

This phenomenon is known as the placebo effect, *placebo* being a Latin word that means "I shall be pleasing."

Research shows that over a third of people in pain get relief from inert tablets that they believe to be painkillers. Headaches, migraines, insomnia, epilepsy, and rheumatoid arthritis are among the conditions that are susceptible to placebos.

In some cases the symptoms may have been psychosomatic in origin, which would account for the good effect of the placebo. It may be that the patient feels gratified by someone taking the illness seriously, or it

---

Lynne

Lynne suffered constant diarrhea and nausea, and became convinced that foods were causing these symptoms. She tried cutting out wheat and milk, and felt a little better for a while, but then the symptoms came back. So she tried cutting out a few more foods, and again felt better—but only for a short while. This led to more and more foods being cut out, until she was on a very restricted diet of lamb, pears, plums, celery, rice, and some fish. Although she still felt ill on this diet, she refused to consider eating other foods, saying that they would make her worse. At the same time she began to suffer panic attacks and feelings of utter exhaustion, which she blamed on sensitivity to perfume and exhaust fumes. There was a danger of her losing her job, so she reluctantly took her doctor's advice and went to see a psychotherapist.

Over the following weeks Lynne began talking to the therapist about things that had happened to her as a child—the violence at home, the constant arguments, and, later, the sexual abuse by her father. For years she had felt very blank and unemotional about these events and had therefore concluded that they had not had any lasting effect on her. In talking to the therapist she gradually began to recognize that she had erased the feelings of terror and anger from her mind, leaving just a sense of numb despair. Bringing these feelings to the surface and acknowledging them was painful and difficult, but when she had done this her relief was tremendous. Her panic attacks stopped, the feeling of exhaustion lifted, and her diarrhea and nausea disappeared. In retrospect Lynne saw that blaming her physical illness on food had been a way of not confronting the real source of her problems.

may simply be the power of suggestion that produces a cure. In other cases there may be a mixture of organic illness and psychosomatic illness behind the symptoms—the two can coexist, one feeding on the other. Again, the placebo could be powerful because it meets some psychological need for attention and treatment.

With diseases such as rheumatoid arthritis, it is less obvious how the placebo effect works. However, the immune system plays an important role in rheumatoid arthritis (see pages 164–66), and this may provide a clue. A new form of treatment, or a new and more enthusiastic doctor, may act as a morale booster that has a beneficial effect on the immune system—the sort of effect that the psychoneuroimmunologists are currently studying. Placebo effects are also seen in allergy, perhaps for the same reason.

A characteristic feature of the placebo effect is that it does not last all that long: usually only a matter of weeks, with two to six months as about the most that can be expected. If a patient responds to a new treatment and is still well after a year, it is unlikely to be due to a placebo effect.

Psychogenic Reactions to Food

The other side of the placebo coin is that people can be made ill by something that they believe will make them ill. Some patients are more suggestible than others in this respect, but a fair proportion of food-sensitive people will react with symptoms if they think they have eaten one of their culprit foods. This reaction in no way invalidates their food sensitivity—it is real, even if the symptoms of the moment are mentally generated or **psychogenic**.

Such reactions are not really surprising, if you remember Pavlov's famous experiment with the dog and the dinner bell. The dog was conditioned by a bell being sounded every time it was fed. After a time the dog would salivate whenever it heard the bell, whether food was present or not.

An experiment with guinea pigs has shown that immune reactions can be conditioned in exactly the same way. The guinea pigs were sensitized to an antigen by having it injected into them, and they were simultaneously exposed to a strong odor. Later the odor alone was enough to make them release large amounts of histamine. If guinea pigs can do this, then why not humans? Certainly those who have ever had a severe, immediate reaction to a food may react in the same way if told that they have consumed some of the same food. And people whose intolerance of a food has long since cleared up may continue to react to that food for purely psychological reasons.

Occasionally people develop psychogenic reactions to food when there is no physical response, usually because they have become convinced that they are food allergic or food intolerant without undergoing proper diagnosis. They may decide that they react to particular foods on the basis of bogus diagnostic tests or elimination diets that are not properly carried out. Thereafter the reactions occur obligingly every time they eat these foods—but the reactions are psychogenic. This response is one of the pitfalls of self-treatment, but it can occur just as readily—if not more so—with treatment by fringe practitioners who use ineffective methods of diagnosis.

Psychogenic reactions of this type are most likely to occur in those whose symptoms are purely psychosomatic, but who prefer to think they are allergic to food, because they see this as being a more respectable sort of illness. The medical neglect of psychosomatic illness and hypochondria must shoulder some of the blame in such situations, because the stigma attached to these disorders owes much to doctors' negative attitudes.

Patients who mistakenly believe that they are sensitive to food often put themselves on increasingly strict diets as their symptoms persist, and they may become seriously malnourished. They are in need of sympathetic professional help to identify the true causes of their malaise, and should be persuaded to undertake psychotherapy or some other form of psychological treatment. Such treatment can be valuable even where foods are a major cause of symptoms (see pages 207–8), so undertaking this type of therapy is worthwhile for a whole range of patients, not just for those whose problems are purely psychosomatic.

Psychogenic reactions to food are important in the diagnosis of food allergy and intolerance, because a challenge with any food may produce symptoms if the patient is expecting symptoms. In order to separate real responses from psychogenic ones, dummy challenges (with foods that are known not to cause any reaction) are included in the double-blind trials. Most patients are expected to respond to some of these dummy challenges, but they should respond to significantly more of the real ones. These dummy challenges are also known as placebos.

Food Intolerance or Psychosomatic Illness?

It will be clear from table 1 that many of the symptoms seen in psychosomatic illness are also features of food intolerance. Indeed, opponents of food intolerance would maintain that most supposed food intolerance is psychosomatic illness. But doctors specializing in the treatment of food allergy and intolerance would disagree. They see innumerable patients who have been told that their symptoms are psychosomatic, or all in their mind, by one doctor or another. Yet a high proportion of these patients respond to an elimination diet. They get better when foods are eliminated from the diet—and they stay better, which is the important thing.

A diagnosis of psychosomatic illness or hypochondria is very largely a diagnosis of exclusion—it requires all other possibilities to be excluded first. With many patients suffering vague, multiple symptoms, food intolerance must be regarded as one of those possibilities. Unless steps are taken to eliminate it from the inquiry—and that must mean a diagnostic diet—then there is no sound basis for saying that a patient's symptoms are psychosomatic.

Things are not necessarily done in this order, however, and for good reason. Many of those in the doctor's office with physical symptoms, such as headache or diarrhea, actually have serious emotional, sexual, or family problems that they want to discuss with the doctor—but they find it difficult to start in on such sensitive topics. Family physicians are trained in the art of discovering what the patient has really come to see them about. If you have symptoms that you think may be caused by food intolerance, you should not feel affronted if the doctor's initial questions seem rather personal and irrelevant to the aches and pains being suffered. Answering the questions calmly and reasonably will do much to convince the doctor that your problems are not psychosomatic.

The question of how many psychosomatic cases the average family doctor sees is an interesting one. One survey concluded that a full third of patients have some psychological element in their illness, with 18 percent showing purely psychiatric or psychosomatic symptoms. Other studies put the figure even higher, some as high as 50 percent. Such studies have received a lot of publicity, so it is small wonder that the average family doctor often suspects a psychological cause rather than a physical one, especially when patients complain of multiple symptoms.

Doctors who are aware of food intolerance and experienced in diagnosing it have a different statistical outlook. They vary in their estimates of how many patients might trace some or all of their symptoms to food, but most say 20 to 30 percent. The surveys described above, which showed large numbers of patients suffering from psychosomatic symptoms, *took little account of the possibility of food intolerance.* Many of those classified as psychosomatic may in fact have been sensitive to food.

On the other hand, more objective methods of assessing psychological disorders have also pinned the *psychosomatic* label on problems such as irritable bowel syndrome and migraine—diseases that are claimed as prime indicators of food intolerance. And forms of treatment that address the mind rather than the body—including psychotherapy and hypnotherapy—have been successfully used to treat them. In the next section we will look more closely at these apparently conflicting claims in relation to one particular disorder, irritable bowel syndrome or IBS.

Mental Factors in IBS

One study that is often quoted by opponents of food intolerance was carried out by Dr. David Pearson of Manchester University and Dr. Keith Rix of Leeds University, both in Britain. They studied twenty-seven patients suffering from irritable bowel syndrome who believed themselves to have food allergy or intolerance. The study found evidence of food reactions in only 15 percent of the patients, compared with 70 percent in another major study. The main reason for this discrepancy was probably their method of testing, which used such small amounts of the test foods that no reactions would be seen in most patients (see page 131).

Dr. Rix, who is a psychiatrist, examined half of the patients. He identified a variety of mild psychiatric problems, principally neurotic depression and anxiety neurosis, in 86 percent of them. (Unfortunately, there was no "blinding" in this part of the study. Ideally Dr. Rix should have seen a mixed group of people, one-third with IBS, one third healthy controls, and one-third patients with some other form of bowel disorder, with no indication of which patient was which. This would have ruled out the possibility of any preconceived ideas about psychiatric causes for IBS influencing his diagnoses.) The conclusion the doctors reached, given the apparently poor response to food testing, was that the psychological problems were affecting the bowel, rather than the other way around, in the majority of patients.

Doctors with an interest in food intolerance take a different view—that the psychological problems, where they exist, are largely a *result* of the illness, or of its rejection by the medical profession, or a mixture of the two. But they would agree that anxiety, tension, or depression can make the physical symptoms worse.

It is not difficult to imagine how a disorder such as irritable bowel syndrome could affect a patient psychologically. For those with diarrhea—one form of IBS—the symptoms are highly disruptive to normal life. Any outing revolves around the need to find a lavatory at short notice, and many outdoor activities, such as hiking or climbing, are virtually impossible. Apart from the pain that many patients suffer, the continual diarrhea does great damage to the self-image, and feelings of self-disgust are common. If the diarrhea comes and goes, there is an understandable tendency to blame "germs" and a neurotic concern about food hygiene may result. Where constipation is the predominant symptom, there may be considerable discomfort—which again is damaging to morale.

Given these difficulties it is hardly surprising that many patients with IBS show signs of neurotic depression and anxiety neurosis. Lack of understanding by family members and doctors is likely to compound the problem. Dr. Joseph Miller, a clinical ecologist working in Alabama, writes:

> These patients are not basically neurotic, but they are less able to cope with daily problems because their symptoms distract and bewilder them. They shop for relief from physician to physician, their self-esteem diminishes, and their anxieties increase when they are told repeatedly that their symptoms are "only due to nerves." They receive symptomatic and supportive care rather than specific treatment. Many . . . become secondarily depressed from the feeling of being hopelessly trapped.

Dr. Pearson and Dr. Rix point out that the level of psychiatric disorder in patients with a variety of other bowel complaints is much lower—only 34 percent, compared with 86 percent. The lack of blinding for the psychiatric assessments (see page 204) throws some doubt on this figure of 86 percent. But even if it is accurate, the differences could be due to other factors, such as the attitude of the medical profession. The other bowel complaints referred to are all recognized conditions that are not dismissed as psychosomatic. Unpleasant symptoms are a lot easier to cope with if you know you have Whatsisname's Syndrome than if you've been told that it's all in your mind.

The idea that the psychological symptoms could be largely a result of the physical symptoms, rather than the cause of them, is substantiated by one of the patients whom Dr. Pearson and Dr. Rix studied. She was sensitive to yeast and reacted to it in very small amounts, so that she produced a positive reaction even with the minute quantities that they used for testing. This patient was put on a yeast-free diet, and given a second psychiatric assessment when her bowel symptoms had resolved. Before the diet her score on the psychiatric assessment was 20— well over the critical score of 12 that indicates significant psychiatric disturbance. With IBS a thing of the past, her score was 1—a marked improvement.

The usefulness of treatments such as psychotherapy and hypnotherapy in treating IBS is entirely compatible with this view. If such treatments could eradicate the symptoms in a large proportion of patients it would be a different matter, but they do not: in most patients they simply reduce the symptoms to a more manageable level. For the patients who respond to such treatment, there is probably a subtle interplay of mental and physical factors—the distressing symptoms lead to anxiety or depression, and the disturbed state of mind makes the symptoms worse. In some patients psychological disorders may be even more important. Mental and emotional problems, which began long before the food intolerance, could make a significant contribution to the symptoms once the gut has become sensitized and overreactive. Even quite ordinary forms of stress can have an exaggerated effect on an irritable bowel. A stressful situation, such as having to catch a train or make a speech, might make a normal person's stomach churn a little, but in the IBS sufferer it can provoke a violent attack of diarrhea.

During psychotherapy or hypnotherapy, patients should acquire new insights into their problems, which can help modify unhealthy ways of thinking and behaving. If the treatment is successful, imbalances between the different arms of the autonomic nervous system—the sympathetic and the parasympathetic—should be corrected. This helps tone down the body's reactions to mental stress and can therefore moderate a symptom such as diarrhea, even though the primary cause of that diarrhea is a reaction to food.

No doubt there are some patients with IBS for whom mental and emotional factors are the major cause of the illness, but the research done at Addenbrooke's Hospital in Cambridge, England (see pages 130–31), and recently confirmed by a team of doctors at the Radcliffe Infirmary in Oxford, show that food intolerance can account for between 50 and 70 percent of cases. When food turns out to be the cause of the symptoms, lasting and complete relief is often possible, which compares favorably with the damping down of symptoms that hypnotherapy and similar treatments offer.

To sum up, *IBS* is probably a general term for a variety of conditions. These look similar, in terms of symptoms, but can be caused in a number of different ways. Some are largely caused by stress or emotional problems, others are due largely to food intolerance or some other physical cause, some are a fifty-fifty mixture of the two. To regard all cases of IBS as psychosomatic, as some doctors still do, is unhelpful to the patient. But it is equally unhelpful for those with IBS to decide firmly that *their* IBS must be due to food and food alone. To consider the possibility of a psychological cause is a sign of strength, not weakness, and to acknowledge such a cause could be the route back to good health.

Mind Over Matter

Thanks to the action of the autonomic nervous system, any disorder of the digestive system can be exacerbated by the emotions—IBS is not unique in this respect. The bronchi and the blood vessels are also controlled by the autonomic system, so they, too, can be affected, aggravating conditions such as asthma and migraine (due to expansion and contraction of blood vessels in the brain). Although the mechanism is not understood, mental stress also seems to make eczema and urticaria worse. Indeed, most of the physical symptoms of food sensitivity can probably be influenced by the mind.

If an illness has multiple causes, it makes sense to attack it on several fronts at once. By coming to terms with basic personal problems and achieving a calmer approach to life, the symptoms of food sensitivity can sometimes be much reduced. It may still be necessary to avoid certain food items or undergo other forms of treatment, but it should speed the body's recovery and make it possible to return to a more normal diet sooner. And in the long run it will help ensure continuing good health.

The approach used can vary considerably. For those who can afford it, a course of treatment with a professional psychotherapist may be the best answer, although it is important to select the person and the approach carefully. At its simplest, psychotherapy consists mainly of talking through past events and present problems with assistance from the therapist or counselor. Hypnotherapy is also useful, except with those susceptible to depression, since this can be brought on or made much worse by hypnosis. A professional hypnotherapist should assess each potential patient carefully and advise against treatment where necessary.

For those who cannot afford this sort of treatment but have plenty of time to spare, co-counseling may represent a viable alternative. After a period of training, cocounselors are paired off, and thereafter act as both counselor and client to each other. The idea may sound strange at first, but it often works very well, and the cocounseling movement has many enthusiastic adherents. Contact information can be found on page 455.

For some people it can be enormously helpful just to write things down on paper. The process of recording how you feel sets up an internal dialogue that can offer new insights into old difficulties. A recent study, published in the *Journal of the American Medical Association* in April 1999, has shown that writing about stressful personal experiences for only twenty minutes on three consecutive days produced a measurable improvement in symptoms among a group of patients with asthma or rheumatoid arthritis. The benefits were still detectable four months later. Yoga or meditation may also be helpful in learning to relax. For the less spiritually inclined, biofeedback offers a scientific route to relaxation.

There is one ailment for which learning to relax is of special importance, and that is asthma. The fear of suffocation that accompanies an asthmatic attack is understandable, but the anxiety itself can make the attack worse—or even bring one on unaided. Asthmatics should learn a relaxation technique and practice it every day so that it can be turned on at will, whenever an attack seems imminent. Hypnotherapy is often used to teach this sort of instant relaxation, and is particularly effective with children. They learn to feel that they are able to control the asthma, which reduces their feeling of helplessness and panic. In the case of children, it is very important for parents and other adults to stay calm as well—anxiety is infectious. For children who are too young to learn a relaxation technique, a reassuring presence and a warm drink can often stave off an attack.

Physical Health—Mental Health

Maintaining good mental health is a vital part of the fight against physical disease, and is especially important in long-term or chronic illnesses such as food intolerance. While some sufferers will quickly be restored to perfect health, for others it may be a long haul. This is particularly true for those with multiple symptoms who have been ill for many years. Patience and perseverance are needed, and a positive frame of mind is essential. The following suggestions should help to improve your general health and maintain a well-balanced mental outlook.

If you are undertaking an elimination diet, you should be cutting out coffee, tea, alcohol, and sugar anyway. Assuming you are not sensitive to these items, you may later reintroduce them, but avoid taking any of them in large quantities, and in particular avoid strong coffee or tea. Caffeine can be very damaging—see pages 213–14. If you smoke, make every effort to quit.

Eat regular, adequate meals and make sure you get enough sleep. Try to keep to a regular timetable of waking and sleeping. Keep your surroundings tidy and well organized.

Get outdoors as much as possible, and get some exercise—preferably fairly strenuous—every day. Feeling fit does wonders for the morale. If you suffer from morning fatigue, getting some exercise before breakfast is often very helpful. It need not take very long, but it should, again, be fairly strenuous—running up and down the stairs a few times will do. You will probably find that you perform very badly and feel dreadful for the first few minutes. Take a rest and try again—it is amazing how much better you do the second time around. Exercising before breakfast seems to clean the slate for the body before it has to deal with a new dose of food.

Try to spend plenty of time with other people, especially people outside your immediate family. If you find yourself endlessly talking about your illness or your diet, as you may begin to do, make a real effort to occupy your mind with other things.

Restrict yourself to one news bulletin a day, or avoid the news and newspapers altogether. The constant exposure to doom and gloom that most of us take for granted can be a source of hidden stress—if you have real problems to contend with, you do not need this extra mental burden. Television programs or books that make you laugh will do you far more good.

TABLE 2 MAIN SYMPTOMS OF HYPERVENTILATION*

Brain	Migraine and headache. Poor memory. Spaced-out feeling, confusion, anxiety or depression, tension, dizziness, panic attacks, hallucinations, delusions, mood swings, phobias, stupor, convulsions. Waking up with symptoms, having vivid or frightening dreams. Fear of sudden death.
Ears	Ringing sounds in ears, vertigo, sensitivity to loud noise, sounds seeming very distant.
Eyes	Blurred vision, double vision, sensitivity to bright lights.
Breathing	Shortness of breath, tightness and aching in chest, frequent sighing or yawning, dry throat, cough, "air hunger" and asthmalike attacks, "lump in the throat."
Heart	Abnormal heart rhythm, chest pains.
Digestive system	Stomach pain, bloating, belching, intermittent diarrhea.
Muscles	Sudden loss of strength, tremors or twitches, exaggerated twitching when falling asleep, cramps, aching muscles.
General	Tingling or numbness in the tongue, lips, fingers, or toes. Coldness or sweating, flushing, poor circulation, fatigue, fainting. Feeling of pressure in the throat, difficulty in swallowing, husky voice, swelling below the jaw ("swollen glands").

*Reproduced by kind permission of Dr. L. M. McEwen.

Hyperventilation

Some of the typical symptoms of food intolerance can also be caused by simply breathing too quickly. When we breathe, we take oxygen into the body and expel the waste gas, carbon dioxide, or CO_2. Our normal breathing pattern keeps oxygen and carbon dioxide at a level to which our bodies are well adjusted. But we have to have some spare capacity in case we want to run for the bus or climb Everest (where the air is less oxygen rich). So we have the ability to breathe faster or take deeper breaths, as required.

The problem, in those who hyperventilate, is that they have gotten into the habit of breathing faster all the time. Yet they are unaware of doing this. The level of CO_2 in their blood falls below the normal level, and this alters the pH (acidity or alkalinity) of the blood, producing a wide range of mental and physical symptoms. The type of symptoms produced by hyperventilation are shown in table 2.

The importance of hyperventilation depends very much on your point of view. Some of those who are dismissive of food intolerance

---

Edith

Edith's medical problems dated back to her teens, but her symptoms had always been rather vague—excessive tiredness, headaches, and indigestion. At the age of thirty-eight she suffered premature menopause, and her health then deteriorated very rapidly. She suffered from migraine, diarrhea with gas and bloating, and stiff, painful joints. Hormone replacement therapy, the standard treatment for symptoms associated with menopause, was tried. She seemed to have more energy as a result, but she developed hives and a vaginal discharge, which turned out to be due to thrush (*Candida* infection). Apart from this she had a great many mental symptoms—floating feelings, panic attacks, irrational bouts of crying, dizziness, and numbness and tingling in her hands and arms.

Her doctor was convinced that most of Edith's problems were psychosomatic, but he referred her to a specialist who was interested in such cases. She immediately recognized the signs of hyperventilation and retrained Edith's breathing pattern, which cleared most of the mental symptoms very promptly. Suspecting that her diarrhea and gas might be due to a yeast overgrowth, she put Edith on a no-sugar, no-yeast diet and a course of antifungal drugs. Her bowels were much improved by this, but Edith still had migraine attacks and trouble with her joints. So she was asked to undertake an elimination diet, which cleared up these symptoms within a week.

On testing foods, she found that wheat brought her stiff joints back while milk and cheese produced a migraine within a few hours. By avoiding these foods Edith has remained very well, and has far more energy in her fifties than she had as a teenager.

see hyperventilation as a widespread cause of vague, multiple symptoms. They claim that large numbers of those who are diagnosed as food intolerant are actually hyperventilators. The belief that they are allergic to a particular food or environmental chemical makes these patients hyperventilate when they encounter it—breathing more deeply is a natural reaction to fear or anxiety. The hyperventilation brings on the symptoms, but the patient perceives them as a consequence of the food or chemical—so the pattern of behavior is reinforced.

Those who specialize in treating food intolerance regard hyperventilation as a somewhat less common problem, but one that can masquerade as food sensitivity. More important, they recognize a group of patients who are both food sensitive and hyperventilators. They suspect that the anxiety caused by the food reactions was originally responsible for the change in breathing pattern, and that the two disorders aggravate one another. A number of these patients are very seriously ill and appear to react to almost every imaginable food and chemical. Some doctors call them **universal reactors**, and they will be discussed more fully in chapter 9.

Another school of thought maintains that a mild form of hyperventilation can be a feature, perhaps a symptom, of food intolerance. According to these doctors, when the incriminated foods are avoided or neutralization therapy is provided (see pages 360–62), the hyperventilation automatically disappears without the patient even being aware of it. They suggest that the adverse reaction to the food has some direct effect on centers in the brain that control breathing.

Anyone who shows a large number of the symptoms listed in table 2 should consider the possibility of hyperventilation. The most characteristic symptoms are numbness, tingling, and a spaced-out feeling. Hyperventilation can be tested for, but not necessarily treated, at home. To test yourself, choose a time when your symptoms are severe, take a fairly large, clean paper bag, and hold it over your mouth and nose. Breathe as you normally would for a few minutes. If you begin to feel better, then it is likely that hyperventilation is the cause of the trouble. By rebreathing expelled air from the bag, you are increasing your intake of CO_2, which raises its level in the blood.

If you are hyperventilating but also have food intolerance, you may find that the hyperventilation clears up spontaneously when you undertake an elimination diet. If it does not, then you need to be retrained into a normal breathing pattern, and your family doctor should be able to refer you to someone (such as a physical therapist) who can do this.

Ken

Ken was in his forties when he was first found to have high blood pressure. He was given drugs, which controlled this well; he had no more health problems for the next four years. Then he experienced pains in the chest, faintness, sickness, and sweating. Suspecting a mild heart attack, his doctor had him admitted to the hospital, but tests were negative and he was discharged after a few days. This seemed to be a turning point for Ken. After leaving the hospital he was tired, anxious, and depressed, apparently losing all interest in life. He also experienced panic attacks from time to time. Hypnosis and electroconvulsive therapy were tried but had no effect, and he became heavily dependent on tranquilizers. Eventually Ken was referred to a doctor who had an interest in dietary factors in disease, and who asked him about his diet. It emerged that Ken drank twenty cups of tea or coffee, both very strong, in the course of the average day. He was told to gradually cut these out, along with all other drinks containing caffeine. Within a few weeks Ken began to feel better, and his depression, anxiety, tiredness, panic attacks, fainting, and sweating are now a thing of the past. Problems due to too much caffeine are fairly common, but not everyone has the sort of symptoms that Ken experienced. Some suffer severe headaches, others abdominal pain, vomiting, or a variety of other symptoms (see below).

Caffeine

One important dietary component that can have a powerful effect on both mind and body is caffeine. This drug is found in coffee and tea, and, in lesser amounts, in chocolate, Coca-Cola, Pepsi, and other cola drinks. Some experts advise a maximum dose of 350 to 500 milligrams per day, but according to others a dose of 250 milligrams a day is potentially toxic. Two to six cups of coffee (depending on its strength), three to seven cups of tea, or seven cans of cola supply this amount. Children are more susceptible to caffeine than adults and should probably not drink more than one or two colas a day. Some individuals are far more sensitive than others and should not consume caffeine at all.

Consuming excess caffeine can produce anxiety, mood swings, tremors, insomnia, abnormal heart rhythms (palpitations), sweating, and weight loss. Hyperventilation sometimes accompanies these symptoms, producing breathlessness, chest pains, tingling in the toes and fingers, dizziness, and fainting. There may also be more serious mental problems such as confusion, panic attacks, and manic episodes in some extreme cases. A court-martial in 1997 heard evidence of how a British army officer who had drunk a gallon of tea every day for twenty years was so badly affected by his addiction to caffeine that he was eventually referred to a psychiatrist. Like many with caffeinism, he was the last to recognize that his excessive consumption of tea did amount to an addiction and was causing serious problems. In this respect, caffeinism resembles alcoholism. Ironically, the officer was a lifelong teetotaler.

Some patients who drink too much caffeine show none of these symptoms, but vomit violently instead—this is particularly common with tea drinkers. Abdominal pain and diarrhea can also be produced by too much caffeine. In children it can produce hyperactive behavior.

Those who drink large amounts of coffee during work hours may suffer from caffeine withdrawal on weekends, or any time they miss their morning cup of coffee. They may be irritable, lethargic, depressed, drowsy, or nervous. Nausea, sneezing, and a runny or congested nose are other possible symptoms, and a headache may follow. Some cases of weekend migraine may be due to caffeine withdrawal.

Another symptom that has been attributed to excess caffeine is the restless-legs syndrome. Extreme discomfort in the legs, and sometimes the arms, leads sufferers to constantly move their legs around in bed, resulting in insomnia for themselves and anyone unfortunate enough to have to share a bed with them. Although not all doctors would agree that restless legs are attributable to caffeine, anyone suffering from this condition should try avoiding caffeine for a while to see if it makes any difference. The amount of caffeine should be reduced gradually, over a period of two to three weeks, to minimize withdrawal reactions. Remember that some painkillers contain caffeine; cut these out as well.

Psychological Effects of Allergy Drugs

Some of the drugs used to treat allergies may have side effects that involve the mind and behavior. It is easy to mistake these for direct effects of the allergy itself, so it is important to be aware of the possible effects of particular drugs. Antihistamines tend to cause drowsiness, but some are better in this respect than others (see pages 433–34). If you or your children are affected, it is worth asking your doctor to change you to another type of antihistamine.

Corticosteroids, if taken in tablet form for a prolonged period, can cause a type of dependency. When they are withdrawn the patient may suffer fatigue, headache, depression, weakness, and aches and pains. These drugs are only likely to cause such problems if they have been taken continuously, at high doses, for some months.

More rarely, psychological side effects may occur with steroid tablets, particulary in those with a history of psychological problems. In the worst cases, there may be paranoia or severe depression, with a risk of suicide. Some people experience an exaggerated sense of well-being (euphoria).

Ephedrine (see page 435) can cause anxiety, insomnia, and restlessness. Although it is much less widely used than it once was, it is still found in some bronchodilators and cough mixtures. Some of these can be bought without a prescription.

Modern beta-2 bronchodilators used for asthma, such as Ventolin, can cause a nervous jittery feeling, trembling hands, flushing, anxiety, and restlessness. Children may become more excitable. A study published in 1999 showed that almost one-third of adult asthmatics, and one-quarter of children, avoided using their inhalers at times because of such problems. These side effects usually wear off quite quickly; if not, ask to try another type of drug, and keep trying different ones until you find something that suits you.

Theophylline, also used for asthma, can cause insomnia, anxiety, and restlessness. There are some reports of it also producing behavioral problems and learning difficulties in young children, but new research suggests it is safe for children over six.

Pseudoephedrine (see page 435) can produce euphoria and delusions if taken in very large doses, and even in normal doses it may cause nightmares and behavioral problems in children. It is widely found in cough mixtures (such as Actifed) and hay-fever medication, some of which can be bought without a prescription.

Ask to speak to the pharmacist at the store where you buy your medication—he or she will be able to tell you if it contains any of these drugs. Consult your doctor before discontinuing any prescribed medicines.

NINE

Chemical Sensitivity

Hazel had been ill, in one way or another, for most of her life. As a child she had pains in her stomach a lot of the time, and shooting pains in her arms and legs. She was sick when she ate certain foods, notably fish. Despite this, she was a bright child and did well at school. At seventeen she suddenly became very lethargic, put on weight, and suffered "swollen glands" (enlargement of the lymph nodes, which are part of the immune system). These symptoms looked just like those of glandular fever, and that was what her doctor diagnosed. But the illness lingered for over a year, and in the end the doctor decided that she must be suffering from depression. Her tiredness was such that Hazel could no longer study and she failed all her school exams. She remained unwell, with recurrent headaches, sleepiness, fatigue, and inexplicable bouts of fainting. Alcohol made these symptoms worse, she noticed, so she gave up drinking at the age of twenty. Her family doctor remained convinced that all her problems were in her mind.

When she was twenty-two Hazel consulted a doctor who felt that her illness might be brought on by something in her diet or her environment, rather than a psychosomatic problem. He tried out an elimination diet and got a reasonably good response. Six common foods were identified as causing symptoms, but even when she avoided all these Hazel was still not particularly well. So she was admitted to a special hospital with controlled environmental conditions (described later, on page 228). Here she blossomed, recovering a great deal of her former vitality and alertness. She was then exposed to various synthetic chemicals in turn, and reacted badly to diesel fumes, cigarette smoke, natural gas, chlorine, and alcohol. Some made her drowsy or faint; others produced a severe headache or nausea. Tap water and filtered tap water also affected her, whereas mineral waters caused no problems.

By avoiding her culprit foods and removing a number of synthetic chemicals (see table 3 on page 220) from her home, Hazel managed to maintain a reasonable state of health once she left the environmental unit.

Problems with Chemicals

Hazel is one of those unfortunate patients who not only have food intolerance but seem to be sensitive to various everyday chemicals as well. A few of these people react to a great variety of chemicals and foods, and are quite severely ill. They are sometimes called **universal reactors** by doctors working in this field. A few cases have attracted public attention, and newspapers invented the misleading name *total allergy syndrome* for the problem, as well as the melodramatic headline ALLERGIC TO THE TWENTIETH CENTURY.

Patients of this sort were first discovered in the late 1940s by Dr. Theron G. Randolph, one of the founders of clinical ecology in America, and they have been reported by many other doctors since. People with a milder form of chemical sensitivity have also been found—they may become dizzy and nauseated if they breathe too many car exhaust fumes, have headaches when there is a strong smell of paint, or develop a sore throat and catarrh when they use particular cleaning fluids. In children, hyperactivity (see page 264) is among the symptoms, and food colorings appear to be common culprits.

The range of chemicals that have been identified as causing problems is enormous—table 3 shows a representative selection. The range of symptoms is also vast, and includes many of those linked with food intolerance: headache, migraine, fatigue, nausea, vomiting, diarrhea, abdominal pain, rhinitis (runny or congested nose), wheezing, coughing, eczema, urticaria (hives), and hyperactivity. Despite these many similarities, patients with chemical sensitivity are noticeably different—for one thing, mental and behavioral symptoms are very common with chemicals. Depression, excessive sleepiness, severe mental confusion, uncontrollable anger, and "drunken," clumsy behavior have all been reported. Another characteristic of reactions to chemicals is that they come on very promptly after the exposure—which helps in the diagnosis.

Recently, the problem of hyperventilation (see pages 210–12) has been diagnosed in some people with alleged chemical sensitivity—particularly the universal reactors. This has led some doctors to dismiss the whole idea of chemical sensitivity and claim that all such patients are hyperventilating. The truth is probably more complex. Careful investigation often shows that these people have a dual problem: they are sensitive to foods and chemicals on the one hand, and they are hyperventilating on the other. Which came first is anybody's guess, but the two are now working together to make the patient even more ill.

Chemical Controversies

The question of chemical sensitivity is no less controversial than that of food intolerance—if anything, it is more hotly debated. But whereas there is good evidence to support the idea of food intolerance (see chapter 6), there is almost no scientific data about chemical sensitivity. Belief that the phenomenon exists is simply based on seeing individual patients who get well when they avoid certain chemical exposures.

A great many doctors feel that chemical sensitivity is improbable—a dubious diagnosis that probably covers up for psychosomatic illness, hyperventilation, or purely psychological symptoms. Convincing them otherwise would take double-blind trials and a plausible explanation of how the sensitivity might arise. Double-blind trials (see page 192) are difficult to perform with chemical-sensitive patients for a variety of reasons. First, it would be impossible to try out many of the gases and solvents blind because they have a powerful smell—the patient would know what was being tested. Second, many of the symptoms produced are highly subjective—headache, confusion, and nausea, for example. These are very difficult to measure objectively.

Looking for a plausible mechanism is slightly easier, but the search has only just begun, and there are few clues to go on at present. Later in this chapter we will consider the various possibilities in this area. First we need to look more closely at chemicals and discover exactly what they are.

What Are Chemicals?

All living things are made up of chemicals—chemicals, water, and nothing else. So are rocks and the air and other inanimate objects. But when people use the word *chemicals* that is not what they usually mean. Colloquially, it means manufactured or **synthetic chemicals**—ones that do not occur in nature, or that only occur naturally in very small quantities compared with the amounts that we manufacture.

Synthetic chemicals are not intrinsically different from naturally occurring ones—their basic chemistry is much the same, although there are some novelties. (One example is chlorinated hydrocarbons—hydrocarbons are fundamental to life, but adding chlorine to them was a human innovation.) What is more, many naturally occurring chemicals are highly toxic: the natural foods we eat are stiff with potentially damaging chemicals—plants, in particular, spike their products with an armory of defensive substances (see pages 17–18), fungi on the plants contribute their own toxins, and the bacteria in our gut add to the number we absorb. Human beings are well equipped to detoxify these natural chemicals with a powerful array of enzymes (see page 21).

For the most part, the enzymes that our ancestors evolved to tackle natural chemicals work pretty well on synthetic ones—as long as they are not overwhelmed by the amount they have to detoxify. However, the initial products of the enzyme reactions are sometimes more toxic than the original chemical. In other words, the body's detoxification enzymes have evolved to deal with a certain range of naturally occurring chemicals—they can go to work on synthetic ones, but on the way to breaking them down they may produce intermediates that are harmful. For this reason, such changes are known as **biotransformation** rather than detoxification.

Chemicals from Oil and Coal

Most of the synthetic chemicals that we come into contact with—including pesticides, fuel, plastics, and most solvents—are made from oil or coal. These are known as **organic chemicals**—which probably sounds like a contradiction in terms to anyone who buys organic vegetables! The word *organic* is being used in two different ways, but with the same etymological root. It means "of living things."

The chemicals that make up living things are all based on chains of carbon atoms, with hydrogen atoms attached to them all along the chain—such molecules are known as **hydrocarbons**. Until 1828 it was thought that only living things could make such molecules—hence the name *organic*. Chemists now know how to make most organic molecules in the laboratory, but the name has stuck.

TABLE 3 SUBSTANCES THAT MAY CAUSE PROBLEMS IN CHEMICAL SENSITIVITY

Gases and airborne droplets	Fumes from chlorinated water and bleach
	Natural gas
	Industrial air pollution
	Aerosols
	Pesticide sprays
Smoke and other combustion products	Tobacco smoke
	Coal smoke
	Fumes from gas or paraffin burning stoves and heaters
	Gasoline and diesel exhaust fumes
Solvents* and other volatile* compounds	Gasoline and oil vapors, also lighter fuel and paraffin
	Perfumes and aftershave
	Scented soaps and toiletries, scented cleaning materials
	Paint
	Varnish
	Turpentine, paint remover
	Disinfectant
	Mothballs
	Air fresheners

In the case of organic farming, the name was originally used to show that crops were grown using fertilizers derived from living things—manure or compost—rather than inorganic fertilizers such as nitrates, which are made by chemical processes. As pesticides became more widely used by most farmers, *organic farming* took on a broader meaning—the crops were not sprayed with synthetic pesticides either. So an organically grown carrot is one that has not been sprayed with synthetic pesticides—despite the fact that these are organic chemicals.

Geologists believe that oil and coal are composed of organic molecules because they themselves are derived from living things. In the case of coal, this is undoubtedly true: it is the partially decomposed remains of forests, which were made up of giant club mosses and other extinct trees. These forests covered the earth about three hundred million years ago. Oil is derived from the remains of microscopic sea crea-

TABLE 3 (CONT.)

Solvents* (cont.)	Polish (furniture, brass, et cetera)
	Formaldehyde (from cavity wall insulation, chipboard, foam rubber)
	Smells given off by: plastics (for instance, when warm), rubber and foam rubber, coated (shiny) paper, newsprint, new fabric
Nonvolatile* compounds	Food additives
	Pesticide residues in food
	Pollutants in water
	Plasticizers (escaping from plastic film and some flexible plastics)
	Waxes (on some vegetables and fruits)
	Medicinal drugs

*A **volatile** chemical compound is one that readily gives off vapor at room temperature—so although it may be a liquid or a solid, some of its molecules escape into the air as a gas.

A **solvent** is a substance in which other things dissolve—water is a solvent, as are alcohol, turpentine, and acetone (nail-polish remover). Solvents are used very widely in the chemical industry and are present in a huge variety of substances. Such solvents are mostly very volatile. It is solvents that give paint and varnish their smell as they evaporate (as they dry). Solvents and other volatile chemicals will mostly enter the body via the nose and lungs, but liquid solvents can also get through the skin.

Nonvolatile compounds mostly enter our bodies in food or drink.

---

tures, and is even older, according to most geologists. A novel theory about the origin of oil suggests that it is actually a product of the earth's core, and not of living organisms at all, but this is not widely accepted.

The origin of these substances is worth considering here, because there is so much misinformation on the subject. It is part of the folklore of clinical ecology that coal and oil are both derived from "ancient pine forests." In fact, both were deposited many millions of years before the first pine tree grew on earth. The club mosses, which created most of the coal seams, are more closely related to ferns than they are to pine trees, and oil—from which most synthetics are obtained—is not derived from plants at all. These distinctions are important, because the ancient-pine-forest myth has led to the idea that chemical-sensitive patients are also likely to react to pinewood and pine products. Perhaps chemical-sensitive patients *are* affected by pine resins—which contain a lot of natural toxins to protect the tree—but it has nothing to do with the origins of coal and oil.

The ancient-pine-forests concept is linked to another myth about chemical sensitivity—that patients who are universal reactors are reacting to all synthetic organic chemicals *because they come from a common source*. In other words, they are reacting to the "coalness" or "oilness" of the chemical, rather than the chemical itself. This theory stretches credibility considerably, because synthetic compounds go through so many chemical reactions, distillations, and purification procedures that they bear little relationship to their raw materials, let alone to each other. And in any case, those raw materials—coal and oil—are not at all similar in their own origins.

Again, these misconceptions are important, because the common-origin idea is the basis for some forms of therapy used with chemical-sensitive patients. Doctors employing the neutralization technique (see pages 360–62) often give ethyl alcohol in **sublingual drops** (under-the-tongue drops) as neutralization therapy for mild forms of chemical sensitivity. Ethyl alcohol, also known as ethanol, is the alcohol we use as a social lubricant in wines, beers, and spirits. But what is used in sublingual therapy is industrial alcohol. This is made by adding water to ethylene gas, which itself is obtained from oil. The theory is that industrial alcohol can desensitize someone to all synthetic organic chemicals, because it is derived from oil. It will be clear from the facts given above that this is highly unlikely. Which is not to say that ethyl alcohol drops do not work—they could help a chemical-sensitive patient by stimulating the liver to produce more detoxification enzymes.

The Chemical Environment

Exposure to synthetic chemicals comes in three main forms—by mouth, through the nose and lungs, and through the skin. The sort of synthetic chemicals we eat and drink are described in appendix 6. Those that we commonly breathe include solvents (see table 3, page 220), exhaust fumes, cigarette smoke, and aerosol droplets. In addition to these, many people are exposed to fumes at work—from industrial processes, photocopier machines, and dry-cleaning solvents, for example. Those living in industrial areas or near rubbish incinerators are exposed to other airborne chemicals from these sources. The third source listed above—the skin—is far less important. The number of synthetic chemicals that get into our bodies through the skin is relatively small, but solvents, such as mineral spirits, can enter in this way, as can oils and solvents, used in cosmetics.

Someone eating an average diet and drinking unfiltered tap water is likely to ingest at least a hundred different synthetic chemicals every day—see appendix 6. Exposure to airborne chemicals will vary more widely, depending on where people live, what work they do, how well ventilated their homes are, and what sort of household products they use. A smoker in the house will increase the variety and quantity of air pollutants considerably. In all, we are probably exposed to at least two hundred different synthetic chemicals every day—and some people will encounter many more.

What Causes Chemical Sensitivity?

Why are some people apparently made ill by everyday synthetic chemicals? There are two types of explanation available, which can be summed up as *allergic explanations* and *deficiency explanations*. The first type of theory proposes that these people make an inappropriate immune response (allergic response) to certain synthetic chemicals, in the same way that a hay-fever sufferer reacts adversely to pollen (see chapter 2). The second type of explanation suggests that these people have some sort of defect that makes them less able to cope with environmental chemicals. It is usually assumed that this is a deficiency in the enzymes (see page 21) that detoxify foreign chemicals. We will look at the evidence—such as it is—for both of these explanations.

The Allergic Explanation

This assumes that the affected person makes IgE antibodies to the synthetic chemical concerned (see page 28), or responds with some other inappropriate and damaging immune reaction. Since the chemicals concerned are too small to act as antigens in their own right, they would have to combine with body proteins and act as haptens (see page 34).

It has been suggested that this can happen with some food additives, particularly preservatives and synthetic colors. These cause chronic urticaria (hives) in some people, and urticaria is sometimes due to an allergic reaction. There are also isolated cases of tartrazine (a synthetic coloring) causing acute asthma attacks, or a severe reaction that resembles anaphylactic shock (see page 33) in some very susceptible people. Other food colorings, particularly the synthetic ones, have been known to cause allergic dermatitis, mainly in food workers exposed to large amounts. The preservative sorbic acid has occasionally caused allergic dermatitis when used in medicinal creams.

In most of these cases, the tests to show that the reaction really is an allergic one have not been carried out. And when a group of patients who were apparently allergic to tartrazine were tested for IgE antibodies, none were found. So it looks as if these are not allergic reactions at all, even though they produce allergy-like symptoms. Doctors suspect that tartrazine produces symptoms in these people by directly affecting the immune response in some way—perhaps by stopping the synthesis of immune regulators called prostaglandins (see page 30), or by triggering mast cells directly. In the case of synthetic chemicals apparently causing asthma, the effect may be due to irritation rather than an allergic reaction. This is well known for metabisulfites and sulfur dioxide (see appendix 1).

These are cases where the symptoms provoked by chemicals at least looked like allergic symptoms. In the majority of chemical-sensitive people, the symptoms are not those commonly associated with allergy. So it seems unlikely that chemical sensitivity is allergic in origin.

The Deficiency Explanation
Some synthetic chemicals are excreted from our bodies unchanged—in urine, for example, or on our breath when we exhale. Some, such as DDT, are stored unchanged in the body's fatty tissues. But these are the exceptions—the vast majority are acted on by enzymes, which change them chemically in biotransformation reactions (see page 219). Ultimately, these reactions lead to the detoxification of the chemical.

In recent years minor enzyme deficiencies have been found in some people; these do not normally make the person ill unless a particular medicinal drug is taken. Studies of such drugs in food-intolerant patients have shown that a large proportion of them suffer from these minor enzyme deficiencies (see pages 299–300). In one study some of the patients also had chemical sensitivities, and when the results for these patients alone were considered, 90 percent were found to be deficient in a particular enzyme system. Such a high percentage is unusual in medical research, and suggests strongly that there is a link between chemical sensitivity and enzyme deficiency. This result was for just one set of enzymes—and hundreds are involved in detoxification.

In another study, described on pages 300–301, certain artificial food colorings have been found to inhibit crucial detoxification enzymes. It is possible that enzyme inhibition by these artificial colors contributes to the problem in people whose enzymes are partially defective. This could account for the frequency with which food colorings have been identified as the source of adverse reactions.

If enzyme deficiencies are at the root of the problem in chemical-sensitive patients, then you might expect them to show the same sort of reaction to small amounts of a chemical as normal people show to large amounts of that chemical. **Occupational medicine**—the study of how exposures in the workplace affect workers' health—is the main source of information here. This branch of medicine studies the effects of brief high-dose exposures (as during an industrial accident) and long-term exposures at a lower level (but still much higher than most people would encounter). It is the latter that are relevant to the chemical-sensitive patient, and they do provide some interesting and revealing parallels.

In the case of organic solvents, for example, the prime symptoms seen in workers exposed to regular but relatively low doses are mental ones. For instance, toluene (found in paints and glues) produces fatigue and vague feelings of malaise, while styrene (used in the manufacture of polystyrene) produces fatigue, a sense of ill health, and irritability. Trichloroethylene (an industrial solvent that is a common contaminant of drinking water) may produce tiredness, dizziness, headache, irritability, and digestive problems. Mineral spirits, which is a mixture of solvents, produces fatigue and general feelings of ill health. These are very much the sort of symptoms seen in many chemical-sensitive patients when they are exposed to organic solvents. (See table 3, pages 220–21.)

It is known from occupational medicine that exposure to two chemicals at once can be far more damaging than being exposed to each chemical individually. This **cocktail effect** commonly occurs when the same enzymes are involved in detoxifying both chemicals—the two then compete for the same enzyme, which is present only in limited amounts. Even chemicals that are broken down by different enzymes may compete: some enzymes need substances known as **cofactors** to help them do their work, so the two chemicals are competing for cofactors rather than for the enzymes themselves. Many organic solvents interact with each other in this way, and it may be the combination of chemicals surrounding them that causes illness in chemical-sensitive patients. Most of the vitamins are enzyme cofactors, and some doctors believe that a lack of vitamins can make people more sensitive to environmental chemicals (see pages 329–32). The alcohol in alcoholic drinks is itself an organic solvent, and it competes with several other solvents for detoxification enzymes, slowing their breakdown. Not surprisingly, perhaps, most chemical-sensitive patients cannot tolerate alcohol—this is often one of the earliest symptoms. Many food-intolerant patients with little or no sign of chemical sensitivity are also unable to drink, which supports the idea that enzyme defects are important to food intolerance as well (see pages 299–300).

The multiple role of many detoxification enzymes would explain one of the curious features of chemical-sensitive patients—the fact that they are usually affected by a whole range of chemicals, not just one. This has nothing to do with the chemicals all being derived from oil and coal (see pages 221–22), as is often suggested. But it could be due to defects in an enzyme that is responsible for detoxifying a variety of environmental chemicals.

In general, enzyme defects are inherited—passed on from parents to children in the form of an abnormal gene. So if enzyme defects are a common cause of the problem, you might expect chemical sensitivity to run in families. No research has yet been done to discover if this is indeed the case. But what about patients who are apparently fit and healthy until they suffer a massive exposure to toxic synthetic chemicals from a crop-spraying plane, for example, or a chemical spill? Many patients with severe chemical sensitivity trace their problems back to such an incident.

It is possible that such people had minor enzyme deficiencies before their damaging exposure, but that these were not causing any symptoms at that stage. Some parts of the liver could have sustained mild damage during their exposure—not enough to cause characteristic symptoms such as jaundice, but enough to leave a legacy of inadequate detoxification systems. Liver damage is known to occur when the breakdown product of a chemical is highly toxic. Because the chemical is being dealt with in the liver, the toxic intermediates (the initial products of the biotransformation reaction) accumulate there. So damage is concentrated in the cells of the liver.

Canaries of the Chemical Age?

One enzyme system involved in detoxification was found to be defective in 90 percent of patients with chemical sensitivity (see page 224). But that same enzyme system is defective in 20 percent of normal, healthy people. This suggests that there is some other deficiency as well in those with chemical sensitivity—perhaps a defect in another enzyme. But it also suggests that many "normal, healthy" people are not as immune from everyday chemicals as they might appear to be. One in five apparently has a potential problem, considering this one enzyme system alone.

Many of the symptoms shown by food-intolerant and chemical-sensitive patients are symptoms that we all suffer from at times— headaches, tiredness, and indigestion, for example. Which is why some doctors feel that such patients are not really ill, simply overreacting to everyday symptoms. But to look at the problem from another angle, none of us lives in an environment free of synthetic chemicals—if we did, would we still suffer from those "everyday symptoms," such as headaches?

Skeptics will argue that the chemicals we are exposed to have all been tested for safety, and should have no ill effects at the concentrations we encounter. But the fact is that such tests are done on single chemicals, never on mixtures. Any cocktail effects will have gone unnoticed in such tests. Given the mixture of two hundred or more chemicals that we may encounter every day, cocktail effects could be very important. It is also the case that the tests use animals such as rats, not human beings. How does a rat tell the experimenter that it has a headache or feels a bit off color? Quite apart from these objections, there are many other doubts about the effectiveness of safety testing. Some of these are discussed in appendix 6, in relation to food additives and pesticides.

Perhaps the chemical-sensitive patient is like the coal miner's canary, carried along in a cage to detect dangerous accumulations of gas in the pit. This may sound alarmist to some people, especially those in the chemical industry who have a large financial stake in the continuing use of their products, but there is worrying evidence that we are being made ill by the chemicals around us. One study of Parkinson's disease, an incurable nervous condition, showed that the use of garden pesticides was associated with a higher incidence of the disease. Another study showed that the children of parents who used pesticide sprays were more likely to suffer from leukemia. Yet these products are supposedly safe for domestic use.

Treating Chemical Sensitivity

For those who think they may be sensitive to synthetic chemicals, the only sound method of diagnosis is to avoid chemical exposure as much as possible and see if the symptoms improve. Individual chemicals can then be tested to discover which are to blame for the symptoms.

Those who are seriously ill may be universal reactors (see page 217), and they will only recover fully if they can be protected from the majority of synthetic chemicals. This is achieved with environmentally controlled units. Ideally, these should be built and furnished using only wood, metals, cotton, and other natural products—no plastics or other synthetic materials, which might release solvent fumes, should be allowed. Air going into the unit is filtered, as is the supply of water used for washing. Springwater only is used for drinking and cooking food. All foods are organically grown, except when foods with pesticide residues are used for testing.

Needless to say, treatment in such units is costly. Fortunately, there is much that can be done at home to reduce the level of chemical exposure. For the majority of patients, these simple measures will be enough to alleviate the symptoms considerably.

Reducing Chemical Exposure

The following measures will reduce the level of chemical exposure experienced. The list begins with the simplest measures and works through to more difficult ones. Try the first three measures for a couple of weeks, and see what effect this has. If there is some improvement, add the next two measures and wait another two weeks, and so on. If there is no improvement, it may be that workplace chemicals or generalized exposures (such as to outdoor air pollution) are the problem. Consider whether this is likely, and if it is, try out the appropriate avoidance measures.

Cigarette Smoke

If you smoke, even only occasionally, you should stop. If other people in your household smoke, try to persuade them to quit, or to smoke outdoors for a while. Wash curtains and other furnishings that harbor smoke residues, and air all rooms thoroughly. If cigarette smoke is unavoidable, you could consider using an air filter (see pages 459–60). Cigarette smoke at work is more of a problem, but if your colleagues smoke, ask your employer to provide you with a smoke-free environment.

Household Chemicals

Clear out all cleaning materials, mineral spirits, turpentine, dry-cleaning fluids, polish, bleach, aerosols, air fresheners, mothballs, and disinfectant.

Rags and dusters with polish, window-cleaning liquid, or turpentine on them should also be removed. Banish all these items to a garage, shed, garden, or balcony for a while. If you live in an apartment, and this is impossible, throw away all those that you do not really need, and store the remainder in large cookie tins or other airtight containers. Stick to an unscented dishwashing liquid (see pages 459–60) for all cleaning purposes.

Painting, gluing, varnishing, soldering, and similar activities are banned for a while. If magazines or books smell strongly (usually the glossy magazines and books with shiny paper), read something else. Do not use felt-tip pens, especially the strong-smelling ones. The rule here is: if it smells, avoid it.

Some furnishings, pot holders, and ornaments have a very strong-smelling varnish coating, particularly cheap bamboo products with a glossy surface. If you have any items of this sort, banish them or put them in an airtight container. Also evict any smelly plastic items—certain plastic bags, for example.

Open all windows whenever you can, to blow away residual smells. If you have gas or coal stoves, and can avoid using them for a while, it would be a useful addition to this list. Make sure electric heaters are clean and free of dust before turning them on.

Avoid places such as dry cleaners and gas stations while you are testing out these measures. Do not use any insecticide sprays in the house or pesticide sprays in the garden.

Perfumes and Cosmetics
Do not use perfume, aftershave, or any strongly scented toiletries for a while. If you have to use deodorant, use the unscented, roll-on variety and try not to breathe the fumes. Do not use aerosols or talcum powder.

Water Pollutants
For details of these, see pages 421–22. You can either buy bottled springwater or use a filter to improve the quality of tap water. Filters do not remove all contaminants, however—see pages 424–30. Rather than investing in a filter, it may be better to use bottled water if you are just avoiding tap water for a few weeks.

Food Additives
Avoid all packaged foods and drinks with additives listed on the label. Remember that "flavorings" count as additives, and that "No Artificial

Additives" can be very misleading—some natural additives are potentially harmful (see pages 414–16). When buying unwrapped bread, cakes, candies, and delicatessan foods ask to see a list of ingredients to check for additives. Do not drink alcohol unless you have homemade wine brewed from pure fruit and sugar (no Campden tablets) or can buy organic wine. Restaurant, cafeteria, and take-out foods are often very rich in additives. Also avoid canned foods, because the phenolic resin that is used to line the can may contaminate the food.

If you are taking any vitamin tablets with colored coatings, give these up—use an uncolored supplement instead. If you are taking medicines that appear to contain colorings, ask your doctor to prescribe an uncolored version.

Pesticide Residues

If you are able to get organic foods and can afford them, then try to use these as much as possible. Growing your own vegetables is by far the cheapest way of avoiding pesticides in the long run, but in the short term it may be possible to get unsprayed produce from someone with a large garden.

Fungicides are also used to prolong the storage life of oranges and lemons. It is a good idea to wash such fruits in hot soapy water and rinse them thoroughly before you grate the peel or add slices of lemon to drinks. Oranges that are to be peeled and eaten should also be washed, because the fungicide is contained in a wax layer that comes off on the hands during peeling and then contaminates the fruit. Some supermarkets now sell unwaxed oranges and lemons, and these do not have extra fungicides applied to the peel after harvesting. (There may, of course, still be residues of sprays used when the fruit was grown, but these should be less concentrated and more easily rinsed off.)

Washing other fruit and vegetables thoroughly will help reduce the amount of pesticide eaten, and peeling fruit will reduce the quantity further. When fruit is cooked in an open pan, some of the pesticides are boiled off, so this can help to lessen the amount that you eat; open the window during this process. For more information on avoiding pesticide residues, see appendix 6.

Formaldehyde

The main sources of formaldehyde in the home are blown-in insulation and particleboard. There is little you can do about the former if it has already been installed. The latter can be replaced or sealed in with gloss paint—get someone else to do this for you, if you can, and stay out of the way until the smell of paint has dispersed. If you have blown-in insulation as well, the only way you can test for its effects is to go away for a while to a house without sources of formaldehyde. Simple stone or brick houses with solid walls are a good bet. Plush modern hotels are likely to be oozing formaldehyde vapor.

Other sources of formaldehyde include foam rubber, new textiles, paper (including newsprint), photographs, leather luggage, antiperspirants, some cosmetics and shampoos, and plywood. It is only worth eliminating these if you have strong reasons to suspect formaldehyde.

Plastics and Other Synthetics

Plastics and other synthetic materials release small amounts of volatile chemicals—a process known as de-gassing. By evicting smelly plastic items (see page 228) you have already gotten rid of the worst de-gassers. Removing those that remain is a fairly drastic step that you should embark on only if you have good reason to suspect chemical sensitivity. Bear in mind that soft plastic items de-gas more than hard items.

With synthetic fabrics, it may be sufficient to just stop wearing them and using them as bedding for a while, to see if this is beneficial. One common source of fumes is the foam backing on carpets—this tends to break down due to constant wear, and formaldehyde (see above) may interact with it to produce toxic airborne chemicals that can irritate the airways, causing symptoms similar to bronchitis.

If you are sensitive to certain plastics, you should avoid keeping food or drinks in plastic containers. This applies to mineral water as well— substances in the plastic bottle can leach out into the water. Choose a mineral water that is available in glass bottles, but do not consume too much Perrier because it seems to cause problems for some people.

Fumes from Natural Gas, Oil, and Other Fuels

The idea that people can be sensitive to natural gas is a contentious one, but it is claimed that some people have made dramatic recoveries after removing the gas supply from their homes. Just turning gas appliances off is not sufficient, apparently—small amounts of gas still escape from the joints of pipes.

The sort of symptoms reported in gas-sensitive patients are faintness, mental confusion, irritability, aggression, lack of coordination, and facial flushing. A vacation in a gas-free house is the best way to test if gas is a problem. Sensitivity to oil fumes, coal smoke, paraffin fumes, and other odors from heating systems can be tested for in the same way.

Exhaust Fumes

For most people a couple of weeks away from it all is the only way to test for sensitivity to exhaust fumes. But for anyone who does a lot of traveling by car or truck, simply reducing the amount of travel can significantly lessen exposure to exhaust fumes. This may be enough to alleviate the symptoms.

Exposure to Chemicals in the Workplace

For anyone working in the chemical, pharmaceutical, engineering, or electronics industries, exposures at work should be a prime suspect. The fact that symptoms come on after work does not rule out occupational illness—the effects can be delayed. Not everyone gets better on weekends, either; sometimes it can take a week or more to recover from the effects of chemicals at work. Taking a long vacation in an unpolluted environment, while avoiding other chemical exposures, is the best way of testing for this possibility.

Hairdressing salons, dry cleaning shops, photo-developing labs, and gas stations are other places of work that may cause ill health. Those working in offices may also be suffering from workplace exposure— to photocopier fumes, for example, or to solvents released by erasing liquids, glue, carbon paper, particleboard, and plywood. Such airborne chemicals are likely to accumulate if the ventilation is poor. Sometimes it is simply dry air that causes symptoms in modern air-conditioned offices. Or it may be fungi and other microorganisms growing in humidifiers and being circulated with the air—typical symptoms in such cases are cough, tightness in the chest, fever, aches and pains, and general feelings of malaise. Whatever the cause, a vacation in a cleaner environment should be sufficient to show if the workplace is the source of trouble. The difficulty here is that simple lack of stress may also alleviate the symptoms—so an improvement while on vacation may be a slightly ambiguous result.

Outdoor Air Pollution

This is only likely to be a problem in heavily polluted areas. Symptoms that regularly appear in close humid weather, or when the wind is in a particular direction, are an indication of air pollution problems. Again, a vacation in an unpolluted environment is the only test.

Living with Chemical Sensitivity

If you find that you are sensitive to various chemicals, then avoiding them is the best treatment. Complete avoidance is often very difficult, but fortunately it is rarely necessary. For most people, reducing the overall chemical load makes them far more robust and able to cope with everyday exposures. So simply avoiding cigarette smoke, household chemicals, food additives, and tap water may be enough to eliminate symptoms or reduce them to a bearable level. You should also avoid exposure to large doses of synthetic chemicals, such as from household timber treatment or crop spraying (see page 317).

There are also other measures that can improve overall health and make the body more resilient. These include correcting nutritional deficiencies (see page 330), getting regular exercise, eating a good, healthy diet, and reducing stress. Tackling underlying problems such as hyperventilation (see pages 210–12) will also help considerably. Try to get outdoors, to somewhere with clean air, as often as you can, and get some strenuous exercise to improve your general health and fitness.

For those with severe chemical sensitivity, creating a chemical-free oasis in the house can be very valuable. For preference, this should be the bedroom, but it should include comfortable chairs, a table, and whatever else is needed for everyday living. A space in which you can do some simple exercises may also be useful if you have difficulty getting exercise outdoors. The idea is to retreat to the oasis whenever you can, thus reducing your overall exposure. The oasis is also useful when you are feeling ill and need to recover.

All synthetic fabrics, plastics, particleboard, plywood, foam rubber, and other synthetic materials are excluded from the oasis. This means old-fashioned armchairs, cotton blankets or a feather comforter, and a traditional type of mattress or a futon. (If you are also allergic to feathers, see pages 459–60.) Nothing that has been painted or varnished recently should be allowed in, nor should cosmetics, cleaning materials, or any of the other items mentioned in table 3. If you must, have a television in the room, but it is best not to watch it for too long, because the warmth of the set causes its plastic components to give off fumes. Books and a radio are a better choice. If the air outside is polluted, an air filter may be a useful addition to the oasis (see pages 459–60).

It is very important for chemical-sensitive patients to keep their problem in perspective and not get unduly paranoid about the world around them. The twenty-first century may seem threatening at times for someone with these problems, but at least you are not likely to be struck down in your prime by cholera, smallpox, or bubonic plague, and there is little risk of being eaten by lions. Life has always had some risks attached to it. Rather than focusing on the hazards of the world around you, try to think what you can do to make your body stronger and more resistant to environmental chemicals.

Above all, make an effort not to develop psychological reactions to chemicals—never assume that you are going to react to a chemical just because you have in the past. If you allow yourself to become fearful of certain chemicals and imagine that they are harming you, you will just be perpetuating the problems rather than solving them.

TEN

Bugs in the System—
Candida and *Giardia*

The *Candida* Question

For several years a strong link has been reported between food sensitivity and overpopulation with a yeast, *Candida albicans*. Again, this is a highly controversial topic, and there is considerable disagreement even among those doctors who treat food intolerance. Some deny that *Candida* is a common problem, while a few claim that it underlies the majority of cases of food intolerance. A third group suggests that there is a genuine problem with unsuitable yeast or bacteria in the gut, but that *Candida* itself is not the guilty party; the real culprits have still to be identified. It is difficult, at present, to decide which of these ideas is correct, but scientific opinion is tending toward the third option.

The Gut Flora

All of us have millions of bacteria and yeasts living harmlessly inside us, natural inhabitants of the large intestine. They are known as gut flora. (A curious name, perhaps, but naturalists used to think that bacteria and yeasts belonged to the plant kingdom; *flora* can mean not just "flowers," but also "plants in general," as in "flora and fauna.")

The gut flora feed on the remains of our meals, but they do us no harm. In fact, we have gotten so used to them being there during the course of our evolution that we would suffer without them. They have become essential to the well-being of the gut.

In the normal, healthy person the gut flora is a balanced community of different organisms. There are hundreds of different species to be found, and the proportions of each vary from person to person, and from time to time. But in general, a particular balance of different species is established, which results in a healthy bowel.

These bacteria provide us with some vitamins and may aid digestion in some way. More important, however, because they occupy all the available surfaces in the bowel, they prevent unfriendly, disease-causing bacteria from gaining a foothold. Of course, they cannot withstand a massive onslaught, such as produces a bout of food poisoning. But in the ordinary way, low levels of harmful bacteria find themselves unable to secure a cozy niche in the face of the regular inhabitants. Not being attached to the gut wall, they are ejected far more quickly.

The members of the gut flora also produce toxins, but our bodies are used to these, and they are broken down in the liver. (This safety mechanism may be ineffective in people with cirrhosis of the liver, who are then poisoned by the toxins their gut flora produce.) As for our immune system, it has learned to regard these microbes as harmless fellow travelers. But it keeps them firmly in their place—within the digestive system. The gut flora are prevented from penetrating the gut wall and making themselves at home elsewhere in the body. Only when the immune system is severely impaired, as in AIDS, do some members of the gut flora threaten to invade the body as a whole.

Bugs in the System

Until relatively recently the gut flora was largely taken for granted by the medical profession. It is still a neglected area, in many ways, and most family doctors probably know little about it. But a few research workers are studying the gut flora in healthy people and comparing it with that in patients suffering from irritable bowel syndrome (IBS) or similar diseases. It would seem that there are differences in the relative proportions of different bacteria. Abnormalities have been identified in IBS, Crohn's disease, rheumatoid arthritis, ankylosing spondylitis, and atopic eczema. Some early evidence suggests that by reestablishing the right mix of bacteria, IBS (or at least those cases in which diarrhea is the main symptom) can be successfully treated. The same success has been claimed with atopic eczema. At present these forms of treatment are still at an experimental stage and not widely available. (The only home therapy that might be tried is eating live yogurt or taking a bacterial replacer; see pages 250–51.)

If there are imbalances, what might have caused them? One answer is a severe bout of diarrhea, which flushes a lot of the resident microbes out of the bowel. Many people date the onset of irritable bowel syndrome to such an infection. A second likely cause of trouble is antibiotics taken by mouth. These could, potentially, kill off useful members of the gut flora and allow others to proliferate. But it seems unlikely that an ordinary one-off course of antibiotics would produce a lasting imbalance—the gut flora should reestablish itself normally afterward. There might be problems, however, with repeated courses of antibiotics (as were once prescribed for acne) or a single course at a very high dose. The main evidence on this point has been gathered by Dr. John Hunter of Addenbrooke's Hospital in Cambridge, England. Dr. Hunter noticed that a number of his women patients had first suffered from IBS after having a hysterectomy. This seemed puzzling, until Dr. Hunter discovered that high doses of antibiotics were always given before such operations, to help prevent infections. An experiment followed in which some hysterectomy patients had the antibiotic treatment while others did not— 11 percent of the first group developed IBS, but none of the second group did.

The *Candida* Controversy

Candida albicans is one of the yeasts that we all have living in the gut, and in women it is also found in the vagina. Normally, its numbers are controlled by other microbes and by the body itself, and it causes no trouble. Where it can become a nuisance is in the vagina, if *Candida* escapes the usual control mechanisms and multiplies excessively. The main symptom is a maddening itch, but there can also be a creamy discharge. This type of *Candida* infection, known as a **yeast infection** or **thrush,** is easily treated by creams or pessaries containing antifungal drugs (yeasts are a type of fungus). There are also drugs that can be taken by mouth; these are useful for anyone who becomes sensitive to the creams or pessaries. Occasionally women become oversensitive to *Candida* itself and may experience the itching even when the yeast is not present in excessive numbers (as defined by laboratory tests). Such cases are more difficult to diagnose, because the laboratory test is negative (which may lead the doctor to make a diagnosis of psychosomatic illness), but they respond to the normal treatments used for vaginal yeast infections.

If *Candida* gets into a woman's urinary tract or bladder, it can produce a form of cystitis—characterized by a burning sensation when passing urine.

Candida can also infect the throat, producing soreness and either tiny red spots inside the mouth or creamy yellow patches that leave a sore area when they are rubbed off. Babies are very susceptible to such infections, especially in the mouth, where *Candida* produces a creamy or gray-colored film over the tongue. In newborn babies the infection is usually picked up from the mother's vagina during birth. The baby's immune system cannot keep *Candida* in its place as well as an adult's, so the yeast flourishes. Some cases of diaper rash are also due to *Candida*.

Diabetic women run a higher risk of developing *Candida* overgrowth in the vagina, because of the sugar in their urine—sugar feeds the yeast. Thrush in the mouth is also more common in diabetics, although the reason for this is unclear.

When the immune system is weakened, *Candida* may become a more serious problem. People with AIDS suffer greatly with *Candida* in the throat and mouth. Others with a severe immune defect may develop *Candida* infections of the eye, kidney, liver, or brain, but such cases are very rare.

Those, then, are the hard facts about *Candida*, with which few doctors would disagree. On other points, there is great controversy.

In recent years *Candida* has come under suspicion as a common cause of diarrhea, gas, and bloating, sometimes with abdominal pain. The main reason for pointing the accusing finger at *Candida* is that these symptoms are sometimes accompanied by itching around the anus and, in women, by recurrent yeast infections. Intrigued by this cluster of symptoms, some doctors tried out antifungal treatments consisting of a low-sugar, low-yeast diet, often combined with antifungal drugs such as nystatin, taken by mouth for several months. For some people this treatment has proved very effective in curing their diarrhea and gas.

This led to the conclusion that *Candida* was definitely a cause of the diarrhea and gas, an idea that is now being critically reviewed. The main evidence against it is that you cannot detect any more *Candida* in the intestines of people who supposedly have candidiasis than in healthy people. The argument often proposed to counter this is that the *Candida* is, for some reason, undetectable by conventional methods. The idea is that *Candida* might grow in a different form, known as a **hyphal** form, which resembles a bread mold—long chains of fungus instead of the single, microscopic cells typical of a yeast. In its hyphal form, so the argument goes, *Candida* clings tightly to the gut wall and so escapes

Jason

From the age of eighteen months onward, Jason developed repeated ear infections and was given many courses of antibiotics. After about six years he began to suffer almost continuously with an upset stomach, flulike symptoms, an itchy bottom, and extremely itchy eyes, which produced a sticky secretion. His doctor prescribed eyedrops for conjunctivitis, which stung Jason's eyes very badly. The following morning all his eyelashes had fallen out. His eyes grew itchier still, and the many different medicines tried were all equally ineffective. He sometimes developed hives as well. The problem continued to worsen over the next seven years. During this time his eyebrows began to itch and within two days, all the eyebrow hair had fallen out. Skin-prick testing produced reactions to a huge range of allergens, including molds, house dust mite, several pollens, and foods. Jason was given corticosteroid eyedrops, which only made the itching worse. The red itchy area spread to his scalp, and his head hair began to fall out. His mother recalls, "I was ready to check myself into the nearest mental hospital to have a nervous breakdown when I came across your book in the library." Having read the book, her first step was to remove all yeast and sugar from Jason's diet to see what happened. To her surprise, there was a noticeable improvement within a few days. His eyes slowly lost the red, inflamed appearance that had begun to seem almost normal for Jason. After eight weeks on this diet his mother tested Jason with a meal containing yeast extract, and the intense itching and redness of his eyes returned. By staying on the no-yeast, no-sugar diet, Jason has remained well. At the outset his mother also gave him garlic and aloe vera every day, which she believed helped him, and he was prescribed a short course of antifungal drugs. Gradually all his symptoms have disappeared. About a year after beginning the diet he underwent a desensitization treatment for yeast sensitivity, and following this his eyebrows and eyelashes grew back. Although there is no proof that a yeast overgrowth caused Jason's problems, it is indisputable that the dietary changes helped him enormously when conventional treatments had all proved ineffective.

detection in the feces. It is true that *Candida* can switch forms in this way, but there is no evidence that it actually does so in the gut. If it did, it would be almost certain to shed yeast-type cells of *Candida* into the feces as well, and these would therefore be detected in abnormally high numbers by the usual tests. Doctors who have made intensive studies of the gut flora, such as Dr. John Hunter, find this theory increasingly unlikely: "If there was a massive overgrowth of *Candida* in these patients, as there is supposed to be, I'm sure we would have found evidence of it by now. The fact is they have about as much *Candida* in the gut as everyone else."

Skin-prick tests and intradermal tests for *Candida* have also been tried for patients with supposed candidiasis, and it is true that some show positive reactions—they are making an immune response to *Candida* antigens. But many healthy people also show positive immune reactions to *Candida*, so these tests do not mean very much. And some people who have been diagnosed as having candidiasis do not react to a skin test. In short, *Candida* is beginning to look like a red herring.

But the fact remains that some people do recover from diarrhea and gas when treated with a low-sugar, low-yeast diet. (And curiously, a number of these patients had previously been eating large quantities of yeast extract.) Nystatin also seems to aid recovery in some of these patients.

It is also true that, for some people at least, there are other symptoms that rear up at the same time. These can include fatigue, poor concentration, irritability, headaches, migraine, aching joints and muscles, hypoglycemia (low blood sugar), premenstrual problems, irregular periods, sinusitis, and urticaria. In very rare cases, psoriasis and asthma also respond to this treatment. How all these symptoms might be caused is another matter entirely, and equally controversial, so we will come back to this later.

If not *Candida*, then what? It is rather like the moment in a detective novel when it becomes clear that the jilted fiancée, despite having the motive, the means, and the opportunity—and being a thoroughly nasty character—is actually innocent. Unfortunately, this is a detective story with no neat ending as yet. But there are two theories currently available—gut fermentation syndrome and gut flora toxins. They are not, strictly speaking, alternative ideas—there are as many similarities between them as there are differences. Only time will tell which is closer to the truth.

Gut Fermentation Syndrome

This theory holds that some people have an imbalance in the gut flora that results in carbohydrates (starches and sugars) being fermented to produce alcohol. Slightly raised levels of alcohol are said to be detectable in the blood, and the symptoms experienced (or some of them, at least) are attributed to this alcohol. The symptoms attributed to gut fermentation syndrome are diarrhea or constipation (or bouts of both), bloating, gas, itching around the anus and genital region, lethargy, poor concentration and memory, inability to think quickly, runny nose or phlegmy cough sometimes with asthma, recurrent sinusitis, and a craving for sugar. It is not suggested that every patient with GFS has all these symptoms, and no one symptom is always present. The spectrum of symptoms described would take in most cases of supposed candidiasis, but would not cover all the symptoms claimed for *Candida*. Proponents of gut fermentation syndrome suggest that other problems could explain these—food intolerance, perhaps, or hyperventilation.

The advocates of gut fermentation syndrome do not suggest which microbes in the gut flora might be at fault. Yeasts are a candidate, but not the only ones. They believe that the antifungal drug nystatin has produced a false lead in this particular mystery. Because it seems to benefit people with diarrhea, it has created the impression that *Candida* or other yeasts are responsible for that diarrhea. Nystatin is an antifungal drug, and yeasts are fungi—it seemed an obvious connection. But as Dr. Keith Eaton, a proponent of gut fermentation syndrome, points out, nystatin affects the body in another way, by stabilizing the membranes that line the intestine. This might produce an improvement in symptoms such as diarrhea even though yeasts had nothing to do with causing the problem.

One related issue should be mentioned here. There is a relatively rare disorder that seems to affect Japanese people more than others, in which the body produces quite large amounts of alcohol from a starchy or sugary meal—enough to become intoxicated. Known as autobrewery syndrome, this disorder is different from the gut fermentation syndrome described here.

Gut Flora Toxins

This is a theory that has been developed, over many years, by Dr. John Hunter of Addenbrooke's Hospital in Cambridge. He believes that, in patients with irritable bowel syndrome, for example, there is an overgrowth of certain microbes in the gut, and a shortage of "good" microbes. This may result from excessive use of antibiotics, a bad bout of diarrhea following an infection, or radiation treatment.

But in Dr. Hunter's view the gut flora disturbance alone is only part of the problem for IBS patients. He suspects that, in addition, they cannot break down the toxins produced by the gut flora as well as they should. So the gut flora produce more toxins than in healthy people, and the toxins cannot be broken down efficiently. This double defect might produce some of the other symptoms that often accompany IBS, such as headaches and joint pains. (What other doctors have called candidiasis would, in Dr. Hunter's view, be cases of IBS.)

As far as Dr. Hunter is concerned, alcohol production is not an important aspect of IBS. He believes that the alcohol levels claimed in gut fermentation syndrome are too small to have much effect—or even to be accurately measured.

There is one very interesting aspect of Dr. Hunter's theory: he believes that it might be the key to *all* food intolerance, no matter what the symptoms. In his view we might explain rheumatoid arthritis or migraine in just the same way. Where a patient has a specific reaction to, say, oranges, Dr. Hunter believes that the patient's gut flora is guilty of making a particular toxin from something that is found in oranges. Alternatively, oranges might contain a particular vitamin or other nutrient that allows certain bacteria to grow at the expense of others, because it is something that they especially need. Those bacteria might produce a particular toxin that the patient cannot break down.

There are only a few documented examples of bacterial toxins that cannot be broken down due to defective enzymes. One is a chemical called p-cresol that seems to play a role in hyperkinetic syndrome in children (see page 300). Another possible candidate is a substance produced by an abnormal bacterium that may play a part in Crohn's disease. This substance seems to attract immune cells into the gut, and thus set up a damaging immune reaction. Whether defective enzymes play a part in allowing this substance to survive in the gut is not known.

An Unsolved Mystery

All this may sound very confusing, with doctors disagreeing about such fundamental matters as whether Disease A and Disease B are the same thing or two entirely different things. If you are feeling puzzled, you may find it useful to read the sections on pages 124 and 125 entitled Safety in Numbers and Different Doctors, Different Patients. They attempt to explain some of the problems involved in identifying diseases, naming them, and categorizing them.

You will, however, probably be more interested in getting well than in the intricacies of medical detective stories! If you have a number of the symptoms listed in table 4 on page 245, then it may be worth trying a no-sugar, no-yeast (NS-NY) diet. Experience shows that this diet can be very helpful for some people, and it will certainly do you no harm to cut out sugar and yeast for a while. The only real inconvenience is that you cannot eat bread, but you can always have soda bread, pita bread, or chapatis instead (although some pita breads do contain yeast, so make sure you read the label).

You will probably find it difficult to decide whether to try this diet or the elimination diet first. It is impossible to say which is more likely to work for you. But there is a good argument for first trying the elimination diet (Stages 2 and 3 of the diet are described in chapter 14), because it produces a much quicker response than the NS-NY diet. If the elimination diet is going to work for you, you will generally know within ten to fourteen days (see page 340). The NS-NY diet may take four weeks or more to produce noticeable effects, and they are generally gradual, whereas the elimination diet tends to produce a dramatic "overnight" improvement, usually after about a week. In general, it would be better to work through the diet described in chapter 14, then come back to the NS-NY diet later if you have not benefited at all.

Notice, however, that the first stage of the three-stage diet described in chapter 14 excludes all sugar anyway. For some people, this alone is enough—there is no need to exclude fruits, starches, and yeast as well. If you get partially well at this stage, you could try out the NS-NY diet next, while continuing with the healthy-eating restrictions on coffee, tea, and so on. If there is no further improvement, you could then go on to Stage 2 of the elimination diet.

Before deciding what to do, please read through the NS-NY diet thoroughly, then read chapter 14 carefully, too. Plan your diet strategy carefully—it may help to write down what you intend to do. Don't rush at it, or follow either of the diets in a halfhearted, indecisive way, swapping from one to the other. You need to be really clear in your mind which diet you are trying out, and what foods you should avoid.

Gerald

As a young man Gerald had suffered a severe bladder infection for which he needed prolonged treatment with antibiotics. Although the infection cleared up, he was left with a mild diarrhea that proved very persistent. Five or six bowel movements a day were not uncommon. Fortunately, Gerald found an office job with a national charity, and his symptoms were only a slight inconvenience. But in later years, as he was promoted to more senior posts, he found that he had to travel more and more to oversee fund-raising projects. The symptoms that he had put up with for twenty years now became a real problem. Sometimes he had to leave important meetings hurriedly and rush to the lavatory, which he found extremely embarrassing. His doctor offered him drugs that would control the diarrhea, but these were only partially effective. Eventually he was referred to a specialist, who took a careful case history and wondered if there might be some connection between the heavy doses of antibiotics he had received as a young man and the continuing diarrhea. He explained to Gerald that by killing off beneficial bacteria in the gut, antibiotics can open the way for excessive growth by yeasts. Gerald was asked to try a diet containing no sugar or white flour and was given an antifungal drug, nystatin. At first there was little change, but after about three weeks his bowel symptoms were much improved. He now has only two or three bowel movements a day, and these are much more predictable and less urgent, which makes traveling easier. A number of activities that were closed to him before—such as camping and sailing—are now a possibility. As a result he gets more exercise and is generally fitter and healthier.

The No-Sugar, No-Yeast Diet

Step 1

There seems to be some unexplained connection between contraceptive pills and the condition that has previously been labeled candidiasis. If you are on the Pill, you should ask your doctor about changing to some other form of contraception. Women who have been on the Pill may have nutritional deficiencies (see page 329) and you may wish to take a nutritional supplement of the kind described in appendix 9. It is a good idea to wait for one to three months after coming off the Pill, to see what effect this has—for some women, the Pill itself is the unsuspected source of vague health problems, so the diet may be unnecessary.

Assuming you continue, the first step should be a sugar-free diet—for some people this is all that is needed. The foods to avoid are shown in table 5 on page 249. If you are taking any medicines in syrup form, ask your doctor to prescribe a sugar-free alternative. Artificial sweeteners can be used if required, but it is best to break the sweetness addiction altogether if possible. Total abstinence from any sweeteners can cure a sweet tooth permanently—which is much better in the long term. After a few weeks on an unsweetened diet, it is remarkable how disgusting anything sugary tastes.

Stay on this diet for at least a month. If there is some improvement, persist for another month or two. If you are no better at all, then go on to Step 2.

Step 2

If the sugar-free diet does not do the trick, the next step is to cut out all fruits as well. White bread and anything made with white flour (such as pastry and pasta) should also be excluded. Whole wheat bread and flour can be eaten instead, because these are broken down more slowly and do

---

TABLE 4 SYMPTOMS THAT MAY RESPOND TO AN NS-NY DIET

Diarrhea or other bowel disturbances
Gas, bloating, abdominal discomfort or pain
Headache or migraine
Fatigue, poor concentration, irritability, slowness of thought
Joint pains, sometimes with swollen joints
Aching muscles
Urticaria (hives)
Itchy anus, with the inflammation sometimes spreading to the
  buttocks and thighs
Premenstrual tension and irregular periods
Psoriasis and other skin complaints
Asthma, but only very rarely
Recurrent *Candida* (thrush) infections in the throat or vagina
Recurrent cystitis not due to bacterial infection
Recurrent fungal infections of the skin
Craving for sweet foods (this can also be caused by hypoglycemia
  (see pages 178–81)

Alan

Alan developed a severe throat infection after swimming in the sea near a polluted stretch of beach. He was treated with antibiotics and his throat healed, but soon afterward he developed red, itchy bumps all over his body—hives. He asked the doctor if the two events might be connected but was told this was most unlikely. The hives got somewhat better in time, but it continued to bother him at regular intervals for the next twenty years. In his forties it grew worse, and he decided to see a specialist. When Alan mentioned that he had taken a lot of antibiotics just before the urticaria began, the specialist suggested that he try a diet with no sugar and very little starch. At the same time he was given a course of antifungal drugs. The hives cleared up promptly and have not returned.

---

not release glucose all at once. But they should only be eaten in small quantities, as should potatoes. The bulk of the diet should be made up of vegetables and high-protein foods such as meat, fish, eggs, and cheese.

Eat plenty of freshly crushed garlic; this is thought to combat yeasts in the gut. Fresh herbs and green, leafy vegetables, such as spinach and lettuce, are also recommended, as they contain antifungal agents. It may also be worth trying an herbal tea called taheebo or pau d'arco—it is said to have antifungal properties, although this has not been verified scientifically. Eating live yogurt may also be worthwhile, because it contains some of the useful members of the gut flora, and may help reestablish a healthy balance among the inhabitants of the gut (see page 241).

Giving up fruit may make you concerned about vitamin C deficiency, but if you eat sufficient quantities of fresh vegetables this should not be a problem. Cabbage, broccoli, and brussels sprouts are rich in vitamin C, and potatoes are a valuable source. It is important not to soak potatoes, which leaches out the vitamin C, and not to overcook cabbage and other green vegetables, because heat gradually destroys vitamin C. Rose hip tea is also an excellent source of this vitamin, as is fresh lemon juice, which is permissible on this diet because it contains little natural sugar.

Again, you should stay on this diet for at least a month, and longer if you begin to feel partially better. If there is good improvement on this diet, fruits and other excluded foods can be gradually reintroduced later, but not sugar. If you feel worse on this diet, then you may have food intolerance—to eggs or cheese, for example.

Step 3

If there is little or no improvement on the Step 2 diet, then cut out all yeast-containing foods as well. These are listed on pages 398–99.

It is sometimes claimed that yeasts in the gut derive nourishment from yeasts in food, but this is not the case. The reason for avoiding yeast is simply that you may be sensitive to it. The distinction is important, because if you are very sensitive to yeast, even the smallest amount can make you ill, so scrupulous avoidance is necessary, especially at first.

If there is a partial reponse to this diet, then it is a positive sign, and you should consider going on to Step 4. If there is no reponse at all, it might be a good idea to try an elimination diet instead at this point, if

---

Louisa

Louisa was about forty-six when she began to be troubled by unsightly red blotches on her face. She worked as an assistant in a dress shop, and it was important that she look chic. She found that she was having to wear more and more makeup to cover the blemishes. Before deciding on the best treatment, the doctor asked her about her health generally. It emerged that she had suffered from mild diarrhea and gas for some years, but had not thought it worth bothering the doctor about these minor problems. She had also been feeling very tired, and had some pain and stiffness in her joints, which she thought was "just her age." Checking through her medical file, the doctor saw that she had been treated for vaginal yeast infections on several occasions. The doctor had no idea what might be causing the red blotches, but he did have a suspicion that the other symptoms might have a common cause. He put Louisa on a diet that excluded all sugar and most starch. She found this very difficult to keep to, as she had a sweet tooth and loved cake. But she persisted, and after two months her bowels were functioning normally, she felt far more energetic, and her joint pains had vanished. At about the same time the red blotches on Louisa's face also disappeared.

food intolerance is suspected. You can always come back to this diet later.

Step 4

This is a very drastic diet, and should not be started without medical advice. Carbohydrates—the "starchy" substances in foods—are restricted to less than three ounces per day. This effectively means no potatoes, bread, flour, rice, breakfast cereals, pasta, or other starchy foods, except for one very small portion each day. The incidental carbohydrates in vegetables, nuts, and other foods will account for most of your daily allowance. High-carbohydrate vegetables such as corn, peas, parsnips, lentils, and broad beans should be avoided. Nuts can be eaten in moderation, but not cashews, which are rich in carbohydrates. Continue to eat plenty of garlic and fresh, green leafy vegetables.

Keeping the Problem at Bay

This diet is not a lifelong cure—the problem can come back if you revert to your old eating habits. Once you are fully better and have been so for some time, you can risk the occasional slice of white bread or sliver of cake. But you should try to eat as little sugar and refined carbohydrate (white flour, pasta, and so forth) as possible. Beware "sugar-free" commercial products such as cakes and jams, especially those from health food shops—often they are made with fruit-juice concentrate and are just as rich in natural fruit sugars as if they were made with cane or beet sugar. Diabetic products are suitable, however. If your symptoms start to return, then you must immediately cut out all sugar again.

If you recovered only on Step 3 of the diet, then you are probably sensitive to yeast. In a few cases this reaction to yeast is permanent, but most people lose their sensitivity after several months of avoiding yeast products. Some people may have to avoid eating yeast every day (see page 364).

Some of those who have been successfully treated will still have residual problems due to food intolerance. Although an elimination diet may be needed to sort this out, going straight on to another restricted diet is not a good idea. It is advisable to stay on a normal, varied diet for a while (while still avoiding sugar and white flour, of course). This will give you plenty of vitamins and minerals, to build you up for the elimination diet. In some cases, it may be a good idea to take a nutritional supplement (see appendix 9).

TABLE 5 FOODS CONTAINING SUGAR

White and brown sugar
Honey
Corn syrup
Molasses
Maple syrup
Malt
Barley sweetener (macrobiotic sweetener)
Jam, including "no added sugar" jam
Chutney and pickles
Cakes
Cookies
Ice cream
Puddings
Chocolate and other candies
Soda and Kool Aid
Any food labeled: corn syrup, dextrose, fructose, glucose, maltose,
    sucrose, or sugar
Baked beans, including "no added sugar" brands
Peanut butter (except sugar-free brands, sold in health food stores)
Some other apparently savory foods contain sugar—some canned
    soups, for example, and some frozen dinners
Some medicines, especially syrups and coated tablets
Dried fruits, which are rich in natural sugars, should not be eaten
Anything that tastes sweet should be regarded with suspicion, unless
    designed for diabetics

Giardia

Giardia was, until recently, thought to be a harmless member of the gut flora, because it was sometimes found in the intestines of apparently healthy people. Only within the past few years have doctors begun to realize that this microbe can cause disease. It is found throughout the world, and about 5 to 15 percent of people are infected. *Giardia* probably originated in the Tropics.

Giardia lives in the gut and produces microscopic hard-walled cysts that pass out of the body with the feces. These can get into food or water, especially in countries with poor sanitary facilities, and thus infect other people. *Giardia* cysts are resistant to chlorine, at least in the amounts usually used for disinfecting water supplies.

For most people who become infested with *Giardia*, there are no symptoms. Such people are infectious however, and if they are involved in food preparation and careless about washing their hands, they may be the modern equivalent of Typhoid Mary, passing *Giardia* on to others.

Those who do suffer symptoms when infected by *Giardia* experience an acute attack of watery diarrhea, with bloating, abdominal pain, belching, and fatigue. This usually clears up of its own accord after a few days; thereafter, the person has no symptoms but may remain infectious. However, some patients continue to suffer milder symptoms. Their main problem is that food is not absorbed from the gut properly. This produces loose, frequent stools, often foul smelling and frothy. There may also be flatulence, pain, nausea, loss of appetite, weakness, and weight loss. Children with this disease—and they are the most susceptible group—are often pale and stunted.

There may also be a milder form of the disease in which there is no diarrhea as such—discomfort, gas, belching, and nausea are the main symptoms in these cases. Hives, joint pains, and feverishness may also be present. Not surprisingly, some of these patients are thought to have food intolerance. Indeed, many do, because *Giardia* seems to be linked in some way to food sensitivity.

Giardia infection can be diagnosed by looking for the parasite in the stools. It is treated by a short course of drugs, the main one used being metronidazole. This can have some side effects, such as nausea and vomiting, but only has to be taken for about a week. Unfortunately, it seems to make yeast overgrowth more likely, so anyone taking it would be well advised to adopt a sugar-free diet during the treatment and for a month or so afterward.

Treating a Disturbed Gut Flora

In theory, the way to treat disturbed gut flora is to repopulate the gut with the good bacteria, and so exclude the more damaging bacteria and yeasts. Unfortunately, a reliable treatment of this sort is not widely available yet. At present the best treatment is to eat live yogurt, which includes one of the most important bacteria in the gut, *Lactobacillus*. There are also commercial preparations of bacteria that are intended to restore the normal flora of the gut. Some of these have been tested and a crucial difference was found between those bought in health food stores or drug stores and those purchased through mail order. The former had often been stored for long periods at room temperature, and, not surprisingly researchers found very few live bacteria in them. The bacterial replacers bought by mail order had only spent two to three days in nonrefrigerated conditions and were as rich in bacteria as the manufacturers claimed.

If you choose yogurt, you can make sure the brand you are buying really is live by adding a spoonful to some warm milk that has been heated to boiling point and then allowed to cool. Keep the mixture in a thermos for six to eight hours. If it has not turned to yogurt, then the original yogurt was not live. The best way of ensuring that your yogurt is live is to make your own—starter cultures are available from some health food stores, or by mail (see page 458).

ELEVEN

Food Problems in Children

The other chapters in this book apply equally to adults and children, but a special chapter on children's food problems is necessary because there are important medical differences between young patients and older ones. Altering the diet is also far riskier for a child than it is for an adult, so there are more difficult decisions to be made before embarking on an elimination diet. This chapter is intended as a supplement to the earlier ones for those with a special interest in children's problems. Parents reading this book with a view to helping their children are strongly advised to read the earlier chapters as well as this one.

Food Allergy and Intolerance in Children

Food allergy generally begins in childhood, while food intolerance can begin at any time of life. Having said that, there is often no clear distinction between allergy and intolerance (see page 10), especially in children. Those with proven allergies, such as asthma or eczema, may show other symptoms that most self-respecting allergists would have nothing to do with—hyperactivity, for example, or muscle aches. If these clear up along with the allergic symptoms when certain foods are withdrawn, is it allergy or intolerance? To avoid the problem, we will use the term *food sensitivity* to cover both allergy and intolerance.

Over the past twenty years doctors have begun to recognize just how many different childhood problems can be caused by food sensitivity. Colic, eczema, asthma, persistent runny nose, glue ear, headaches, migraine, and even behavioral problems have all been traced back to cer-

TABLE 6 SYMPTOMS THAT MAY BE DUE TO FOOD SENSITIVITY IN CHILDREN

The page numbers show where these problems are discussed in detail.

Digestive system
Vomiting
Colic, in babies (page 254)
Persistent diarrhea (page 263)
Diarrhea with blood or mucus in the stools (page 182)
Poor appetite and failure to grow, in babies
Stomachaches, in older children

Nose, ears, and lungs
Rhinitis (runny or congested nose) (page 44, page 78)
Glue ear (page 45)
Asthma (page 47, page 74)

Skin
Eczema (page 52, page 79)
Urticaria (hives) (page 50, page 114)

Nervous system
Headaches (page 168)
Migraine (page 132, page 169)
Epileptic fits, where these accompany migraine (page 177)
Hyperkinetic syndrome (hyperactivity) (page 264)

Other symptoms
Aching joints (page 163)
Muscle aches (page 163)
Rheumatoid arthritis (page 164)
Some types of kidney disease (page 99)

tain foods or food additives. These discoveries have a bittersweet taste for the many mothers who have been told by their doctors that they themselves were at the root of such problems—because they were overanxious, inexperienced, nervy, overindulgent, or whatever. This sort of diagnosis is usually based on minimal evidence and does untold harm to the self-confidence of mothers at a time when they most need help and support. Anxious, inexperienced mothers can be the source of a child's mysterious health problems, of course, but there is increasing evidence that it is commonly something in the diet or the environment. There is also evidence that children who show food sensitivity in their early years are more likely to develop other health problems later, often continuing—or reappearing—in their adult lives. Helping these children adapt to their environment is therefore important, and putting their symptoms down to poor mothering, without any evidence, is irresponsible and potentially damaging.

It is now believed that babies can be sensitized to food even before they are born, because a few food molecules, from food the mother eats, can reach the baby in her womb (see page 310). More important, food molecules get into the mother's breast milk, and babies that are exclusively breast fed can become ill because of the sort of food the mother is eating. Although sensitivity to cow's milk is by far the most common problem in babies and children, all sorts of other foods have been implicated. These relatively recent discoveries have meant that food sensitivity can now be recognized and dealt with far more effectively. They have also suggested ways in which parents can reduce the risk of food sensitivity in their children, as explained in chapter 13.

The common features of food sensitivity in children are listed in table 6. Of these, asthma, eczema, and rhinitis (runny or congested nose) are all examples of classical allergies and are therefore dealt with in chapter 3. Glue ear, which frequently follows on from rhinitis, is also described there. Treating these conditions is discussed in chapter 4, although anyone who is interested in investigating the role of food should also read Investigating Food Sensitivity in Babies and Toddlers, beginning on page 275. Symptoms that fall outside the allergic camp and that also affect adults—such as headaches, migraines, nausea, diarrhea, and rheumatoid arthritis—are discussed in chapter 7.

Colic

Colic is a sharp pain in the stomach or intestines of a baby that causes uncontrollable crying. This crying is more common in the evening, and the baby may draw his or her legs up and become very red in the face. Because the attacks are most common in the first ten to twelve weeks of life, the term *three-month colic* is often used.

The Colic Controversy

Of course, it is not always easy to tell why a baby is crying—there may be many different causes. Even the question of how much crying is natural is contentious. The following quotations illustrate the widely differing views of this common problem:

> During the first few weeks of life the average baby sleeps a great deal but, when awake, cries lustily and often. . . . It is only from about six weeks of age onwards, when the baby is becoming aware of his or her surroundings, that there are some wakeful periods without crying. . . . There is no reason why the simple milk diet (whether natural or otherwise) of the normal baby should cause tummy ache. If the baby cries uncontrollably for several hours each evening, it is more likely that the cause is so-called 3-month or 10-week colic (sharp tummy ache). But, although some doctors consider that the baby has genuine physical pain, others believe that this is an example of the baby reacting to the tensions of the mother at the end of a hard day: and they believe that the crying stops after 10 to 12

TABLE 7 SOME MINOR SYMPTOMS THAT MAY ACCOMPANY COLIC*

Frequent regurgitation of food (posseting)
Loose stools
Gas and bloating
Constipation
Poor appetite, stops feeding and screams after a few minutes
Stuffy or runny nose; nose rubbing
Frequent sneezing, coughing, sniffing, or snorting
Noisy breathing
Frequent hiccups
Frequent ear infections or colds
Bad breath
Dry, cracked skin; rashes; eczema
Constant scratching or rubbing
Sweatiness, slight fever, or cold hands and feet
Redness around mouth or anus, or on cheeks
Swelling around eyes

*Adapted from *Food for Thought* by Maureen Minchin, with permission.

weeks because by then the mother has become more competent and confident in her handling of the baby, and has communicated this new calmness to the baby. (*The Macmillan Guide to Family Health*, edited by Dr. Tony Smith)

We in the West regard infant crying as normal, and in a thousand different ways condition our children to associate babies with bawling. But in societies where infants are exclusively breast-fed from birth and in contact with their non-allergic, non-food-bingeing, non-smoking mothers, "colic" is unknown and infant crying is seen as a sign of distress, which warrants immediate attention. And that is exactly what it sounds like to the new mother, until she is persuaded by others, against every instinct she possesses, that this is "normal" or "naughty." . . . Crying, colic and night-waking are only a tiny portion of the range of symptoms which experienced mothers report as disappearing and reappearing with dietary changes—changes in maternal diet for the breast-feeding mother, or changes in infant diet directly. These symptoms range from minor oddities [see table 7 on page 255] to serious problems. In the series of mothers followed up, those who consistently reported the minor symptoms were regarded as neurotic or overprotective. Yet these same mothers found that over months there was often a gradual increase in the severity of symptoms. . . . The question should be asked, would the serious symptoms ever have appeared had the mother identified and avoided the dietary allergen responsible? Mothers were almost never taken seriously until the child had gross symptoms. . . . Maternal anxiety is an appropriate response to the experience of living with a crying baby—but what physiological mechanism exists to explain the notion that anxiety causes colic? In my experience, babies are remarkably placid through all sorts of family rows, so long as they are warm and well fed; while they will infallibly disrupt the most harmonious scene if they have a pain. (*Food for Thought*, Maureen Minchin)

Jamie

Claire's eight-week-old baby, Jamie, was apparently healthy but cried a lot of the time, and seemed to be in pain. Because Claire was breast feeding, her doctor asked about her diet and found that she was a vegetarian. She explained that she had been eating more cheese and drinking an extra pint of milk a day to make sure she got enough protein during pregnancy and breast feeding. The doctor suggested that she might avoid milk, cheese, and butter for a while, to see if this had any effect, and prescribed some tablets to give her extra calcium. He persuaded her to eat a little fish to make up for the missing protein. A couple of days after starting this diet, Jamie's crying was noticeably less and it became easier to get him to sleep each evening. Claire was delighted at the improvement. She tried drinking a glass of milk, to see what would happen, and twenty-four hours later Jamie, following a feeding, suffered, a severe attack of colic. After that Claire stayed on a milk-free diet for six weeks. She then introduced a little milk and butter into her diet and found that Jamie could now tolerate this.

Is there any scientific evidence for either of these opposing views? The main piece of evidence for the "tense-mother/crying-baby" idea is that first babies tend to cry more than subsequent ones; doctors infer from this that the mother's inexperience is an important factor. However, there are no data to show that first babies really do cry more—it is just a subjective impression. One study that investigated this idea found that there was little difference between first babies and later ones. Even if a first baby does cry more, the link with maternal anxiety is still only a speculative one, and there are other, far more plausible explanations.

The evidence for the second point of view is limited, but certainly stronger than that for the first. A Swedish study of nineteen bottle-fed babies with colic found that more than 70 percent improved when changed to formula feeds that did not contain whole cow's-milk protein. The same research team found that cow's milk in the mother's diet could cause colic in breast-fed babies.

Another trial carried out in New Zealand, and widely quoted in the medical literature, apparently failed to find any link between the mother's diet and colic in breast-fed babies. In fact, there were several serious flaws in this trial, and its findings have been widely misrepresented anyway. Twenty mothers were involved, and the main focus of the trial was the role of cow's milk in causing colic. The mothers were asked to avoid cow's milk, and were then challenged with it in a disguised form, so that they would not know when they were drinking milk and when they were drinking the control substance. Soy milk was used for this control without any investigation of whether the babies might be sensitive to soy proteins. The mothers were given milk with soy to drink for two days or soy only for two days. There was an interval of two, four, or six days between each milk challenge. Experience suggests that this may not be long enough to detect changes in the baby's symptoms—although some babies recover within twenty-four hours of the mother eliminating offending foods from her diet, others can take many days, sometimes as much as two weeks, for their colic to settle down. The whole trial only continued for twelve days.

Interestingly enough, the researchers did notice a link between the foods the mother ate and her baby's symptoms. They observed that the colic was worst in those babies whose mothers ate all the commonly implicated foods such as milk, eggs, chocolate, nuts, and fish. The fewer foods the mother ate from this list, the less severe was the colic. They concluded that the mother's diet "may influence the likelihood of infantile colic in breast-fed children, but that the source of the colic cannot be attributed to a single dietary component [that is, milk]. It may however involve a variety of foodstuffs." *Despite this clear statement of their findings, this paper is widely quoted as showing that there is no link between colic and maternal diet.*

Other evidence supporting the second point of view comes from a retrospective study of sixty-eight children with proven sensitivity to cow's milk. When the medical history of these children was investigated, it turned out that a very high proportion had persistent screaming and colic as babies. This is only circumstantial evidence for a link between food sensitivity and colic, of course, but it is of interest. And it gives support to the idea that treating the colic is important, because the children in the study all had serious health problems as a result of their sensitivity to milk—problems that might have been avoided if they had been taken off cow's milk at an earlier age.

One aspect of colic is difficult to explain from either viewpoint: the fact that the symptoms tend to disappear or diminish at about three months of age. The traditional explanation is that all mothers with colicky babies—regardless of what sort of people they are or what else is happening in their lives—suddenly become more confident and relaxed at this point. This seems implausible to say the least, but is there an alternative explanation that is compatible with food intolerance? One possibility is that the colic represents an initial crisis reaction as the child is exposed to large amounts of cow's-milk or other foreign proteins. The child later adapts to the problem foods, and the colic apparently clears up, but sensitivity continues in the form of other, less acute symptoms such as eczema, asthma, or diarrhea. There is ample evidence from case histories that this might happen—and the retrospective study described above supports the idea.

Lactose—The Sugar Found in Milk

Before considering what can be done about colic, we need to look at the question of lactose and lactose intolerance. Lactose is the main sugar found in all animal milks, including human breast milk (the name means "milk sugar"). Unlike most sugars, it does not taste sweet—if it did, milk would be quite sugary to the taste buds, because it is loaded with lactose.

In order to break down lactose, we have an enzyme (see page 21) known as lactase (the *-ase* ending denotes an enzyme) in our intestines. Almost all babies have this enzyme, although there are rare cases in which the enzyme is entirely lacking. (These babies are likely to be detected soon after birth, because they are made seriously ill by any sort of milk, cow's or human.) Adults tend to lose this enzyme unless they continue taking cow's milk and milk products from the time they are weaned onward. In China and Southeast Asia, where milk and cheese are not part of the diet, most adults are lactase deficient, but they can regain the ability to produce lactase if they persist in drinking milk.

If a child or adult lacks the ability to deal with lactose, the sugar passes through into the intestine, where it provides a bonanza for waiting bacteria. They consume the sugar, giving off gas and toxic products as they grow and multiply. These toxins then cause unpleasant symptoms such as pain and diarrhea. They may be at the root of colic, which is why lactose intolerance is important here.

Following a bout of diarrhea—due to an infection or whatever other cause—the digestive processes in our intestines take a little while to get back to normal. During this recovery period, the gut lining often produces far less lactase than usual. This happens in both children and adults, and it may cause a continuation of the diarrhea if milk is consumed after an infection. Formulas without lactose are available, and your doctor may be able to prescribe one for you temporarily if your baby has had gastroenteritis and continues to have colic or diarrhea afterward. In the case of breast-fed babies, it is probably better to continue breast feeding, even though breast milk contains lactose. In general, children and adults should not be given too much milk to drink if they are recovering from a stomach upset. Yogurt and cheese (but not cottage cheese) are usually tolerated because they contain far less lactose. Soy milk is lactose-free.

It is also possible that some small babies have insufficient lactase to cope with very large feedings—they can digest small feedings, but if their morning feeding is larger than usual, the extra lactose overwhelms their capacity to cope with it. This could explain why some babies only have colic in the evening, when the morning feeding reaches the intestines and the bacteria that live there begin to feed on the undigested lactose. This theory has recently been investigated scientifically, and the results suggest that it could well be correct.

In the past it was often assumed that all babies who could not tolerate milk were lactase deficient, and this idea is still current in some quarters. It is now known that most children who are sensitive to cow's milk are actually reacting to the proteins it contains. But the diarrhea produced by this reaction may, in turn, cause lactase deficiency. Doctors refer to this as **secondary lactase deficiency**. There are readily available tests for lactase deficiency, but these do not distinguish between true lactase deficiency (or **primary lactase deficiency**) and secondary lactase deficiency. More complicated tests can distinguish the two, and these show that primary lactase deficiency is actually very rare. So if you are told that your baby is lactase deficient after some routine tests, you should be prepared to question the diagnosis and ask your doctor to help you investigate the possibility of food sensitivity, as described in the following section.

What to Do about Colic

The first and most important step is to get your baby examined by a doctor, who should check for serious problems such as gastroesophageal reflux—acid passing from the stomach up into the gullet (esophagus), and thus causing pain or intestinal obstruction. Assuming that there are no such problems, and that your doctor can suggest no other likely causes for the excessive crying, then it is worth investigating the possible role of food.

Bottle-Fed Babies

Try giving smaller, more frequent feedings as an initial step. If the baby has slight difficulties with lactose (see above), then this may be the answer. Should this produce no improvement, then follow the measures described on pages 275–78.

Breast-Fed Babies

There are two main possibilities to be considered here: temporary lactose intolerance and other forms of food sensitivity.

If your baby has colic only in the evening, then a temporary deficit in lactase, due to the morning feeding being larger than usual, is a possibility (see page 260). There are various ways to reduce the amount of milk in the morning feeding, and these are worth trying. The simplest approach is to let the baby feed first from one breast only and then from the other—rather than to keep switching breasts. This reduces the amount of milk produced overall. If this has no effect, try expressing some milk before the morning feeding; refrigerate or freeze it for use later. For advice on how to express milk, contact one of the breast-feeding advice groups whose addresses are given on pages 454–55. Another method is to give the baby a small amount of boiled water from a bottle before the morning feeding, so that he or she feels full more quickly, or to feed from one breast only. This will tend to reduce your supply of milk overall, so you should only do it if you know your milk is plentiful.

For the baby who does not respond to this, or who has colic at any time of day, food intolerance should be investigated (see pages 278–81).

Smoking and Babies Don't Mix!

One significant measure that any mother with a colicky baby should take is to stop smoking and get her partner to stop. Whether you are breast feeding or bottle feeding, cigarette smoke will make your baby more prone to colic. In the case of breast-feeding mothers, some of the toxins from the cigarettes that enter the bloodstream are passed into the milk and have a direct effect on the baby's delicate stomach lining.

Prevention of Colic

If you are pregnant or planning to have a baby, there are measures you can take that could well reduce the chances of colic developing. The most important is to make sure that the baby is not given supplementary or complementary feedings while in the hospital. It might also be worth avoiding certain foods and drinks while breast feeding. For more details on this, see pages 310–13.

Insomnia

A recent report suggests that babies who cannot be persuaded to sleep are suffering from a form of food intolerance. A group of these babies was studied, all were being bottle fed. When ordinary cow's-milk formula was replaced by hydrolysate they began sleeping better, and when they went back onto ordinary formula the insomnia returned. If insomnia is a problem for your baby, ask the doctor if hydrolysate could be prescribed for a while. There are more details about hydrolysates on pages 275–76.

This problem can also occur in toddlers and young children. In such cases the children tend to take a while to fall asleep, and then awaken repeatedly during the night. Other possible causes for this—and there are many—should be investigated first, but if these investigations reveal nothing and the problem cannot be explained or treated, then it is worth investigating the possibility of food intolerance. A simple elimination diet is the recommended form of diagnosis but this should, of course, be supervised by a doctor.

To return to babies, some breast-fed babies awaken frequently and seem to be hungry every two hours. The most likely reason for this is that there is too little milk available, that the stomach is very small and cannot take in enough milk at any one time, or that the baby is undergoing a growth spurt that requires more food. Occasionally, however, food intolerance may be to blame. One breast-feeding mother, who also happened to be a pediatrician, found that when she stopped eating all dairy products and beef her baby slept for four to six hours after a feeding, woke up smiling, and did not seem eternally hungry. A day or two after she reintroduced milk to her diet, the baby was again waking up with a howl every two hours and feeding voraciously. Repeated double-blind testing (see page 192) confirmed this surprising finding—that the breast milk soothed him initially but then caused unpleasant symptoms that woke him up two hours later. It seemed that he was experiencing an intolerance reaction to cow's-milk allergens in the breast milk about two hours after a feeding. Whether this reaction occurs in a significant number of babies or just a few rare cases is unknown. (It is interesting that the same mother had exactly the same experience with a subsequent baby, and that both children had a full allergic reaction when later given a drink of cow's milk.) If your breast-fed baby seems to fit this picture, you could try cutting out milk or other potentially allergenic foods from your own diet, but you must have your doctor's blessing, and you will probably need a nutritional supplement.

Diarrhea in Babies and Children

Diarrhea in babies and children can have a great many causes, the most obvious one being infection with bacteria, viruses, or other microbes. But if infections and other possible causes (such as cystic fibrosis) have been ruled out by your doctor, then you should consider the possible role of food.

Diarrhea due to food sensitivity can come on suddenly and acutely, or it may start gradually and slowly get worse. There may be physical damage to the gut wall, which can be checked by taking a tiny sample and examining it under a microscope—this is known as a **biopsy**. However, there can also be diarrhea due to food without any major damage to the gut. Where there is visible damage, this may indicate celiac disease (see pages 104–7) or infant colitis (see page 182). The latter is characterized by blood and mucus in the stools. The doctor will wish to eliminate both these possibilities before looking at other forms of food sensitivity.

An acute reaction to food may be difficult to distinguish from a viral infection that produces an attack of gastroenteritis, because the virus cannot always be detected in the baby's stools. Even if there has been an infection, this does not rule out the possibility of food sensitivity. Diarrhea of any sort can sensitize the gut so that foods previously eaten without trouble now produce symptoms. Drinking milk makes the situation worse, because there is often a transient lactase deficiency (see page 260).

When diarrhea is due to food sensitivity in infants and children, the culprit food often turns out to be cow's milk. When milk sensitivity occurs, problems with other foods may follow, because the structure of the gut wall is altered by the reaction to milk. It becomes leakier, which allows other food molecules through—and the body may then react adversely to these as well. Often the reaction to other foods is only temporary; if they are eliminated from the diet for a few months, they can be eaten again without difficulty. The reaction to milk tends to be more persistent, but most children who are sensitive to milk as babies can drink it once more by the time they are three or four. For a small number of people, however, the milk sensitivity will be lifelong.

What to Do about Diarrhea

Acute attacks of diarrhea should be taken very seriously indeed, especially in small babies. They can lose so much water from the body that they become seriously ill. In extreme cases they can suffer brain damage or die. The signs of moderate to severe **dehydration** are little urine, which is very dark and smells strongly (or no urine at all), sleepiness, dry sunken eyes, fast breathing, and dry mouth. If you see these signs, you should get medical help without delay: the baby needs special treatment to replace the lost water and salts. This treatment may be given by mouth (when it is known as **oral rehydration therapy** or **ORT**) or directly into the bloodstream in more serious cases. In mild cases of dehydration, there are mixtures of salts that can be used for ORT at home. These are marketed under various names, including Pedialyte. Older children and adults can also become dehydrated during severe attacks of diarrhea, and ORT can be useful for them as well.

Given that the doctor has ruled out infection and other likely causes for the diarrhea, then food sensitivity should be considered.

As new foods are introduced into a child's diet, there may be temporary bouts of diarrhea in response to them, although these do not necessarily develop as soon as the new food is eaten. Such transient diarrhea is sometimes given the name *toddler diarrhea* and is characterized by loose stools that contain some undigested food. Toddler diarrhea usually clears up by about two years of age, and the usual medical advice is to leave it untreated. Given what we now know about food sensitivity, this is not necessarily the best advice. There seems to be a general pattern in some children, particularly with illnesses such as colic and eczema, of symptoms disappearing but other symptoms appearing later in their wake. If this is also true of toddler diarrhea then it might be better, in the long run, to identify the offending foods and avoid them for a while. In one study, six out of twenty-one children with toddler diarrhea proved to be food sensitive. Follow the procedure outlined on pages 281–82.

The Hyperkinetic Syndrome

This is a typical day in the life of a hyperactive child, as described by an exhausted mother to Dr. Doris Rapp, a pediatrician working in Buffalo, New York:

In the morning Matthew was stuffy and tired. He was cranky and would get upset over homework not done, cry, call himself stupid, and pester his sister. When he arrived home from school, he immediately took off his shoes and did somersaults throughout the house. He thumped and jumped about the house, or would lie and watch television with his hands and feet tapping and banging away constantly. At dinner he rapped his fork and knife on the plate, picked up and handled things on the table, turned the salt shaker upside down, kicked the table and his sister, and intermittently, throughout the meal, jumped up to do somersaults in the living room. After supper he would try to do his homework. He would get upset because he forgot some books and say he was stupid. He'd write two or three words, rip up the sheet because of an error and do this about five or six times. He'd cry, get upset again, and the next morning either lose or forget his homework. At bedtime he would say that his muscles and belly had ached all day (a problem since his early years) and it would take an hour and a half to get to sleep. He'd roll and toss all night with bad dreams and talking. During the day he talked constantly about anything and would not listen. He never ate more than half a meal, never had an appetite. His nose was usually stuffy.

The proper name for Matthew's condition is the *hyperkinetic syndrome;* although *hyperactivity* is often used as a diagnostic label, it is actually just one aspect of that syndrome. Other terms used for this collection of symptoms are *minimal brain dysfunction* and *attention deficit disorder.* The symptoms are listed in table 8.

Estimates of the prevalence of hyperactivity range from 1 to 20 percent. Boys appear to outnumber girls by about five to one, but it may be that girls with the problem are less overtly hyperactive and tend to display more subtle symptoms, such as inattention, speech disorders, and mood changes, which may not always be identified as hyperkinetic syndrome.

The aggressive, destructive behavior that is often seen in hyperkinetics usually develops later than the other symptoms, and may be largely a response to feelings of frustration that stem from the other symptoms. Hyperactive children may grow out of it in time, but this takes a long time and their behavior tends to get worse before it gets better. Their

Joanna

Joanna's problems began as a baby. Her mother found it very difficult to get her to take her bottles, she never seemed to be hungry. She had a bowel movement very rarely—sometimes only once a week. When she was six months old Joanna was taken to the hospital for tests, but the doctors could not work out what was wrong. Their final verdict was that she was "extremely independent and will refuse to eat until she is able to feed herself." Her mother found this an astonishing pronouncement to make on a six-month-old baby, but she had to accept what they said and continue to struggle with Joanna's health problems alone. As Joanna grew up, the symptoms continued. Because her bowel was emptied so rarely, she suffered severe abdominal pains and couldn't bend down, even to tie her shoelaces. The pressure on her bladder from the overloaded bowel resulted in Joanna wetting herself several times a day. School proved to be an ordeal, with the other children teasing her constantly about her problems. Joanna was admitted to the hospital again when six years old, but the doctors again concluded that there was nothing physically wrong with her. They decided that she was deliberately "holding in" her feces and referred her to a child psychiatrist. It was then that Joanna's mother came across an earlier edition of this book. Reading the book, and remembering the problems she had trying to get Joanna to take bottles as a baby, her mother tried removing all milk and dairy products from the child's diet. Within twelve hours her stomach pains cleared up, and over the next few weeks she began to experience daily bowel movements. Wetting herself several times a day soon became a thing of the past, and Joanna also felt much happier. "It is hard to believe, after six and a half years of hell, it took something so simple to make her well," her mother said. Although diarrhea is more common in food sensitivity, a small minority of children do show constipation, as in Joanna's case.

inability to concentrate or order their thoughts means that they generally do not learn much at school, even though they may be quite intelligent. Some have difficulty in writing and spelling. There is evidence of criminality and psychotic behavior in some hyperkinetics when they reach adulthood, so it is advisable to try to sort out the problem sooner rather than later.

The Causes of Hyperkinetic Syndrome

One of the early theories about the causes of hyperkinetic syndrome put it down to brain damage, but research has failed to find any evidence of this. In fact the problem seems to be determined genetically, which means that the tendency to hyperkinesis is passed down from parent to child.

One study carried out in Canada showed that 20 percent of cases could be attributed to true IgE-mediated allergy to food. From the case histories compiled by allergists treating such children, it seems that most are sensitive to a great variety of things, including pollens, house dust, food additives, and household chemicals. So it may be that IgE-mediated allergy plays a role in more than 20 percent of cases, when other types of allergen, besides food, are taken into account.

Hyperkinetic children may also have deficiencies in certain enzymes that break down the toxic compounds found in food or produced by bacteria in the gut. The evidence for this is described on page 300. It is quite probable that both IgE and enzyme deficiencies are important in causing the symptoms.

The role of food colorings, preservatives, and other additives in hyperkinetic syndrome has received a lot of publicity. This idea was first put forward by Dr. Ben Feingold of San Francisco, who also suggested that aspirin might be to blame, along with naturally occurring salicy-

---

TABLE 8 FEATURES OF THE HYPERKINETIC SYNDROME (HYPERACTIVITY)

Overactive, excitable
Unable to keep still; constantly fidgeting
Poor concentration; short attention span; never finishes anything
Sudden mood changes; unpredictable, explosive
Cries easily; has emotional outbursts or temper tantrums
Gets into fights; is aggressive or bullies other children
Cannot cope with being criticized; seems depressed
Talks too fast, or is difficult to understand
Often irritable or unhappy
Easily distracted, impulsive
Quickly becomes frustrated
Clumsy and poorly coordinated
Touches everything and breaks things easily
Unaffectionate to others; has poor self-image
Sleeps badly
Constantly thirsty

lates (aspirinlike compounds) in fruits and vegetables. His diet excluded all these items and he claimed that 70 percent of children improved considerably on this regime. Subsequent studies have not endorsed this, but they seem to show that there is a more modest level of improvement. For a small percentage of children, the Feingold diet makes a dramatic difference.

It would appear from more recent studies that food additives are important in a great many children with hyperkinetic syndrome, but that it is unusual to find a child for whom additives are the sole problem. Most also show sensitivity to various commonly eaten foods, pollen, dust, other common allergens, and chemicals. The role of natural salicylates seems to be a minor one. When food and other allergens are considered as well as additives, 50 to 80 percent of children respond, although not all of them are completely cured. Sensitivity to unavoidable synthetic chemicals, such as solvents and the contaminants of natural gas, may account for the partial success with some patients.

In one recent study carried out in Britain, impressive results were obtained with a group of boys who were both hyperactive and habitual criminals. Ten boys, age seven to seventeen, were chosen for the study, and put on a very restricted diet of lamb, turkey, vegetables, and fruit. Six improved dramatically, and two more improved after the third week on the diet. Their hyperactive and aggressive behavior improved and, for the five who stuck to the diet, criminal behavior has also stopped so far.

Although Feingold's theory was not entirely right, he was correct to single out food additives for blame—they do seem to play a disproportionate role in hyperactivity compared with other types of illness such as asthma or eczema. This suggests that enzyme deficiencies may contribute to hyperkinetic syndrome, because such additives need to be detoxified by the body's enzymes. They may also prevent some enzymes from working properly (see page 300). The involvement of additives may explain why the incidence of hyperkinetic syndrome seems to have increased dramatically in the past twenty years—a period that has seen the meteoric rise of junk food, fast food, and instant everything. All these convenience foods tend to be rich in colorings, flavorings, preservatives, and other additives.

Recognizing Hyperkinetic Syndrome

The first step for parents is to decide whether their child's behavior really is abnormal. As Dr. Philip Graham of the Institute of Child Health in London points out:

All normal children show some degree of aggressiveness, disobedience, and antisocial behavior: all at times show sadness, depression, anxiety, and social withdrawal. All are at times unusually active and distractible. What makes a child a cause for concern is the severity and persistence of the problematic behavior in question.

Although a child like Matthew clearly shows abnormal behavior, others with hyperkinetic syndrome may only be mildly affected. In such cases it may be quite difficult to distinguish hyperkinetic syndrome from normal behavior—emotional upset and misconduct may be due to family tensions, lack of discipline, an unsettled home life, difficulties at school, or a great variety of other causes. It is very tempting for parents to attribute their child's awful behavior to some simple external cause when the real problem lies within the family. Conversely, some parents may find lively, childish behavior disruptive and label it hyperactive when in

---

David

David was very restless as a baby and slept little. By the time he could toddle he was a constant worry to his mother, because he was into everything and could not be left alone for a minute. Getting him to bed in the evening was almost impossible, and when he was forced to do something he did not want to do he could throw violent tantrums. Like many children, David was fond of sugary foods and liked ice cream, soda, chocolate, and potato chips. Since he was still only three it was relatively easy to exclude all these items and other common foods, such as milk and eggs, from his diet. On this diet he showed a dramatic improvement. He began to sleep through the night, and became much less active—for the first time he could sit down and watch a television program through to the end. When he had been on this diet for ten days he was tested with various foods. After eating a small square of chocolate he became very aggressive and rushed around the house frantically banging doors and kicking furniture. Then he became dopey and fell into a deep sleep that lasted for several hours. Similar reactions occurred when he was given sugar, milk, and oranges. Avoiding these foods has produced a great improvement in his behavior.

fact it is perfectly normal. Parents may not always be the best judge of what is wrong with their child, and it is a good idea to discuss the problem with a sympathetic teacher, doctor, or child psychiatrist, keeping an open mind about the possible causes of the problem.

Even if the child *is* showing hyperkinetic syndrome, the problem may be emotional rather than dietary, but certain clues point to food or additives as the triggers. Physical symptoms, such as muscle aches, stomachaches, rashes, headaches, or bowel problems, usually accompany the mental symptoms in those who are sensitive to something in their diet or environment. (Such symptoms can also be produced psychosomatically, however; see page 195.) A pale, flushed, or blotchy face is another indicator, and an intense thirst is seen in many of these children. In general, it seems that those with atopic symptoms—hay fever, perennial rhinitis, asthma, or hives—are far more likely to respond to dietary treatment.

Differences in behavior between home and school are not uncommon in hyperkinetic children, but they do not really help in deciding whether the problem has dietary origins. The perceptions of parent and teacher are not always the same, for one thing. Parents may be more critical of their child's behavior than a teacher, or less critical. Or it may be that one environment is overstimulating for the child—a classroom full of other children with colorful posters covering all the walls may be so distracting for a mildly hyperkinetic child that he or she behaves far worse than usual. Such children need special teaching in a quieter and less stimulating environment. Children who behave well at school but badly at home may be responding to family tensions, or they may find it easier to accept discipline in the more formal atmosphere of a school.

For some children, however, differences in food and chemical exposure between school and home may explain different behavior patterns. It is worth investigating what the child eats for school lunch, or how much candy is consumed at breaktime, if school behavior tends to be worse. For children who show chemical sensitivity, cleaning materials, disinfectants, floor wax, fumes from the heating system, marker pens, and other items used in school may be to blame. Conversely, items used around the home, such as perfumes, aerosols, and air fresheners, may make the child more unmanageable than at school. But it makes sense to consider other explanations first, because family problems are far more likely to be the source of trouble than household chemicals.

What to Do about Hyperkinetic Syndrome

Hyperkinetic syndrome can begin in infancy. Babies who sleep little and cry frequently often go on to become hyperkinetic. If there are no obvious reasons for the baby showing this disturbed behavior, then the role of diet should be considered. Follow the guidelines given on pages 275–84.

For older children, there are more complex issues to think over before deciding on a course of action. Restricted diets are socially disruptive and can sometimes be nutritionally inadequate, especially if the child is sensitive to a variety of foods. With mild behavioral symptoms, it may be better to cope in other ways than to try a dietary approach. For a child who is very disruptive, however, there is little to lose by trying a diet. Although it might seem impossible to get cooperation from such a child, given his or her usual behavior, this should not put you off. If the child does respond, the early stages of the diet may produce a remarkable improvement that makes the subsequent stages a great deal easier for all concerned.

Do not attempt any diet without consulting your family doctor or specialist. If your child is seeing a child psychiatrist who is totally unsympathetic to dietary ideas, then ask your family doctor to refer you to someone else—an allergist, for example, or a more open-minded psychiatrist—who will be prepared to supervise an elimination diet.

Specialists may have their own preferences regarding the diet, but if not, the three-stage diet given in chapter 14 can be used. Once they get to Stage 2, children may need a calcium supplement to compensate for the lack of milk in the diet, and the doctor can prescribe this. Children who also have asthma should be tested cautiously. *Any child who has had severe allergic reactions or asthma attacks in the past should not be tested for foods at home: the reaction can occasionally be life threatening.*

Drugs used to control behavior, such as amphetamine derivatives, can be continued during the diet. If there appears to be an improvement in behavior then you can try delaying the medication, or reducing the amount, but keep an eye on the situation and be prepared to top up the dose if necessary. *Needless to say, you should talk to your doctor before making any changes to the child's medication.*

Although in some children there will be a dramatic response to the diet, in others the reaction may be more subtle. Bad behavior may seem a lot worse on a day when the washing machine has flooded the kitchen floor than on a day when everything has gone well. To help you assess your child's reaction to the diet objectively, you should keep a scorecard

TABLE 9 SAMPLE SCORECARD FOR A HYPERACTIVE CHILD

Dates: From . . . .   To . . . .

Scores: 5 = very bad, much worse than usual
4 = bad, worse than usual
3 = about the same as usual
2 = a little better than usual
1 = much better than usual
0 = no sign of this behavior

Symptoms	Mon	Tues	Wed	Thur	Fri	Sat	Sun
Fidgeting							
Aggressiveness							
Crying							
Overexcitement							
Touching everything							
Inability to concentrate							
Aching muscles							
Stomachache							
Thirst							
Anxiety							
Unclear speech							
Total							

NB The symptoms shown here are just given as examples. When drawing up your own table, you should include each of your child's symptoms, making the list as long or as short as it needs to be.

of symptoms for each day. An example of such a sheet is shown opposite, but the exact symptoms written in the left-hand column will vary for each child. Draw up your own scorecard and get enough photocopies made to last for two or three weeks. Start filling them in at least a week before you embark on the diet so that you have a baseline from which to judge the effect of the diet. Make sure you sit down and fill the form in every evening, after your child has gone to bed, and try to be objective. You will learn most from the diet if you can time it so that there are not too many parties, outings, or other disruptive events, especially during the retesting period.

Always bear in mind that *the diet may not be the answer.* If you pin all your hopes on it, you may see improvements where there are none, and in the long run this could be very damaging to your child. Be careful, also, not to give the child the impression that the diet will make everything all right. A child may be so anxious to please you that he or she tries extra hard to be good. Psychogenic reactions to food testing (see pages 201–2) can occur just as easily in children as in adults, and if they know they're expected to go wild when they try milk, they may well oblige. Throughout the diet, try to keep an open mind about the outcome, and do not put any ideas into the child's head about what might happen.

On the other hand, you do need children's cooperation, especially if they're old enough to go out and buy candy or other foods for themselves. Rather than forcing a diet on them, you should explain that it might help and ask if they would like to try it. You need to impress on them that it will only work if it is done properly—there must be absolutely no cheating.

Sean

Sean, age thirteen, was on the point of being expelled from school for his aggressive behavior, uncontrollable temper, and vandalism. Although he was obviously intelligent, he could not concentrate in class and disturbed other pupils. He had been referred to a psychologist, but none of the forms of therapy that had been tried made much difference. Then, by chance, the psychologist discovered that Sean drank cans of cola all through the day, and ate a huge amount of chocolate. Sean admitted to feeling shaky and unwell when he hadn't had a can of cola for several hours.

The psychologist referred Sean to an allergist, who found that the boy also suffered from stomach pains and a constant runny nose. By eliminating cola and chocolate from his diet, Sean recovered from these physical symptoms, and his behavior improved considerably. He was allowed to stay at school and began to catch up on the education that he had missed. Five years later he is still well—though he still has to keep off chocolate and cola—and about to go to college. Not all disruptive, aggressive children respond so well to diet, but a significant percentage do.

Because food additives can be important in hyperkinetic syndrome, you need to be aware of other ways in which they can be consumed. The colorings in toothpaste are identical to certain food colorings, so white toothpaste should be used. Put any colored toothpaste well out of reach. Medicines also contain colorants, often in very large amounts, which is why you should try to discontinue syrups and tablets during the diet (as long as your doctor agrees) or get coloring-free alternatives. Try to stop your child from chewing things, and from licking sticky paper or stamps. Bear in mind that there can be additives in unlabeled food such as bread from a bakery and hamburgers, french fries, or other take-out and restaurant food. For more details on additives see appendix 6.

The timing of responses in the diet varies. Most children recover within a week or two on the initial stages of the diet, but others take up to three weeks. Foods should only be tested after there is a noticeable and sustained improvement. If this does not occur, then revert to the normal diet and consider other options. It may be that your child has chemical sensitivities—reading chapter 9 should help you assess this possibility. Be prepared to reconsider the likelihood of emotional stresses and strains.

The procedure for testing foods is slightly different for hyperkinetic syndrome. Although a few children may take up to a week of daily feeding with the culprit food before they respond, this is probably fairly unusual. The response time for most is between fifteen minutes and four hours. Reintroduced foods should be fed in the morning, and again in the afternoon if there was no reaction, or only a slight reaction, to the first feeding. A normal-sized portion should be eaten, except with children who have asthma or urticaria, then try a very small amount first, in case there is a severe reaction. If there is no reaction to the food by the morning after, then it can be incorporated into the diet, and testing begun on a new food. As always in an elimination diet, it is important not to eat too much of any one food.

Assuming the diet is effective and you discover what foods or additives cause the problems, then you have to decide on a plan of action. Again, you should discuss this with your doctor. Avoiding the foods in question may be quite difficult, especially at school or with friends, and you may wish to reconsider other options, especially if your child is not affected all that severely or reacts to a great many foods. Drugs are one option, and you should discuss the pros and cons of these with your doctor. Another, more controversial form of treatment is neutralization therapy.

Although not accepted universally within the medical professions, there are many reports of it being used successfully for the treatment of hyperactive children. For more details see pages 360–62. A recent study suggests that enzyme-potentiated desensitization (see page 362) could also be helpful for children whose hyperkinetic syndrome is linked to food intolerance.

If you decide on avoidance of the food, bear in mind that the child's sensitivity may disappear in time. The culprit foods should be retested at one- or two-year intervals, to see if they still produce the same symptoms.

Although most children remain well as long as they stick to their diet, a few seem to relapse after a few years for no apparent reason. It may be that they have developed new sensitivities to foods, or that they are becoming sensitive to synthetic chemicals. In general, children with hyperkinetic syndrome are likely to fare better if their exposure to synthetic chemicals (see pages 218–19 and 303–4) can be minimized. They should also be encouraged to get plenty of outdoor exercise and eat a good healthy diet.

Investigating Food Sensitivity in Babies and Toddlers

You should check that your doctor approves of the measures suggested here. Do not make any substantial changes to the child's diet, or your own (if breast feeding), without medical supervision.

Bottle-Fed Babies

If your baby is being fed with cow's milk or cow's-milk formula and you suspect that this may be the cause of the symptoms, then ask your doctor to prescribe a "milk-free" formula (not always strictly milk-free). These are of three types: **soy-based formula; comminuted chicken formula;** and **hydrolyzed formula** or **hydrolysate,** such as Alimentum and Nutramigen. The hydrolysates are made up of cow's milk, cornstarch, and other foods, but treated with digestive enzymes (see page 21) so that the milk proteins are partially broken down. This makes them a great deal less allergenic, although they still cause problems in some children who are highly sensitive to cow's milk. For these children there are some new products on the market called **whey hydrolysates.** These are made from the whey of cow's milk—the liquid part that is produced when the milk is curdled or separated. (The other hydrolysates, made from the milk solids, are called **casein hydrolysates,** as their main protein is casein.) Since whey proteins are less allergenic than casein, these hydrolysates are potentially useful for highly allergic babies, but even they have produced serious problems occasionally.

With hydrolysates generally, some are designed for treatment of an existing allergy, others for preventive use in bottle-fed babies who are at high risk of developing milk allergy. The ones used for treatment are more highly digested than those used for prevention.

Do not expect instant results, especially if the baby has diarrhea or colic—it may take up to two weeks for the baby's digestive system to return to normal. If there is no improvement, discuss the situation with the doctor, and consider trying another type of "milk-free" formula—it may be that one works for your baby while another does not.

In general, there is evidence that children who have developed a sensitivity to cow's milk may become sensitive to soy proteins as well if they consume them in large quantities. For a young baby who has several more months of formula to come, the hydrolysates are thus a better choice than soy formulas.

Should the baby recover on one of these alternative formulas, then test cow's-milk formula about a month later, to see what effect it has. It may be that the switch to an alternative formula happened to coincide with a spontaneous recovery. Or the sensitivity to cow's milk could have cleared up thanks to a month of avoidance. Either way, the baby can now return to ordinary cow's-milk formula.

For babies who seem to react badly to all the different formulas, the possibility of some other cause, such as an infection, should be reconsidered. If all such causes have been ruled out and there is strong evidence for food sensitivity being at the root of the problem, then breast milk is the best solution. Inquire about the possibility of donated breast milk from a milk bank—you may be fortunate enough to live in an area where such a bank has been established. Alternatively, there is relactation—returning to breast feeding. This is not possible for everyone, and it is not something to be undertaken lightly, but it may be the only answer for some babies. Help can be obtained from breast-feeding advisory groups (addresses are given on pages 454–55). Mothers who choose this course of action should not drink cow's milk themselves, nor should they eat butter, cheese, yogurt, or soy.

For the older baby, early weaning may be the answer, although it involves the risk of sensitizing the child to even more foods or—if all high-risk foods are avoided—failing to give the child an adequate diet.

Early weaning is only recommended if the baby is suffering quite badly and you have exhausted all other possibilities. It would not be appropriate, for example, in the case of a colicky baby who is otherwise well and growing normally. If you decide to try early weaning, remember the following points:

1. Certain foods seem to contain more potent allergens than others. Do not give the child eggs, fish, chocolate, wheat, oranges, peanuts, or other nuts for at least the first six months, and preferably for the first year of life. If you introduce them before a year old, do not give them every day. Test beef and chicken cautiously, because these can cross-react with milk and eggs, respectively. If they seem to cause no problems, you can include them in the child's diet.

2. Formulas commonly contain corn and tapioca, as well as cow's milk, so your child may have become sensitive to these. Avoid these foods for at least six months and then try them carefully. Corn comes in many guises, including cornmeal, cornflakes, corn oil, corn syrup, sweet corn, corn-on-the-cob, and popcorn. Some medicines contain corn syrup: ask your pharmacist for advice if you are concerned about avoiding all corn products.

3. No food should be eaten in very large quantities, and it is best not to give any one food every day. This means using your imagination and buying some fairly unusual items. Foods such as millet and sweet potatoes make a good basis for baby foods, and if the baby does become sensitive to them, at least they are no trouble to avoid in later years. Appendix 5 lists the main "rare foods" and describes how to prepare them.

4. Do not force the child to eat any food that is obviously disliked. Most children reject new foods the first time they are offered, but if your child clearly finds a food disagreeable even after trying it three or four times, then don't serve it again. A dislike of the taste is sometimes an early sign of sensitivity.

5. If a child is not eating eggs, milk, or fish, there is a risk of protein being in short supply. Make sure that you include other protein-rich foods, such as lamb, pork, and other meats. Beans are a good source of protein, but they are also rather indigestible and cause gas; chickpeas (see pages 410–11) are less of a problem and have a milder taste.

6. Your child will probably need a calcium supplement, and the overall diet should be checked by a pediatric nutritionist to see if it contains enough other minerals, as well as vitamins. Ask your doctor to arrange this for you.

Breast-Fed Babies

With breast-fed babies who are thought to have food sensitivity, the first step is to check that it is not something other than breast milk causing the problem. Think about what else the baby consumes, and if possible eliminate everything except breast milk, including medicines (with your doctor's approval), vitamin drops (which often contain artificial coloring), nipple creams containing peanut oil (see page 74), fruit juices, and any solids. If the baby needs to continue taking medicines or vitamins, ask the doctor to prescribe something that does not contain any coloring or other unnecessary ingredients. You may need to give boiled water to compensate for fruit juices or other extra liquids that you have withdrawn.

If this has no effect, the next step is to compile a list of suspect foods from those that you are eating. Keep a record of everything you eat, including the quantities and times of eating as well. Make a separate record of your baby's symptoms, along with their time, duration, and intensity. Continue this for a week or two, then compare the two records to see if there are any likely suspects. The time interval between the mother eating the food and the baby suffering symptoms can vary from one to several days.

Don't make the mistake of thinking that the problem must be cow's milk just because this is the food problem that we hear about most often in babies. For the exclusively breast-fed baby, it could be any food. However, babies who have received supplementary bottle feedings (see pages 311–12) are more likely to react to cow's milk than anything else. Even if you have never given a bottle feeding yourself, it is possible that the baby received one from a nurse while in the maternity ward.

The foods that are most likely to cause problems are those that you always eat in large quantities or binged on during pregnancy, those you have a craving for, and, paradoxically, those that you actively dislike but eat because they do you good. You should also be suspicious of foods that are known to be potent allergens. Apart from milk, these are: eggs, peanuts, other nuts, wheat, chocolate, fish, oranges and other citrus fruits, chicken, and beef. If you eat a lot of any of these foods, then add them to your list.

Anything with a druglike action, such as coffee, tea, wine (especially red wine), beer, spirits, or other drugs, is also a prime suspect, especially in the case of colic. Try cutting out all these druglike items, plus cow's milk, for two weeks and see if the baby improves. Eat extra protein from other sources and take a calcium supplement, which your doctor can prescribe.

If there is no improvement, then you should try eliminating all the other suspect foods that you have listed. Avoid them for two weeks, but substitute other foods that will fulfill your nutritional needs. Remember to cut out all the hidden forms of foods, especially with ubiquitous foods such as milk, eggs, and wheat. Read the labels on packaged foods carefully and see appendix 3 for some of the synonyms used, as these can be deceptive. Avoid all restaurant or take-out food during this time, too; it's difficult to know what you are eating.

If you have cut out more than two or three foods, and your baby gets better, then you will probably wish to test the foods to see which ones were the cause of the trouble—often it will just be one food. Wait until the baby has been well for about a week and then reintroduce each food in turn, beginning with those least likely to cause trouble, and testing cow's milk last. Eat a normal-sized portion of the food to be tested every day for a week. If the baby remains well, discontinue that food and go on to test another one, again eating it every day for a week. Make a note of which foods cause symptoms and which do not. When all have been tested, those that produced no symptoms in the baby can become part of your normal diet again.

It is possible that the baby will remain well and not respond to any of the foods—a brief period of avoidance can sometimes clear up the sensitivity. If this happens, continue with your normal diet, but be careful not to eat too much of any one food.

If cow's milk does turn out to be the problem, you can try drinking sheep's or goat's milk instead, after a few weeks. But keep an eye on the baby's symptoms—he or she may have problems with these milks, too, because of cross-reactivity (see page 375) between the proteins. If so, give up all animal milk for a while and try soy milk instead.

Above all, make sure you are getting enough protein, vitamins, and minerals, and avoid any drastic changes in your diet. If your list of suspect foods is very extensive, it may be better to split them into two groups and try eliminating each group in turn. Consult your doctor to see if your diet is adequate.

Janice, Ben, and Amy

Janice had suffered a range of health problems for years, including irritable bowel syndrome, migraine, and severe premenstrual tension. She could no longer drive, because she had had two car accidents: "I was just fuzzy in the brain, I couldn't function. I found it difficult to even get out of bed in the morning and get the children to school." She was then about thirty-five and had suffered migraines since childhood, but the other problems had only come on in her thirties. Her son, Ben, developed asthma at five years old, along with glue ear, producing deafness. Amy, her daughter, developed eczema and glue ear. Janice thought about food intolerance, and, suspecting that it might be the source of her own health problems, went onto a very simple diet of fruits, vegetables, milk-free margarine, meat, and fish. The improvement was prompt and dramatic. A year later, when both children were quite severely deaf due to glue ear, Janice decided to try the diet out on Ben. "We had to go back to the doctor a week later for a checkup, and he was amazed. There was almost no trace of asthma, and Ben's hearing was normal. The doctor had to accept that the diet had done the trick. If Ben has to break the diet for some reason, the symptoms always come back." When Amy, too, went on the diet, her eczema and glue ear both cleared up. The doctor advised Janice that their food intake be checked by a nutritionist, to make sure that the children, in particular, were getting all the nutrients they needed. "It's hard work, because I can never use convenience foods, but we are all so healthy that I think it's worth it," Janice concludes.

If none of this works, then you could try a full elimination diet as a last resort—but you must ask your doctor first. The elimination diet is fairly stringent and there is a risk that you'll become undernourished, because milk production makes heavy demands on your body. You should eat plenty of meat and fish while on the diet to ensure you get enough protein, and a vitamin and mineral supplement may be necessary. Chapter 14 outlines the procedure for the elimination diet—you should have already completed the equivalent of Stage 1, so you can go straight into Stage 2.

If you manage to resolve the baby's problems but find yourself on a quite restricted diet, then you should retest foods after a month or two. It may be that the baby's sensitivity has cleared up of its own accord; you can then return to normal eating. If the symptoms recur, go back to the restricted diet.

Older Babies and Toddlers

For older infants who are taking some solid food, try cutting out different foods in turn, but replace them with others that are equally nutritious. Begin with the most common offenders: milk, milk products, and chocolate. Cut out beef at the same time, because this can sometimes cross-react with milk. If the child is eating any food or drinks containing additives, these should be avoided as well. Next try eggs and chicken, then nuts and peanuts, then citrus fruits, then fish. Omit each food or set of foods for about two weeks before going on to the next set.

If the child gets better when certain foods are excluded, then they should be reintroduced to check that they were the source of the trouble. Begin with a very small amount and watch carefully for reactions—these can sometimes be severe. Particular care is needed for children with atopic eczema (see page 80). Some doctors recommend that no foods should be reintroduced until the child is more than a year old, to minimize the risk of future sensitivity. This is probably a good idea, but it means that you may never know if the food you avoided was indeed the guilty party, because the child is likely to have outgrown the sensitivity by the time the food is eaten again.

If these measures are unsuccessful, then it may be worth carrying out an elimination diet, as described in chapter 14. *In no circumstances should you do this without help and advice from your doctor*—restricting the diet of small children can be very dangerous.

In the case of eczema, it may be better to start with a simplified form of the elimination diet. Rather than cutting out a whole range of foods, concentrate on the foods that are known to be problematic in eczema: milk, eggs, beef, chicken, food additives, oranges, lemons, and other citrus fruits. These should be avoided during the exclusion phase of the diet (see pages 341–42) and then, if the eczema clears up, tested in the normal way during the reintroduction phase (see pages 346–49). If there is no response to the exclusion phase, then cut out nuts, fish, wheat, tomatoes, lamb, peanuts, and soy as well. Should this produce no results, then you could consider trying Stage 3 of the elimination diet (see page 349), but only if the eczema is bad enough to justify this, *and* if your doctor agrees.

Staying Well

Once you have established a diet on which the child remains well, be careful not to allow too much of any one food. Have your child's food intake checked by a nutritionist—this is something that your family doctor should be able to arrange for you. Incidentally, the most common deficiencies in children on restricted diets are in calcium and iodine. Calcium is most likely to be deficient if there are no dairy products in the diet. It is also found in nuts, seeds, peas, beans, lentils, broccoli, and green leafy vegetables, so give your child plenty of these. Or you can get calcium gluconate tablets from your pharmacist. Iodine may be in short supply if dairy products, meat, and grains are not eaten. Other rich sources include fish (particularly sardines, salmon, tuna, and haddock), shellfish, pineapple, eggs, peanuts, lettuce, spinach, green peppers, and raisins. Some table salts have added iodine—look on the label. Seaweed is an extremely rich source and can be used as a supplement, but it is important not to eat too much, as excess iodine is also damaging.

Most children do grow out of their sensitivities gradually, and it is important not to keep them on a restricted diet any longer than necessary. Retest foods once or twice a year to see if they are still a problem. If the child has ever had a severe reaction, or suffers from asthma, then the retesting must be done very cautiously. Parents who have had one food-sensitive child will want to minimize their chances of having another, and some useful preventive measures are described in chapter 13.

Keeping Things in Perspective

It is natural to worry about children, especially when they are ill, but worrying too much can be very harmful to them. Children need to feel safe and secure about the world they grow up in, and it is unwise to give them the idea that everything they eat or come into contact with is a potential threat. Parents of allergic children have to walk a tightrope—on the one hand they need to warn their child about things to avoid, but on the other they must not make the child overanxious. Sometimes they must conceal their own fears to avoid alarming the child.

In some families the question of the child's health becomes entangled with other problems—a tense relationship between husband and wife, for example, or friction with grandparents or other relatives. It is not uncommon for one parent to use the child's illness for his or her own purposes in these domestic problems. For the child's sake, it is vital to

Stephen

Stephen was a little boy with a constantly runny nose and occasional attacks of "tummyache." He had never been particularly well behaved, but after his parents separated he grew much worse. When a teacher described him as hyperactive, his mother, Angela, felt food or food additives might be to blame. So she tried Stephen on an elimination diet. His runny nose cleared up, and he seemed to feel better generally. Angela also thought that his behavior improved, although the teachers were unsure.

The testing phase of the elimination diet did not go smoothly, because Stephen was uncooperative. As a result—and because any bad behavior was taken as a positive reaction by Angela—he seemed to be reacting to a lot of the food and additives that were tried out. Angela devised a very restrictive diet on the basis of these tests, and persuaded the school to help in getting Stephen to stick to it. But she was less successful with Stephen's father, Bob, who had Stephen to stay for one weekend every month.

Bob liked to indulge Stephen, since he saw the boy so little. He let him have all the treats that were forbidden at home—chocolate, chips, sodas, and more. When Stephen returned home his runny nose had usually returned, and he often behaved very badly. Angela saw both these as an outcome of the broken diet, ignoring the fact that many children whose parents have separated are disturbed after a visit to the noncustodial parent, becoming difficult and aggressive. Angela did not want to acknowledge that the breakup of the marriage had affected Stephen badly, because this would have made her feel guilty for not keeping the family together.

She became ever angrier with Bob for not taking the diet seriously, and tried to prevent the monthly visits. She had long wanted to sever all contact with Bob anyway, so the conflict over the diet became a means to this end. Her conviction that food and additives made Stephen hyperactive was now unshakable, even though he behaved pretty badly most of the time, regardless of what he ate. Angela had a vested interest in her fixed belief, which was now an obstacle to getting to the real root of Stephen's behavioral problems.

try to keep these issues separate from the question of illness and treatment. If there is disagreement over how seriously ill the child is, or how the illness should be dealt with, try to discuss these matters quietly when the child is not there, and agree on a common approach. Arguing things out in front of the child may give him or her the idea that the illness can be used to manipulate difficult family situations—which can create yet more trouble in the future. Talking the matter over with a sympathetic doctor, teacher, or other professional may be helpful.

As children grow older and start going to school, it is very important that they feel as normal as possible. Anything that makes them different is likely to lead to teasing by other children. So you should try to minimize restrictions on diet and environment as much as possible. If you can keep your home free of allergens and other offending substances, your child's health may be good enough for him or her to tolerate limited exposure at school. This may be less damaging overall than the psychological effects of feeling alienated from normal school life by constantly having to avoid certain classes or not eat school food. Make sure your child gets enough exercise, so that he or she is fit and not overweight. This will make integration with other children a great deal easier. A well-adjusted, happy child is less likely to be physically ill (see chapter 8), so it is important to get the balance right.

If the child is allergic to certain foods, and if the reaction is not too severe, then the drug cromolyn sodium (see pages 431–33) may be useful, although it does not work in all cases. The drug can be taken before special events such as birthday parties or holiday dinners, and allows the child to eat forbidden foods without any symptoms. Unfortunately, it is not usually effective if taken long term.

Munchausen-by-Proxy and Meadow's Syndrome
Baron von Münchausen was an eighteenth-century Hanoverian soldier who greatly exaggerated his prowess in war—and his battle scars. *Munchausen syndrome* is the name given to attention-seeking patients who feign illness or deliberately fabricate symptoms. There are instances, fortunately very rare, of mothers simulating illness in their children in order to get medical attention. This is known as Munchausen-by-proxy or Meadow's syndrome, after Professor Roy Meadows, who first described two cases in 1977. Doctors are far more aware of this possibility in children than they once were, and any parent attempting to fabricate symptoms is likely to be found out very quickly.

The question of Meadow's syndrome in relation to food sensitivity is a difficult issue. Various doctors have described cases of children whose parents believe them to have food sensitivity, but where no consistent reaction to a food can be shown. If those parents seem overanxious or overprotective and have obvious emotional problems of their own, then the cases have often been labeled as Meadow's syndrome.

Eleven such cases were reported in 1984, in an influential article that has colored the outlook of many doctors and led to the belief that Meadow's syndrome is quite common in relation to food sensitivity. However, there were several important differences between the cases described in this article and Meadow's syndrome proper. For one thing, the children involved all had genuine symptoms, and there was no suggestion that the parents had attempted to fabricate any symptoms. Unlike Meadow's syndrome mothers, these women did not seem to relish their child's hospital stay, nor were they willing to subject them to any investigation, however painful and unpleasant. Such differences are important and must raise serious doubts about the conclusions reached— was the label *Meadow's syndrome* really justified? These parents may have been disturbed or overwrought, but this does not necessarily mean that they were mistaken about their child's illness. The elusive nature of the reactions seen in food intolerance makes it difficult to rule out this diagnosis without very thorough testing, and there seems to have been undue reliance on skin-prick tests in this study, despite the fact that these are unreliable indicators in most cases of food sensitivity. Despite the doubts over this study, the idea of Meadow's syndrome has become a popular one, especially among those doctors who are skeptical of food intolerance generally. This is unfortunate for parents, especially when such a diagnosis is made without proper testing for food sensitivity, and without any firm evidence of fabrication. There undoubtedly are cases of parents who exaggerate their child's ills and are determined to blame them on some physical cause when family tensions and emotional problems are actually the true source of the symptoms. But unless there is gross exaggeration or fabrication of symptoms, these should not be described as Meadow's syndrome.

From a parent's point of view it is important to be honest about family problems, to yourself, to your partner, and to others. Seeking help from a professional counselor when things begin to go wrong may help avert more serious problems. Try to insulate children from arguments, and to protect them from tense and difficult situations until they are old enough to cope with them. Children are just as susceptible to psychosomatic illness (see page 195) as adults are, and sometimes physical symptoms are an expression of their distress. If your child is ill, try to think about that separately from your other problems, and deal with it as rationally as possible. Be prepared to consider the possibility that it is nothing to do with food. Never exaggerate the child's ill health to anyone, and resist the temptation to manipulate other people by imposing special diets or other restrictions. Facing up to your own problems, and trying to resolve them, may be the best thing you could do for your child.

It has to be said that the existence of self-help books, such as this one, is regarded as part of the problem by some doctors. Munchausen syndrome is usually seen among those with some medical knowledge, such as failed medical students or nurses. Consequently, some doctors believe that ignorance is bliss—if medical knowledge were more widespread, there would be more cases of Munchausen and Munchausen-by-proxy. So books that seek to inform the public about illness are simply adding to the problem.

Our own viewpoint is that genuine cases of Munchausen or Meadow's syndrome are very rare, because these people are seriously disturbed. If they had not had medical knowledge, their mental problems would have surfaced in some other form. In the same way, many suicides jump from tall buildings—but removing all the tall buildings in the country would not stop people from killing themselves. Presenting ordinary, well-balanced men and women with medical knowledge does not turn them into cases of Munchausen syndrome; if it did, the problem would be far more widespread. On the other hand, lack of knowledge about food sensitivity has led thousands of children to suffer unnecessarily from symptoms such as colic, diarrhea, asthma, eczema, and migraine. Improving their lot is, in our view, far more important.

We hope that parents using this book will read it carefully, try to understand it fully, and use the information responsibly. Above all, consult your doctor and make every effort to work with him or her. The human body is very complex, and the human mind even more so—a book such as this can only provide a glimpse of the factors that may be involved in your child's illness. If you feel that the doctor regards you as an overanxious or difficult parent, then try to stay calm and state your case clearly. Remember what Kipling said: "If you can trust yourself when all men doubt you, but make allowances for their doubting too. . . ." It is "making allowances" that is difficult, but bear in mind that the doctor does see parents who are genuinely harming their children, either mentally or physically, and it is part of his or her job to consider all the possibilities in every case.

TWELVE

What Causes Food Intolerance?

The simple answer to the question, "What causes food intolerance?" is, "No one knows." Which is not to say that no one has any ideas about the subject—there are ideas and theories in abundance. There is even a certain amount of evidence for some of them. At present we are at the stage of picking through the ideas, looking at the meager evidence, and trying to make some sense of it all. Consequently, this chapter is rather like a detective novel with the last page missing. Those who like simple, cut-and-dried explanations would do well to go on to chapter 13 without delay.

One thing is clear: there is no single, straightforward mechanism behind all types of food intolerance. Even in the individual patient there may be more than one abnormality causing the symptoms. In fact, it is possible that there has to be more than one malfunction for the illness to materialize—in other words, the causes of food intolerance are like straws being added to the proverbial camel's back. One or two deficiencies in the body's functioning, or its environment, are tolerated. It takes several factors working together to produce the actual symptoms of food intolerance. This would explain why all patients are different in terms of the symptoms they show and the progress of their illness—because each person has a unique combination of circumstances leading up to that illness.

Is the Immune System Involved?

At the beginning of this book we defined *food intolerance* as "any adverse reaction to food, other than false food allergy, in which the involvement of the immune system is uncertain because skin-prick tests and other tests for allergy are negative. This does not exclude the possibility of immune reactions being involved in some way, but they are unlikely to be the major factor producing the symptoms." Because food intolerance has long been thought of as an "allergy," most research into its causes has centered on the immune system. It is only in the past ten years or so that other possible reasons for intolerance have been investigated.

Despite extensive research, the evidence for immune-system involvement is fairly limited. The general consensus of opinion now is that immune reactions may have some role in food intolerance in some people, but they are only part of the story—something else must be going wrong as well.

Oral Tolerance—How the Immune System Copes with Food

One line of research into food intolerance has investigated what normally happens to food in the healthy person. There is no reason why the immune system should not attack food molecules just as enthusiastically as it attacks invading germs—after all, food is chemically different from our own bodies, and the immune system relies on just such differences to recognize unwelcome aliens.

At one time it was thought that the gut wall rigidly excluded all food molecules, but this is not the case (see pages 23–24). In fact, the body *learns* not to mount a major immune attack on food. Certain parts of the immune system "examine" the foreign substances absorbed from the gut and "make a decision" about how the body should respond to each of them. No one knows at present exactly how it distinguishes dangerous microorganisms from harmless food molecules. But the smaller size of food molecules and their lack of stickiness is probably important— microbes have a habit of clinging to cell membranes, which is a potential giveaway.

Once the immune system has recognized a given molecule as food rather than foe, it produces a type of cell known as a **T-suppressor cell**, which is specific for that molecule and tones down the immune response to it. T-suppressor cells can also influence the type of antibody produced in response to a particular molecule. Some **isotypes** of antibodies (see page 28) produce inflammation when they bind to their antigen (in this case, the food molecule). One isotype does not—it is called immunoglobulin A or **IgA**, and it plays an important part in the body's response to food.

When microbes get into the blood from the gut, they are met by IgG and IgM antibodies. These bind to their antigen (a molecule on the surface of the microbe) and thus form **immune complexes**. Once bound, both IgG and IgM summon the body's defensive forces for an all-out attack, which may cause local damage to the body's own tissues, seen as inflammation. IgA is different—it has a "softly, softly" approach. Although it binds to its target to form immune complexes, it does not provoke inflammation. Circulating immune complexes containing IgA are mopped up by phagocytes or "eating cells"—the body's garbage-disposal team—without any fuss (see illustration titled "How Eating Cells Work," on page 292).

It will be clear that IgA is the ideal antibody for disposing of food molecules that accidentally make it through to the bloodstream. The process that leads to the body producing more IgA to food molecules and less IgG is called the **induction of oral tolerance**.

The idea that this process breaks down in food intolerance is an attractive one. At present, there is some evidence to support it, but not a great deal. It does seem, however, that patients with food intolerance make more IgG to food molecules in the blood, and less IgA. They may also produce a little IgE, so that the immune complexes could trigger off mast cells (see page 30).

Getting through the Gut Wall

There is evidence that people with food intolerance have leakier gut walls than healthy individuals—so they let more undigested food molecules through. This has major health implications that will be considered later, but how does the gut become leakier in the first place?

Inflammation, produced by immune attack, can make the gut wall leakier. One source of inflammation is disease—any gut infection that produces diarrhea may inflame the gut wall. In babies, such infections are often the start of food intolerance.

Alternatively, foods themselves might provoke inflammation of the gut wall, if there is a localized allergic response to them. This is not something that most allergists would agree with—they see IgE/mast-cell reactions to foods (see page 32) as all-or-nothing affairs that produce immediate and unmistakable symptoms. The idea that there might be a small-scale, localized IgE reaction whose main effect is to make the gut more permeable is not widely accepted. The main evidence in its favor is the effect of a drug, cromolyn sodium, on some patients with food intolerance.

The effects of this drug have mainly been studied in migraine patients. If such patients undertake an elimination diet, a large proportion of them get better (see pages 172–73) and can then identify one or more foods that provoke their symptoms. Each time a culprit food is eaten it will provoke a migraine—but not if cromolyn sodium is given in advance. Cromolyn sodium is known to stabilize mast cells and prevent them from releasing their inflammatory mediators. And the drug is not absorbed from the gut in any appreciable quantity. So the logical conclusion is that it prevents reactions to culprit foods by blocking mast-cell reactions in the gut wall. (Unfortunately for those with migraine, cromolyn sodium is not the instant cure that it might appear to be from these studies—see pages 432–33.)

There is a third way in which the gut wall might be made leakier. We all produce a special type of IgA antibody called secretory IgA or **SIgA**, which pours out into the gut, where it binds to its target antigen. By binding to antigens and locking them into immune complexes, SIgA effectively makes them much bigger. The bigger they are, the more difficult it is for them to pass through the gut wall. So SIgA reduces the number of food molecules that cross the gut wall—and the number of microbes, because SIgA is made to these as well. Like IgA in the blood, SIgA does not cause any inflammation.

There is some evidence that people with food intolerance have less SIgA than healthy people. However, there are patients who have severe deficiencies of SIgA, and, although they are ill in other ways, they show no more signs of food sensitivity than the population at large. This suggests that SIgA deficiency alone is not enough to cause food intolerance.

The Role of Immune Complexes

If more food molecules get through the gut wall, more immune complexes will form in the blood. There are certain diseases that produce an excessive load of immune complexes in the blood, too many for the eating cells to cope with. This results in **serum sickness**. The unpleasant symptoms of serum sickness are due to immune complexes depositing in small blood vessels (see page 97).

It has been suggested that some symptoms of food intolerance might come about in the same way. The reduction of IgA antibodies in the food-molecule immune complexes, and the presence of inflammatory antibodies such as IgE, would be likely to make the problem worse. The two main symptoms that might arise in this way are joint pain

How "eating cells" work

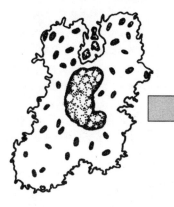 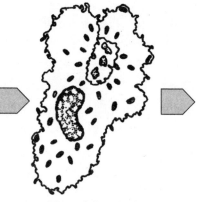

The phagocyte or "eating cell" can engulf bacteria coated with antibodies, immune complexes, and dead body cells.

Bags of enzymes inside the cell pour their contents over the items that the cell has "eaten."

and migraine. At present, however, firm evidence for this is lacking. In both cases there are certain to be other mechanisms at work as well (see pages 169–75).

Too Many Messengers?

There is one other way in which the immune system might be involved in food intolerance. All immune cells use small messenger molecules, known as **lymphokines**, to communicate with each other. One cell will produce a particular messenger molecule when it is stimulated, and this will make another cell become active, or divide rapidly to produce more cells, or respond in some other way.

One important messenger molecule is **interferon**, whose main job is to combat viral infections. Interferon makes cells resistant to viruses. Some of the less beneficial effects of interferon only came to light when it was used as a medicine. Hepatitis B is a debilitating viral disease that is very difficult to treat. The discovery of interferon led to its use in treating hepatitis B, because it can stimulate the body to mount a more effective attack against the virus. But the patients who were receiving

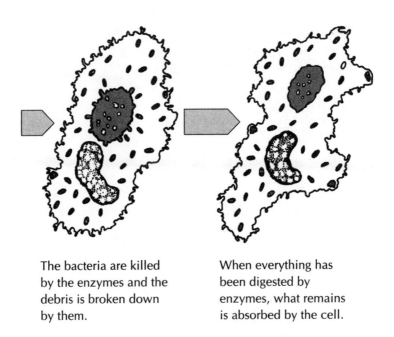

The bacteria are killed by the enzymes and the debris is broken down by them.

When everything has been digested by enzymes, what remains is absorbed by the cell.

large doses of interferon suffered from unpleasant side effects, including severe fatigue, headaches, dizziness, abdominal discomfort, bowel disturbances, nausea, and joint pain.

This list of side effects is remarkably similar to the symptoms of a mysterious and controversial illness that goes by the name of **post viral syndrome (PVS), chronic fatigue syndrome (CFS),** or **myalgic encephalitis (ME).** In looking for the causes of this illness, most doctors have concluded that it must be psychosomatic. However, most cases seem to follow on from a viral infection of some sort, and 50 percent of patients show a high level of antibodies to viral proteins. The parallel with interferon side effects suggests an alternative explanation to the psychosomatic one—that the immune system has overreacted to a viral infection and is continuing to produce excessive amounts of interferon. Alternatively, other lymphokines might be responsible for producing the symptoms—several others have similar effects.

If this is the case—and there is no definitive proof that it is—then interferon might also play a role in food intolerance. Perhaps there is some unknown immune reaction to food that stimulates the body to produce interferon, or other lymphokines, in damaging amounts. It is interesting that many PVS patients have been greatly helped by an elimination diet—it would seem that reactions to food are contributing to their symptoms. Some have also been helped by a no-sugar, no-yeast diet and antifungal drugs—see chapter 10.

Viral Infections

Viruses themselves might also play a part in food intolerance; it is known that they can alter our immune responses in subtle ways. Some people date their food intolerance to a bout of influenza or other viral infection.

Viruses in the gut could alter the structure of the gut wall, simply by binding to its cells—they might even do this without causing any noticeable signs of infection. Such viruses could make the gut wall leakier for a while by changing its structure.

The Exorphin Puzzle

A good half of patients with food intolerance have cravings for the food or foods that make them ill, and eat such foods to excess. Addictive eating is an aspect of food intolerance that does nothing to improve its credibility with orthodox physicians—yet it has been observed repeatedly and reported in respected medical journals. It exists and cannot be ignored. Within the past few years, a possible mechanism for this strange behavior has emerged in the form of chemicals called **exorphins**. To understand what exorphins do (or might do) we must first look at the **endorphins**.

Endorphins—Built-In Painkillers

Pain is all about survival. We have specialized nerves, known as pain receptors, to help us avoid damaging ourselves—on sharp objects, for example, or by overextending our joints. But there has to be a way of turning pain off when it no longer serves a useful purpose. For that reason we have endorphins or natural opioids.

Endorphins are natural painkillers, released during intense pain or strenuous exercise, or when some stressful event evokes our flight-or-fight response (see page 196). There are receptors for these molecules on cells in the brain. When the endorphins bind to these, feelings of pain are reduced, and a sensation of well-being ensues. (In fact, there are about four or five different types of endorphin receptor, and they have different effects—although blocking pain is the main one, there are others as well.)

Morphine, heroin, and other opiates happen to be chemically similar to endorphins and bind to the same receptors—hence their use as drugs. They are addictive because they suppress the body's natural ability to produce endorphins. When they are stopped, the addict suffers agonizing withdrawal symptoms.

Hooked on Food?

The endorphins are all **peptides**—short chains made up of amino acids. Proteins also consist of amino acid chains (see page 26), but the chains are much longer. When foods are broken down in the gut, the proteins are split into shorter lengths—in other words, into peptides. By chance, some of those peptides consist of a very similar sequence of amino acids to the natural endorphins. Such peptides are therefore called **exorphins** (exogenous morphinelike molecules). In the laboratory these exorphins have been produced from milk, wheat, corn, and barley, using human digestive enzymes. Other foods have yet to be investigated.

Further laboratory experiments show that exorphins can bind to the natural receptors for endorphins—but whether they actually do so in the body is another matter. First they would have to get through the gut wall and into the bloodstream. They would also have to evade protein-cracking enzymes in the liver; endorphins have a special chemical structure at the end of the molecule that prevents such enzymes from attacking them, but exorphins do not.

So can the exorphins have any effect on the body? One experiment suggests that they can. A partially digested sample of wheat protein was fed to human guinea pigs, and produced certain measurable changes in bodily function. The experiment was then repeated, with a drug called naloxone being given before the wheat. This drug is known to block endorphin receptors, and prevents peptides from binding to them. When naloxone was given first, the wheat protein had no effect.

Many more experiments are needed before we can reach any firm conclusions about exorphins, but the results so far suggest that they might influence our mood. There is certainly no question of anyone getting high on a glass of milk or a slice of bread—the amounts involved are too small for that—but these foods might induce a sense of comfort and well-being, as food-intolerant patients often say they do. There are also other hormonelike peptides in partial digests of food, which might have other effects on the body.

Rebecca

Rebecca began to have problems with severe sore throats when she was in her teens. At the same time she suffered "swollen glands" (swelling of the lymph nodes), producing painful lumps in her groin, armpits, and neck. The pain was often so bad that she had difficulty walking. She also felt bloated, with a noticeable puffiness around her face and neck, and she suffered spells of dizziness, when she would sometimes pass out. Eventually, her tonsils were removed, but this did not bring much improvement. Her throat was less sore, but it was still painful and swollen. In her early twenties Rebecca married, and although she was very happy with her new husband, her symptoms began to get worse. She frequently felt as if she had flu coming on, with aches and pains, headaches, and swollen glands. Severe catarrh, recurrent mouth ulcers, and stomach pains were also making life difficult.

All these problems came to a head when she was twenty-five and they moved. Looking back, Rebecca thinks it was the stress of moving that precipitated a crisis in her state of health. All her symptoms became more frequent and more severe, and she felt as if her body was "totally out of control." She also developed some new problems, including aching joints and bouts of severe depression. She had to give up her part-time job, and even simple tasks around the house became impossible.

Rebecca had seen many different specialists over the years, and none had been able to do much for her. But at this point she

If foods can produce these peptides, then why do they only affect certain people? It is possible that the leakiness of the gut wall is important here—if more peptides get through, more are likely to get to the receptors before they are broken down by enzymes. Any deficiency in those enzymes would also increase the person's vulnerability to exorphins.

Enzymes and Food Intolerance

Enzymes make chemical reactions happen, as described on page 21. The two main types of enzymes that concern us here are digestive enzymes and detoxification enzymes.

heard something about "food allergies" from a friend, and asked her family doctor if he thought this might be worth investigating. The doctor was skeptical but made an appointment for her to see a specialist, who put her on a strict diet, starting with a three-day fast. Then she went on a diet of lamb, pears, and mineral water. Within a week she felt so much better that she could scarcely believe it. Almost all her symptoms had gone, except for a few aches in her joints. "I had been ill for so long, I'd forgotten what it was like to be well—it was an amazing feeling," she recalls.

The long process of testing foods then began. Eventually Rebecca identified the following culprits: most types of additives, wheat, oranges, lemons, butter, strawberries, and alcohol. Eating any of these would produce swollen lymph nodes, depression, headache, stomach pains, aching joints, and general flulike symptoms within a few hours. It took her a long time to test all foods and establish a workable diet, but she now enjoys very good health and can eat a variety of foods. She can even tolerate small amounts of wheat and her other culprit foods occasionally, but has to avoid additives.

Cases such as Rebecca's are rare but they raise some interesting questions about what causes food intolerance. The swollen lymph nodes suggest that her immune system was affected by her reactions to foods, even though her symptoms were not those you would associate with allergy.

Digestive enzymes are mostly found in the gut, where they break food down into smaller molecules (see pages 23–24). The purpose of digestion is to reduce food molecules to their basic building blocks, which can then be used by the body to construct its own molecules— rather like demolishing an old house and then using the bricks to build something else. There are also some digestive enzymes (mostly protein-splitting enzymes) within the gut wall and in the liver; these complete the digestion of food molecules after they have been absorbed.

Detoxification enzymes are charged with destroying or disarming all the toxins that get into our bodies. Some of these toxins are found in food, where they mostly serve defensive purposes (see pages 17–18).

Others are produced by the bacteria living in our gut—the gut flora. To add to this natural load, there are a variety of synthetic substances that have to be detoxified, including alcohol and nicotine, medicinal drugs, food additives, and pesticide residues in food. Most of the body's detoxification enzymes are found in the liver, but there are also some in other parts of the body, such as the surface of the blood platelets—the tiny "cells" in the blood that help it clot.

Detoxification enzymes respond to the body's particular needs—if more toxin is taken in, then more of the appropriate enzymes are produced to cope with the added load. An obvious example of this is alcohol—the more we drink, on a regular basis, the more it takes to feel inebriated. Give up alcohol for a few months and a wine cooler is enough to make you tipsy. In effect, the body has become much more sensitive to the effects of alcohol, because the liver has scaled down its production of the necessary detoxification enzymes.

Although this works for alcohol, it is by no means certain that it works for all toxins—the body may only have a limited capacity to cope with some toxins, and increasing the load may not increase the detoxification enzymes. Even with alcohol there is a limit—the task of detoxification eventually becomes too much for the liver, which begins to fail. When this happens, the vital role that the liver normally plays becomes apparent—alcoholics suffer badly from the effects of natural toxins, especially those produced by gut bacteria, which they can no longer detoxify.

Enzyme Defects

In some people certain enzymes are either in short supply or fail to work properly because their structure is abnormal. Such people are said to have enzyme deficiencies. Some deficiencies have no obvious effects, because there are other enzymes that can cover for the missing one—the body often has more than one option, especially when it comes to digestion and detoxification. Other deficiencies are far more damaging, because the enzyme is the only one that can do a particular job. Toxic substances build up in the body if it fails to work.

Enzyme deficiencies have been known of for many years. The more serious ones become noticeable soon after a child is born, or after it is weaned, and can kill or severely disable the child unless treated. The usual treatment is a special diet that excludes foods that the child cannot deal with. The most widespread enzyme deficiency of this type is phenylketonuria; all babies are tested for this soon after they are born.

Another example of a major enzyme deficiency is a shortage of the enzyme lactase, which breaks down the sugar in milk (see page 259). Both of these enzyme defects are very rare—phenylketonuria only affects one baby in twelve thousand. A third type of enzyme deficiency has only been recognized relatively recently, and the frequency is, as yet, unknown. This defect prevents the breakdown of fructose—the sugar found in fruit and in table sugar. Luckily, children born with this deficiency soon develop a strong dislike of anything sweet, so they remain well as long as they are not forced to eat such foods. Parents should bear in mind that some apparently savory foods actually contain sugar, and the child's dislike of a food should be their guide. If a child has fructose intolerance, it may be helpful to tell the school that he or she should not be forced to eat any food that is actively disliked, as the reaction can be very unpleasant.

In recent years it has become clear that there may be other, less noticeable, forms of enzyme deficiency. Some of these have come to light when certain patients reacted very badly to particular medicinal drugs. It turned out that they were less able to detoxify them than most people. Special chemical probes have been developed in an effort to detect such patients—these are nontoxic compounds that are processed by the same enzymes and can readily be measured. The probe is given to the patient, and the level is later measured (in the blood or urine) to see how thoroughly the drug has been broken down.

When these probes are tried out on people with food intolerance, they produce interesting results. Such people are much more likely to be deficient in some enzymes than healthy people are—they do metabolize the drugs, but more slowly. However, there is no single enzyme that is defective in all food-intolerant individuals—or if there is, it has yet to be found. With enzyme defects, as with everything else, it looks as if food intolerance is a mixed bag.

One interesting factor to emerge from these experiments concerns patients who are sensitive to synthetic chemicals, as well as food (see chapter 9). In this group an even higher percentage are enzyme deficient than among those with food intolerance alone. For one enzyme, 90 percent of such patients were deficient, compared with 80 percent of those with food intolerance and 20 percent of the population at large. Interestingly enough, a high proportion of those with food allergy—64 percent—also showed a deficiency.

The fact that some apparently healthy people are deficient in these same enzymes is revealing. This clearly shows that a single enzyme defect of this type could not be the sole cause of food intolerance. Those who suffer from food intolerance must have other underlying problems as well—perhaps a shortage of another enzyme, a leaky gut wall, or some other problem entirely. It is tempting to speculate that people with multiple sensitivities (foods and chemicals) are defective for a whole range of enzymes, making them much more susceptible to environmental factors. But at present, there are too few studies of enzyme deficiency to know if this is likely.

Enzymes, Colorings, and Hyperactivity

One discovery about enzyme deficiencies is particularly intriguing, because it may explain the link between hyperactivity in children and food colorings (see page 268). Hyperactive children appear to be deficient in an enzyme known as phenolsulfotransferase-P or **PST-P**. This enzyme detoxifies various compounds, including a substance called p-cresol that is produced by bacteria in the gut. No one has any idea how p-cresol might cause hyperactivity, however it is a phenol, and phenols are known to be toxic.

What is interesting about PST-P is that it can be inhibited by certain food colorings—in other words, the enzyme no longer works if those food colorings are present. If a normal, healthy child eats coloring of this type in moderation, it will not do any apparent harm, because that child's PST-P is fully active to begin with. But for a child with defective PST-P, the same amount of coloring could reduce the level of PST-P activity to damaging levels.

It is interesting that a high proportion of patients with migraine, who are affected by dietary triggers such as cheese and chocolate, also have a defect in PST-P. Wine, like some food colorings, appears to inhibit PST-P, and this may contribute to the effects of red wine in triggering migraines. It is likely that enzyme defects play a part in migraine, because migraine sufferers tend to be defective for certain enzymes, but exactly what goes wrong is far from clear. The chemicals that are under suspicion of triggering migraine—tyramine and phenylethylamine (see pages 170–71)—are not detoxified by PST-P. Tyramine is detoxified by a related enzyme called PST-M, but this is generally not lacking in migraine sufferers. This is a puzzle that can only be sorted out by more research. For more on enzyme defects in migraine, see pages 173–74.

Bugs in the System

Our digestive tract is home to a great many bacteria and other microbes, which do not cause any disease, and are actually important for good health. They are known as gut flora. Some doctors believe that the composition of the gut flora becomes disturbed, and that this condition might contribute to food intolerance (see chapter 10).

A Modern Epidemic?

Is food intolerance becoming more common? It is impossible to answer this question, because there is little agreement on how common food intolerance is today (see pages 124–26) and no way of finding out how common it was in the past. But the general impression among doctors who treat food intolerance is that it has become increasingly widespread. There is little hard evidence to support this, apart from a few epidemiological studies. One of these concerns Crohn's disease in Africa. It shows that Crohn's disease—which has been linked with food intolerance in a proportion of sufferers (see pages 158–61)—is virtually unknown in rural areas, but becomes more common when people move into towns.

Crohn's disease is a serious and debilitating illness—most of those with food intolerance have much milder symptoms. Indeed, many people in the early stages of food intolerance may scarcely be aware of being ill: headaches, indigestion, persistent tiredness, and occasional diarrhea are all reported as the early symptoms by those who later become more seriously ill and then discover they are sensitive to food. Symptoms of this sort are everyday problems that most people tend to accept as part of life. But are they? Or have these things slowly crept up on us all, so that we have scarcely noticed a gradual decline in health? In her autobiographical book *Lark Rise to Candleford*, Flora Thompson recalls life in her native farming village during the 1880s:

> There were two epidemics of measles during the decade, and two men had accidents in the harvest field and were taken to hospital; but, for years together, the doctor was only seen there when one of the ancients was dying of old age, or some difficult first confinement baffled the skill of the old woman who, as she said, saw the beginning and end of everybody. There was no cripple or mental defective in

Carol

Carol was an active woman in her fifties who had a part-time secretarial job and was a voluntary worker at the local hospital. With a large family of children and grandchildren to worry about, she tended to ignore the odd aches and pains that she suffered. But as the years went by these grew worse, and finally began to interfere with her life. She had difficulty getting out of bed in the morning, her joints were so stiff, and it was only by the evening that she really loosened up and could move around normally. As well as joint pain, she began to suffer from diarrhea and gas, which was worse whenever she drank alcohol. Headaches became more regular until she had them almost every day, and she often had severe pains in her face due to sinusitis. She also suffered repeated vaginal yeast infections and an itchy rash between the toes that looked like athlete's foot. Her doctor put Carol on a sugar-free diet and prescribed an antifungal drug, nystatin. This made her feel much worse initially, but after a month her bowels were functioning normally, her joints were less stiff, and her headaches were less frequent. Since she was still not completely well, the doctor asked her to try an elimination diet, avoiding cereal grains, dairy products, and eggs. Carol was impressed by the change this brought about—she felt much better, less tired, and able to be cheerful without making an effort. She also lost some excess weight that she had accumulated. On testing, it turned out to be eggs and wheat that caused her problems. Having improved so much, she was now able to notice the specific effects of certain other foods. For one thing, she noticed that foods containing a lot of additives made her feel tired and unwell, with vague muscle aches. Cleaning the house also produced these sort of symptoms, and she found later that solvents, such as mineral spirits and dry-cleaning fluid, regularly had this effect.

As this case shows, there are often several different factors at work in individual patients. It is not unusual for food intolerance to go hand in hand with abnormal gut flora (see chapter 10) and sensitivity to synthetic chemicals. How these three problems might interconnect is still unknown.

the hamlet, and, except for a few months when a poor woman was dying of cancer, no invalid. Though food was rough and teeth were neglected, indigestion was unknown, while nervous troubles, there as elsewhere, had yet to be invented.

Contrast this with the general state of health of people today. As Dr. Ronald Finn of the Royal Liverpool Hospital observes: "It is depressingly rare to come across someone who is entirely well."

Doctors who are involved in treating food intolerance, as Dr. Finn is, may not be impartial observers, of course. But others have noticed the same general trend. The American psychiatrist Dr. Arthur Barsky calls it the "paradox of health." He points out that while in 1900 a man's life expectancy was 47.3 years, now it is almost 75 years—yet we feel we are less healthy. In the 1920s only 10 percent of recognized illnesses could be treated successfully; now the figure is more than 50 percent, but we are all preoccupied with illness. Why should this be? Dr. Barsky believes that it is all a question of attitude. One factor, in his view, is our "heightened awareness of health" due to "medico-media hype"—in other words, if people knew less about their bodies they would feel better.

An alternative explanation, which psychiatrists such as Dr. Barsky seem not to consider, is that people really are ill, with vague, long-term symptoms that are not life threatening and do not, therefore, reduce their life expectancy. Perhaps such problems have only become widespread within the past fifty to one hundred years—this could explain the "paradox of health" that Dr. Barsky describes. Such illness might simply be due to the increased stress of modern living, but the circumstantial evidence suggests that food intolerance could also be important.

Modern Life

A lot of things have changed in the past century. Of all the momentous changes that have occurred, is there anything that might have made people more susceptible to food intolerance? On the basis of what we already know about how food intolerance begins, there are several obvious candidates.

Chemical Exposure

The main one, in our view, is the increasing exposure to synthetic chemicals—food additives, pesticide residues, exhaust fumes, solvents, industrial pollutants, and the like. It is known (although only from case histories) that a single massive exposure to a toxic chemical, such as a pesticide, can bring on a severe form of food intolerance. It is also the case that a small proportion of people with food intolerance are unduly sensitive to everyday chemicals (see chapter 9). What is more, if those people can reduce their chemical exposure, they often find they can tolerate the foods to which they are sensitive normally. It seems likely that these people have certain enzyme deficiencies that make them vulnerable to synthetic chemicals and intolerant of certain foods—but if the chemical stress can be reduced, they are able to cope adequately with those same foodstuffs. Such people would not have been ill if they had lived a century ago, but they are ill now, because the environment around them has changed.

Environmental chemicals could also be a factor in others with food intolerance—even those who are not overtly sensitive to everyday chemicals. It is possible that chemicals in food and drinking water affect the gut wall, making it leakier—there might be no obvious effect from the chemicals alone, but they could create the right conditions for food intolerance.

Such chemical exposure might also play a part—along with other factors—in the rising levels of true allergy. We have already seen that patients with food allergy are more likely to be enzyme deficient than those with no allergy or intolerance (see pages 299–300).

Antibiotics

If changes in the gut flora are an important factor in food intolerance, then the use of antibiotics must undoubtedly shoulder some of the blame. The major antibiotics have only been in widespread use since the 1940s, and no one would deny their major contribution to medicine. Indeed, a short course of antibiotics is unlikely to do anyone much harm. It is prolonged use or a very high dose that is most likely to affect the gut flora. In some situations the antibiotics are not strictly necessary—in treating acne, for example, or in repeated childhood "infections" that are not really infections at all, but undiagnosed allergies. Antibiotics are often prescribed for viral infections, despite the fact that they do not kill viruses.

It is interesting that links are now emerging between true food allergy and the gut flora. There have been several different studies, but one of the best, published in *Clinical and Experimental Allergy* in 1999,

Increasing use of synthetic chemicals by farmers

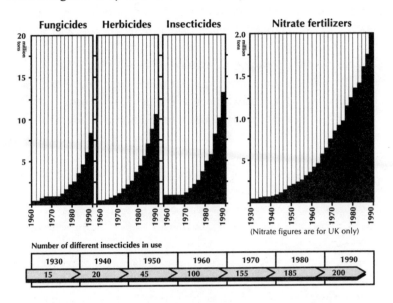

Number of different insecticides in use

1930	1940	1950	1960	1970	1980	1990
15	20	45	100	155	185	200

was based on research involving children in Sweden and Estonia. In both countries, those with food allergy had a different pattern of gut flora inhabitants, with fewer lactobacilli and more coliforms and *Staphylococcus aureus*. Other research has suggested that rising rates of allergy in general could be due to the eradication of intestinal worms, a medical advance that, some people now believe, may also be a contributing factor in Crohn's disease. Separate lines of research have now found that antibiotic use in babies under two is linked to an increased chance of asthma by the age of seven. Some antibiotics—the macrolide antibiotics andcephalosporins (erythromycin)—are linked with a greater subsequent asthma risk, according to a British study from 1998. This could be due to an effect on the gut flora or some impact on the maturing immune system.

Bottle Feeding and Early Weaning
The change from breast to bottle has been one of the major changes of the past fifty years. Although there is now a partial reversal of this trend, many babies are still bottle fed, and many more are given additional, or complementary, feedings from a bottle.

Several studies show that babies born into atopic (allergic) families are less likely to develop food allergies if they are exclusively breast fed for at least six months (see pages 310–11). During the first few months the immune system is not fully developed, and the oral tolerance mechanism described above does not seem to be fully functional. To make matters worse, the baby's gut is excessively leaky to allow protective antibodies from the mother's milk to get through to the bloodstream. These factors conspire to make the baby vulnerable to food allergy.

If food intolerance involves some type of immune reaction—even though it is not the major factor involved—bottle feeding and early weaning could also be a factor in causing food intolerance. So far there is not much hard evidence for the value of breast feeding in preventing food intolerance, because very little research has been carried out in this area. But there is good evidence that breast feeding is helpful in preventing colic.

The Pill

Oral contraceptive tablets—the Pill—have been in widespread use since the 1960s. Some doctors believe that the high incidence of food intolerance in women is related to this, and there are individual case histories that link the onset of food intolerance with starting the Pill. Unfortunately, there are no studies to show if this reaction is common. One of the difficulties with the Pill is that its ill effects are usually very much delayed—and even after stopping the Pill there may be lingering effects for months or even years. So the link with the symptoms may be far from obvious.

There are various ways in which the Pill might lead to food intolerance. It appears to have an effect on certain detoxification enzymes in the liver, and this could make women more susceptible to toxins in food, as well as to environmental chemicals. The Pill also seems to affect vitamin and mineral status (see pages 326–27), and some nutritional deficiencies may make food intolerance more likely. In the case of migraine, the hormones in the Pill have a direct action on the blood vessels and are well known as a cause of migraine.

THIRTEEN

Preventing Food Sensitivity

There is little doubt that food allergy runs in families, and food intolerance may do so as well. But this does not mean that illness is inevitable.

It is clear, in food *allergy* at least, that the environment is important, especially in the first year of life. What a child inherits is a *predisposition* to allergy. The sort of conditions a baby encounters immediately after birth (and, perhaps, before birth) will decide whether he or she actually develops allergies. Parents who know that their child is likely to suffer from allergies can take steps to reduce the risk.

With food *intolerance,* the case for prevention is less clear-cut. But where one member of the family suffers adverse reactions to food, it is worth considering various simple measures that may help others escape the same fate.

The Allergy Risk

The risks of a child developing allergies can be gauged, very roughly, from the health of the parents. If one parent has allergic symptoms, the chance of the child being atopic—predisposed to allergy—is 20 to 35 percent. If both parents have allergies, the likelihood rises to 40 to 60 percent. Where both parents are affected in the same way—if both have atopic asthma, for example, or both have rhinitis (runny or congested nose)—then the chance is 50 to 70 percent.

If neither parent has allergies but one or both come from families with a history of allergic disease, then there is also an increased risk of the child being affected. However, almost a third of atopics are born into families where no allergic symptoms have ever been noticed. So predicting which babies will be prone to allergies by looking at their families is, at best, an inexact science.

A more accurate prediction can be made by laboratory tests that measure the amount of IgE (see page 28) being produced by the child. The level can be measured by taking a sample of blood from the new-born baby, or by measuring the IgE level in blood from the umbilical cord. A high level indicates that a child has a greater chance of going on to develop allergies. Measuring a group of immune cells called T-suppressor cells, as well as the level of IgE, provides the best possible test for susceptibility to allergy. If both are high, the likelihood of allergy is more than 90 percent. However, both these tests require very sensitive chemical analysis, and they are unlikely to be available in most hospitals.

If your child happens to be given skin tests or specific IgE tests (RAST) at some stage, he or she may show up as having high IgE levels to certain foods. What should you do if the test for a particular food is positive but your child eats the food without apparent ill effects? You may well be told to ignore it, but in the opinion of many experts this is bad advice. One study of such children has shown that, within seven years, they usually go on to develop allergic reactions.

Preventive Measures for Food Allergy

The aim of the preventive measures described here (and summarized in table 10) is to reduce the child's exposure to potent allergens, and other factors that can trigger allergy, during the early phases of life. The measures are relevant to any immediate (IgE-mediated) reactions to food and to more delayed reactions such as asthma or eczema. In general, however, the former are more difficult to prevent, because the child can become sensitized by minute amounts of food. In the case of asthma, rhinitis, and eczema, a mixture of allergens may produce symptoms: the effect of allergens in food may be exacerbated by inhaled allergens such as pollen or by allergens touching the skin. For this reason, any preventive measures must include inhalants and contactants as well as foods.

TABLE 10 PREVENTIVE MEASURES FOR ALLERGY

These measures can help to prevent allergies developing in babies born into atopic (allergic) families. See the text of this chapter for further details.

- Don't eat too much of any one food while pregnant. It may also be worthwhile avoiding foods that are potent allergens (listed below), but there is no firm evidence that this is of benefit during pregnancy. Restricting your diet during breast feeding is much more important for the baby.
- Give up smoking before becoming pregnant. Once the child is born, make sure that no one smokes in the house.
- Breast feed for the first year if possible. Give nothing but breast milk for the first four to six months.
- If breast feeding is not possible, discuss with your doctor the possible alternatives, such as donated breast milk or hydrolysate formulas.
- While breast feeding, avoid eating foods that are likely to cause allergic reactions: milk, eggs, peanuts, fish, shellfish, citrus fruits (oranges, lemons, et cetera), wheat, beef, and chicken. To this list, add any food to which a previous child is allergic.
- After four to six months introduce some solid foods, but withhold those listed above until nine to twelve months. Withhold peanuts until the child is three years old.
- Introduce these foods gradually, one at a time, so that reactions can be noted. Do not give new foods when the child is ill.
- For the first year have no furred pets, keep dust mite infestation to a minimum, and keep the house free of molds (see page 86 for details). If the child has an infection, take special care to keep allergens to a minimum.
- When possible, avoid exposing the baby to air pollution. If you have a gas stove, change to an electric one or ventilate the kitchen thoroughly while cooking.
- Avoid unnecessary surgery and antibiotics during the first year of life.

Breast Feeding

A baby's immune system is not fully developed at birth. To protect it against infection in the first few months of life, a mother's milk contains antibodies to commonly found bacteria and viruses, and the baby's gut is leaky to allow these antibodies through into the bloodstream. Because the gut is so permeable, undigested food molecules also get into the blood in far greater quantity than in an older child or adult. At the same time, the control reactions that regulate damaging immune reactions are not yet up and running. In particular, the system that prevents the manufacture of IgE to harmless antigens is not fully effective.

Any food that the baby eats or drinks during the first three or four months of life will be absorbed into the bloodstream in appreciable quantities. Some unknown mechanism prevents babies from mounting damaging immune reactions against the proteins in their mother's milk— although there are cases of babies apparently being allergic to their mother's breast milk, these are *extremely* rare. Presumably, the process by which the baby learns to tolerate the breast-milk proteins happens before birth, while the baby is still in the womb.

A bottle-fed baby, or one who receives solids before three months of age, is exposed to large quantities of foreign proteins entering the bloodstream, and there is ample evidence that these can cause allergic reactions. Even a baby who is never bottle fed is not entirely safe. Proteins from the mother's food can be absorbed intact from her gut and pass into her breast milk. Although the quantities involved are small, there is little doubt that these can sensitize an atopic child. In fact, the most violent reactions to cow's milk are seen in children who have been sensitized via breast milk, rather than those who have been bottle fed from birth. This might seem like a good argument for bottle feeding on the face of it, but bear in mind that these violent reactions are rare, whereas the less severe but very troublesome symptoms that might result from bottle feeding are far more widespread.

The advice generally given to parents of high-risk babies is to feed nothing but breast milk for the first four to six months of life. Weaning should then be conducted at a very gradual pace, with breast feeding continuing until the child is a year old if possible. If breast milk is still supplying most of the baby's food needs, then the amount of solid food eaten can be much less. In addition, factors in the breast milk are thought to give useful messages to the baby's immune system regarding appropriate reacations to the new food allergens it is encountering.

When it comes to introducing new foods, those with low allergenic potential should be given first, and the foods that most often produce allergic reactions withheld for a time. The main problem foods are eggs, milk, fish, shellfish, peanuts, wheat, rye, barley, nuts, (peanuts and other nuts), soy, citrus fruits, and chocolate. Beef and chicken should also be kept off the menu, as they share some allergenic proteins with milk and eggs, respectively. A working party set up by the World Health Organization has suggested that such allergenic foods should not be given before the child's first birthday, and peanuts withheld until the child is three, but some doctors feel that avoiding them for six to nine months is adequate.

When they are introduced, new foods should be given gradually, one at a time, so that any adverse reactions can be related to particular foods. Infections and bouts of diarrhea make the child more easily sensitized, so new foods should not be introduced if the child is ill.

Because food molecules pass into breast milk, it is important for the mother to watch what she eats while breast feeding. She should avoid eggs, cow's milk, peanuts, and fish, and should restrict her alcohol intake, especially of red wine. It might also be worth avoiding soy, tree nuts, citrus fruits, wheat, barley, and rye. Calcium gluconate tablets can be prescribed to make up for the lack of calcium in a milk-free diet—or she can try goat's or sheep's milk, in limited quantities. If any previous children are highly allergic to specific foods, then these, too, should be excluded from her diet, and should not be given to the new baby in the first year.

If all these restrictions seem too much to bear, then take a middle road or allow yourself some days off. The important thing is to breast feed and to keep it up for as long as possible—six months if you can. Anything that puts a mother off breast feeding is a bad idea. Quite clearly, the best course is to breast feed and keep high-risk foods out of your diet, but there are times when we have to accept that we can only manage second best. If the dietary restrictions become so tiresome that you want to stop breast feeding after a couple of months, then drop the diet rather than the breast feeding.

Maternity Wards

Ironically, the most difficult place to ensure that a baby is given nothing but breast milk may be in a maternity ward. The practice of giving supplementary or complementary feedings is still common in some hospitals, and can be very damaging in the first few weeks of life. These feedings are of infant formulas based on cow's milk, which are likely to be allergenic for the susceptible child. At this early stage in life the baby is very vulnerable to sensitization by foreign proteins. One study looked at over seventeen hundred babies, of whom fifteen hundred received supplementary feedings and two hundred did not. There were thirty-nine cases of cow's-milk allergy, and all of these were in babies given supplementary feedings.

Giving supplementary feedings can also have more insidious effects that may lead to the baby having to be entirely bottle fed. Extra feedings from bottles upset the subtle balance of demand and supply that is established between a breast-feeding mother and her child. A rubber teat works differently from a real one, and babies who are given bottles do not always suck properly at the breast. Their appetite is also diminished so they suck less hard, and the mother therefore produces less milk. This sets up a vicious circle that may end with the mother being told that she "does not have enough milk" and must therefore bottle feed.

Where there is a hospital policy of not putting babies on the breast during the night, breast milk can be expressed and stored, to be given from a bottle by a nurse. This method can also be used at home for times when breast feeding is not a practical proposition.

Preparing for Breast Feeding

The mother who wishes to ensure that her baby is solely breast fed needs to be prepared in advance. Because breast feeding is thought of as natural, it is often assumed that it comes naturally. Unfortunately this is not true, and many mothers give up because they have not been shown how to breast feed properly, or because they have sore nipples or other problems. Pregnant women should prepare themselves for breast feeding by strengthening the skin of the nipple. Begin in mid pregnancy by rubbing gently with a washcloth every day for a week, then graduate to a rougher cloth, then a soft toothbrush, and finally a firm brush. This is the best possible insurance against cracked nipples. Further advice and help with breast feeding can be obtained from several organizations whose addresses are listed on pages 454–55.

Before going into the hospital, inquire about its policy on night feeding and supplementary feeding. Make it very clear to the nurses and your physician or midwife that you do not wish your baby to have anything but breast milk. You may need to put a notice on the crib to reinforce the message; you won't be awake all the time, and some nurses just love giving babies bottles. Ask whether you will be able to have your baby with you and feed on demand—this is far more conducive to successful breast feeding than a system that is ruled by the clock. Another factor in establishing a good working relationship with your baby is starting breast feeding within four hours of birth. Where a baby or mother is very ill, this may not always be possible, but you should ask that the baby be put to the breast as soon as possible.

If breast feeding is not possible, for whatever reason, then the mother should not feel guilty about the situation. There *are* alternatives that carry less risk of allergy than standard infant formulas. These are mixtures known as hydrolysates (see pages 275–76), which are available by prescription.

Formulas based on soy (see pages 275–76) are sometimes used with children who are known to be sensitive to cow's milk. These tend to be prescribed because they are a great deal cheaper than hydrolysates, and they may be very effective in clearing up symptoms that are due to cow's-milk sensitivity. However, there is always the risk that a child will develop allergic reactions to soy proteins, which are themselves noted allergens. This is especially likely if the mother has eaten soy, which she may well have done, since soy flour is increasingly common as a hidden ingredient in many foods. As part of a prevention program, soy-based formulas are not necessarily that much better than standard milk-based formulas—hydrolysates are definitely preferable.

There is little doubt that prolonged breast feeding and careful, gradual weaning are the most important factors in diminishing the risk of allergy in newborn babies. There are also good reasons for believing that breast feeding reduces the likelihood of food intolerance, as well as having more general benefits such as protecting babies from infection. Trying to breast feed for as long as possible is something that would benefit any child. (Recent studies suggested that it led to higher IQ and less obesity in later years, for example.) As a matter of national health care policy, the many remaining obstacles and discouragements to breast feeding should be removed and the promotion of formula feedings in maternity wards should stop, as the World Health Organization has recommended.

Preventive Measures during Pregnancy

Although the baby in the womb is nourished by the mother's blood, the blood of mother and baby do not mix. Instead, they both pass through tiny blood vessels (capillaries) in the structure known as the placenta. The capillaries carrying the mother's blood lie directly alongside those carrying the baby's blood, and vital substances such as glucose and oxygen can pass from one to the other through the capillary walls. It used to be thought that larger molecules, such as undigested food proteins, would not be able to get through, but it is now known that they do. Such food molecules could sensitize high-risk babies even before they're born.

In the light of this discovery, some doctors believe that women whose children are likely to be atopic should restrict their diets during pregnancy. However, the few studies that have attempted to test this idea have produced largely negative results. Given the difficulty of eating a restricted diet during pregnancy, it is probably not worth doing so for such uncertain gains. But anyone who is concerned about allergies in their children—having had one severely allergic child already, perhaps—could omit certain foods that are highly allergenic. The list should include cow's milk, eggs, peanuts, fish, and wheat, plus any foods to which the earlier child is allergic. It is, of course, essential that you consult your doctor to ensure that you are getting enough nutrients. A calcium supplement will probably be required.

The more of a food that is eaten, the more passes into the bloodstream. So eating huge quantities of one type of food during pregnancy is probably bad for the unborn child who may be predisposed to allergy. There have been no scientific tests to prove this, but not bingeing during pregnancy, or while breast feeding, would seem to be a sensible preventive measure.

Smoking during pregnancy has been shown to increase the risk of allergy, quite apart from its other damaging effects on the fetus. It is advisable to give up well before conception, and to maintain a smoke-free house once the baby is born—see the next section. Putting on excess weight during pregnancy is also a risk factor for allergy in the child.

Pure Air

The more allergens babies are exposed to during the first year of life, the more likely they are to develop allergies. The first three months are by far the most crucial. Airborne allergens are just as important as food allergens for the high-risk child, and reducing exposure to the main ones may help your child escape the miseries of asthma or rhinitis in later years.

The major domestic allergens are house dust mite, molds, and particles of animal skin. Suggestions for eliminating these are given on pages 85–87. If children have not shown eczema or any other allergic symptoms by their first birthday, then pets can probably be allowed into the house again, but watch for symptoms and bear in mind that these can take some time to develop.

The other major airborne allergen is pollen, which is best avoided by planning the time of birth (if you can!). In temperate climates a baby born in the winter has the best chance of escaping hay fever. If one or both parents is a hay-fever sufferer, this particular form of family planning may be worthwhile.

Apart from allergens, there are various nonspecific irritants that can make allergies more likely. Tobacco smoke is one, industrial air pollution another. A study in Sweden found that asthma and hay fever were more common in children living near a paper factory than those living in an unindustrialized area. Children whose parents smoked showed more allergic problems, and so did those whose houses were built on badly drained land. The researchers concluded that these houses had more molds growing in them. The highest risk of asthma and hay fever was in children who were exposed to the mold allergen and to both forms of pollution—factory fumes and tobacco smoke.

Infections of the throat and chest by a type of virus called RSV can sometimes trigger allergic reactions. This virus affects immune cells in the area, making IgE production more likely. All babies get colds and coughs, of course, and only about one in ten colds is due to RSV. It is difficult to avoid such infections, but if a vaccine against RSV becomes available in the next few years, as is likely, then children from allergy-prone families would undoubtedly benefit from vaccination. In contrast to RSV, other types of infestion push the immune system away from allergic reactions. Infection by harmless soil bacteria are thought to do this, explaining why grubby kids who frequently play outdoors are less likely to get asthma than those who are always washed and neat.

Any severe form of stress can also trigger allergies in the susceptible child. Serious illness or surgery during the first year of life is one such stress, and unnecessary surgery is best postponed.

Keeping Things in Perspective

None of these preventive measures is foolproof, unfortunately. Some children go on to develop allergies, come what may. So a philosophical outlook is essential—do what you can to protect the child from allergens and irritants, but accept that it may sometimes be impossible. Above all, try not to get too anxious. A child needs to see the world as a safe and welcoming place, not one that is fraught with dangers. If your anxiety is obvious, it may do a great deal of psychological harm.

Once the child is a year old, the risk of sensitization is far less, and you should be able to sit back and reap the benefits—an allergy-free child. There is no need to continue stringent preventive measures unless there is a clear need for them—if the child obviously reacts to house dust mites, for example, then you will have to continue measures to combat them, but if there are no problems then you can allow your standards to slip a little.

If your child develops allergies anyway, try not to blame yourself or other people—you can never know for sure what went wrong and it is pointless to guess. Take comfort from the thought that your child's allergies might have been much worse if you had not gone to so much trouble—in the Swedish study described above, it was notable that the different risk factors added up to give an even greater risk. Your preventive measures must have subtracted some aggravating factors and made your child's illness less severe than it might otherwise have been.

Preventing Food Intolerance

The measures so far described for preventing food allergy are very largely based on scientific trials. Because food intolerance is less well recognized than food allergy, it attracts far less funding for research, and no comparable studies have been carried out. The preventive measures that we suggest here are commonsense ones, based on an understanding of what factors might cause food intolerance. If one member of the family already shows food intolerance, following these guidelines may be worthwhile for those who are presently in good health.

Diet and Drugs

Since commonly eaten foods are the most frequent offenders in food intolerance, varying the diet is recommended. In particular, avoid eating milk and wheat too often—try to restrict these foods to just one meal a day. Avoid eating large quantities of the other high-risk foods, notably eggs, orange juice, and peanuts. Never consume huge quantities of a particular food at one sitting—sausage-eating competitions are not for you.

Try to cut down on the number of cups of coffee and tea you drink each day, and make them a little weaker. The evils of caffeine are listed on pages 213–14, and both drinks contain a variety of other chemical constituents that can irritate the stomach lining or cause changes in the body chemistry.

Avoid anything that increases the permeability of the gut wall: excess alcohol, highly spiced food, and raw pineapple or papaya. Certain drugs also make the gut leakier, notably aspirin and other similar drugs (nonsteroidal anti-inflammatory drugs; see pages 443–45)—these are used mainly for treating rheumatoid arthritis, osteoarthritis, menstrual pains, and headaches. You should take these only if you really need them.

Other Factors

One thing that is thought to trigger food intolerance is a heavy exposure to toxic chemicals. Such exposures are usually accidental and unforeseen, of course, but there are some avoidable ones. If a house is to be sprayed with insecticides to eradicate termites, or with fungicides for wet or dry rot, then it is advisable to move out for at least a week, to allow time for the fumes to disperse. The company doing the spraying may claim that this is unnecessary, but there could be a risk of becoming ill after spraying, even though you are not directly exposed to the spray. The fumes travel throughout the house, so even if only one part is being sprayed you should try to find somewhere else to stay for a while. This is particularly important for young children. Another hazard that can be very largely avoided is direct exposure to pesticides used on crops. If you see fields being sprayed, keep your distance, especially if they are being sprayed by a plane. The spray can easily drift. If you have a choice, don't buy a house next to a large arable field. Avoid using sprays in your own garden, and keep household chemicals to a minimum (see page 228).

Finally, the general health measures listed in appendix 5 are recommended to anyone who might be at risk of developing food intolerance. Above all, don't ignore symptoms such as recurrent headaches, regular bouts of indigestion, or persistent fatigue. Living on aspirin, antacids, or strong coffee is going to make the problem worse rather than better, and experience suggests that the decline into severe food intolerance is a very gradual one that begins with symptoms of this sort. Treating a mild form of food intolerance—the early stages—is a great deal easier than trying to tackle entrenched symptoms and multiple sensitivities. The longer you leave it, the more difficult it may be.

The Elimination Diet

The purpose of the elimination diet is to ask your body questions about the foods it has to cope with and give it a chance to tell you which ones make it ill. In order to hear the answers, you need a period of "silence"—that is, a period with no symptoms at all. This is why you must exclude all foods that are likely to be causing problems at the outset. Eliminating different foods one by one rarely works, because most people are sensitive to more than one food. They must all be eliminated at once for the symptoms to disappear—to create the silence you need. (The main exception to this rule concerns very small children who are eating a limited number of foods anyway, and are unlikely to be sensitive to a great many of them. See pages 275–84 for details of investigating food problems in babies and toddlers.)

All elimination diets fall into two parts. First you avoid any food that might be causing trouble and see if the symptoms clear up—we will call this the **exclusion phase**. If the symptoms do disappear, then foods are reintroduced, one at a time, to discover which ones produce the symptoms. This is referred to here as the **reintroduction phase**.

The elimination diet sounds simple enough, although in practice there can be pitfalls and the results are not always clear-cut. This chapter has been carefully planned to help you avoid as many of those pitfalls as possible, and to give you the clearest possible answers with the least amount of change in your diet. It is very important that you work through it carefully. You should read the whole chapter first, then reread each section and understand it thoroughly before you begin.

Do not be put off by the constant references to things going wrong. Only a minority of people will encounter problems such as these, but when they do arise, extra advice is needed—which is why the possible pitfalls seem to loom very large in this chapter.

There is no point whatever in following an elimination diet half-heartedly—it simply won't work. You cannot have a day off in the middle, unlike a weight-reducing or health diet—it is a diagnostic diet, not a treatment in itself. If you stop for a day—or even a meal—you will not get a clear result.

It is also a mistake to rush into it: if you do, things are more likely to go wrong. You may feel impatient to be well again, but try to think ahead. Imagine how you might feel in six months' time, if you are only partially better, or little improved, because the elimination diet has not worked out properly. If you had taken it more slowly, you might have been fully recovered; even if it had taken an extra few months, this would have been thoroughly worthwhile, because it could mean many years of really good health in the future. Doing the diet again is often very difficult. The process itself can change you—in particular, you may acquire new sensitivities to the foods eaten during the exclusion phase, simply because they are eaten more regularly and in greater amounts than before. If you are already sensitive to a wide range of foods, acquiring new sensitivities may prevent you from having a second go at the elimination diet—you need a basic set of foods to which you have no reaction in order for the diet to work. This is an extreme situation, of course, but it is worth bearing in mind that it can happen. The important thing is to get the elimination diet right the first time.

Variations on a Theme

Although all elimination diets work on the same principle, doctors differ considerably in the sorts of food they allow during the exclusion phase. The objective is to avoid all foods that are likely to cause problems. In essence, this means all foods that are eaten frequently, because these are the most likely culprits (see pages 143–44). However, the safeness of foods is also taken into consideration—some foods seem less likely to cause problems than others. The question is: How far do you take this? Some patients will be sensitive to twenty or more foods—to get better, they need to avoid almost everything they normally eat. But these patients are a tiny minority. Most patients will be sensitive to between two and five foods. For them a rigorous exclusion phase is not necessary—they simply need to avoid the most frequent offenders, such as wheat, milk, eggs, citrus fruits, yeast, chocolate, and additives. On the whole, the latter group have a much easier task ahead of them in discovering which foods make them ill, so doctors tend to think more about the unfortunate patients with multiple sensitivities. With them in mind, they devise diets that eliminate most commonly eaten foods, even if this means putting the patients with just a few sensitivities through an unnecessarily arduous regime. The approach to elimination diet that we recommend is a flexible three-stage procedure that provides the best possible diet for each type of patient. This is described beginning on page 335. First, however, we will consider the different types of diet that are commonly used by other doctors.

Different Types of Elimination Diet

The most drastic form of the elimination diet is to fast for the first five days, taking nothing but bottled springwater. This method has several drawbacks. Fasting requires a great deal of willpower and it is bad for anyone who is underweight and in poor health. Even for those who are not underweight, major metabolic changes occur during fasting, as the body begins to break down its fat reserves. These metabolic changes, and others that occur when food is reintroduced, may themselves produce symptoms. For these reasons, we would not recommend fasting except in certain very difficult cases.

One step up from fasting is the **lamb-and-pears diet**, probably the best-known type of elimination diet. It originated in the United States, where lamb is not widely eaten and sensitivity to it is unusual. Lamb is more commonly eaten in many other parts of the world; in Britain and New Zealand, for instance. In such countries, some doctors use a turkey-and-pears or turkey-rice-and-pears diet.

While these very simple diets are useful when someone has a great many sensitivities, they are unnecessarily strict for most people. Again, they require a lot of willpower, and they involve eating huge quantities of two or three foods, which is never a good idea.

The next step up from here is the few-food diet or the rare-food diet. On a **few-food diet** the exclusion phase consists of a dozen or more foods that most people do not eat all that often. The exact foods chosen vary from one doctor to another, but they tend to include things such as parsnips, turnips, and carrots, which most of us do not eat in great quantity. The allowed foods also vary from patient to patient, because the doctor will ask you if you eat any of the foods on the allowed list often—if you do, these must be excluded, too. Most doctors have a second version of their few-food diet, with a different list of allowed foods; patients who do not get better during the first exclusion phase are switched to the second diet, in the hope that they will fare better. Of course, there is always a chance that both lists will include one or two foods that cause symptoms.

The **rare-food diet** is an extension of the few-food idea, but instead of eating uncommon foods such as turnips or parsnips during the exclusion phase, you are asked to eat exotic items such as cassava or buckwheat. Since these items may never (or only rarely) have been eaten before, they are very unlikely to cause any reaction. In a sense the rare-food diet is an improvement on the few-food diet, because if you fail to get better during the exclusion phase, you probably aren't food sensitive. With the few-food diet there is always some doubt—perhaps you are sensitive to parsnips, even though you only ever ate them for Sunday lunch? The drawbacks of the rare-food diet are principally cost—exotic foods are expensive—and the problem of getting such foods for those who do not live in a large city. The foods have to be prepared differently and the taste may take some getting used to, but on the whole they are at least as palatable as turnips! For those with multiple sensitivities who can afford the exotic foods and have access to them, this type of diet is well worth considering.

The final step takes us to the least-rigorous form of elimination diet, in which most fruits, vegetables, fish, and meats are allowed, but wheat and other cereals, milk, eggs, and other common offenders are excluded. This diet is quite good enough for many people, but those with multiple sensitivities tend to slip through the net because they are still eating some foods that cause symptoms.

One other form of elimination diet should be mentioned here. This uses elemental diets during the exclusion phase, rather than any foods. **Elemental diets** are made from various ordinary foods, but these are treated to break down the food molecules into smaller pieces. They are similar to the hydrolysate formulas used for babies who are sensitive to cow's milk (see pages 275–76) but they are designed to be eaten—or rather drunk—by adults. In theory, the molecules that remain in the elemental diet are too small to cause any allergic reactions or other problems. In practice, some people with established food sensitivity do react to them, because the fragments of molecules they contain are too reminiscent of the original molecules. For many people, however, they are very effective.

Various drawbacks are associated with elemental diets. First, they taste dreadful. Second, they are very expensive. Nevertheless, they might be useful as a last resort for someone who is intolerant of a great many foods and has therefore not succeeded with an elimination diet. You should not try an elemental diet without the approval and help of your doctor. Some of the companies selling elemental diets direct to the public in the United States also publish information about "food allergy," which is, to put it politely, confused. Follow your doctor's advice rather than any information sheet or diet recommendations that come with the product.

A Three-Stage Approach

Doctors are obliged to deal with patients quickly and efficiently. If they use an elimination diet as a diagnostic method, it must be a fairly simple diet that can be given to everyone and does not need a lot of explanation. One advantage of self-help is that the diet can be tailored more closely to the individual patient's needs, and toward this end we have devised a three-stage plan that we believe offers the best form of diagnosis for every type of patient.

The plan is outlined briefly in this section, and then described in more detail beginning on page 335. You should try each stage of the plan in turn, and only go on to the next stage if you are no better. The vast majority of readers will probably not need to go beyond Stage 1 or 2. The main advantage of this three-stage approach is that it should not involve giving up any food unnecessarily, and if you have a simple problem—such as getting too much caffeine—it will lead you to it simply and quickly. There is little point spending a week eating nothing but lamb and pears when all you really needed to do was give up coffee or cut out milk.

Stage 1 of the plan is a one-month healthy-eating program. During this stage the foods and drinks that have a druglike action on the body are eliminated, namely coffee, tea, colas, cocoa, chocolate, and all forms of alcohol. The unpleasant (and often unsuspected) effects of caffeine are described on pages 213–14. Sugar and sugary foods are also excluded, because these can cause problems in some people, by making their blood-sugar levels go up and down wildly (see pages 178–81). Finally, histamine-rich foods (see pagse 113–14) and all types of additives are excluded, since these are sometimes a source of problems.

If you get better during this first stage then you have gotten off very lightly, because you have not had to cut out any foods, in the strict sense of the word. Even if you do not recover at this stage, there are still substantial advantages. If you are food sensitive, the withdrawal symptoms that occur when you cut out the offending foods can be quite grim (see page 146). Suddenly cutting out caffeine, alcohol, and sugar at the same time is just plain masochistic—it makes much more sense to kick these habits first.

You may also discover that you can feel partially better by just eating healthily and avoiding everyday "drugs." This information could be useful later, when you have to decide how to cope with your food sensitivities—you will know how much of your illness is due to food and how much is due to other items.

Stage 2 of the program is a simple form of elimination diet that just excludes the most common offending foods—this is the least-rigorous form of exclusion phase. Most people will probably find the answers to their problems here.

Stage 3 of the program is a more drastic form of elimination diet, designed to detect those with sensitivities to many different foods. The exact form of this exclusion phase can vary to suit individual needs—we suggest either a few-food diet or a rare-food diet, or a combination of the two.

Related Foods

Before embarking on an elimination diet, some understanding of how foods can **cross-react** with one another is necessary. Foods derived from two related plants (or two related animals) will have similar proteins. They do not have to look like one another to be alike chemically—our own proteins are 99 percent the same as those of the chimpanzee and the gorilla, our nearest living relatives. In the same way, the potato and the tomato may look quite different, but the plants they come from are closely related.

If you are allergic to one sort of food, you may show a reaction to food from a related source, because the IgE antibodies that bind to the first protein will also bind to a similar related protein. Cross-reactions also seem to occur in food intolerance, although the mechanism is not understood in most of these cases.

Biologists use various methods to work out how closely two animals or plants are related. Having done so, they express these relationships by grouping creatures together in a hierarchical scheme—very closely related creatures belong to the same **species**, related species belong to the same **genus** (plural **genera**), related genera belong to the same **family**, related families belong to the same **order**, and so on. There are often further subdivisions within each level, such as the **subfamily** and the **tribe**, which are subdivisions of the family.

How is this sort of classification scheme relevant to food sensitivity? The practical experience of thousands of patients suggests that they can cross-react to related foods, although they do not always do so. It also seems, from this collected experience, that the **family level** in biological classifications is a useful one in deciding which foods will cross-react—although sometimes you have to look at higher or lower levels to understand the cross-reactions that are seen. For example, all cereals are grasses and belong to the grass family, Gramineae. Some food-sensitive people react to all cereals—to all members of the family. But others react only to wheat or corn, the two most commonly eaten cereals in the West. Many who react to wheat also react to rye and barley, and sometimes oats. If you look at the classification of the Gramineae, you'll find that wheat, rye, barley, and oats all belong to the same subfamily, the Pooidae, and wheat, rye, and barley are in the same tribe, the Triticeae. Corn is in a different subfamily, and rice in a different subfamily again, so there is less likely to be a cross-reaction between wheat and these cereals. This nicely explains the observation that wheat-sensitive folks are more likely to tolerate rice than any other commonly eaten cereal.

It has to be said that this is an unusually neat example, and most of the cross-reactions that are seen (or suspected) in patients do not match so well with the biological classification (see appendix 4). For many foods, the use of the family group to predict cross-reactions is more a matter of faith than science, but it is still the most useful guide we have. There are also some unexpected cross-reactions that do not tally with classification schemes but may be explained in other ways (see pages 376–78).

If you have reason to suspect any food before starting on your elimination diet (because you eat it in large amounts, for example), you should check the food-family list (see pages 371–75) to discover which family it belongs to. All its relatives should be excluded during the first phase of the diet, along with the food itself. But do test these foods later, and do not expect a reaction just because foods are related. While cross-reactions are fairly common with some foods, notably cereals and shellfish, they are very rare with others. For example, tests have shown that most people who are allergic to peanuts are not affected by other legumes such as beans, peas, or soybeans. Anticipating a reaction to a food is always a mistake, because it can lead to psychogenic symptoms—those created by the mind. And that could lead you to avoid foods unnecessarily.

The food families may also be useful later, in planning your everyday diet—just as you should not eat too much of any one food, you should not eat too much from any one food family either.

Preparing for the Elimination Diet

Seeing Your Doctor

The first and most essential step is to see your doctor, describe your symptoms fully, and ask for a medical checkup. As explained in chapter 7, many of the symptoms of food intolerance can be due to other causes, and some of these may be serious—your doctor can examine you for such problems. It is particularly important to investigate the possibility of celiac disease (see pages 104–7) *before* altering your diet in any way. Should there be nothing obviously wrong, then the next logical step is to try an elimination diet. Explain to the doctor that you want to do so, and ask for advice. He or she may well have reservations about elimination diets, and you will be better prepared if you have read all or most of this book and understand what is involved. *If the doctor feels that you should not alter your diet for medical reasons, you must take this advice.*

Keeping a record

As soon as you can, start keeping a daily record of your symptoms. This might seem rather unnecessary at this stage, but it will prove very useful later. The main purpose is to give you a detailed picture of how you felt before you began the diet—a baseline with which any later state of health can be compared. It is remarkable how quickly the memory fades—especially the memory of illness. If you only make a partial recovery, as some people do, you may later forget how awful you felt at the outset and begin to think that the improvement is very small. Looking back at your symptom record is often a startling reminder, and it can help strengthen your resolve to persist with the diet. It is also valuable if friends or relatives start to question the usefulness of what you are doing—you may need to prove to yourself that you really are better. This point is stressed by one of our readers, describing his success with the diet:

> The importance of keeping a diary should be emphasized, particularly concerning symptoms. After a few days of improvement it is amazing how easy it is to forget how bad things were—and hence to be tempted to give up the diet.

At the same time, you could also make a record of what you eat. Some people are more conscious of what passes their lips than others, and when you come to plan your diet you need to be aware of what foods you eat very regularly. Keeping a food diary for a week or two can be quite an eye opener. It will also get you into the habit of reading ingredients labels and watching out for synonyms (see appendix 3).

Smoking and the Pill

If you smoke, now is the moment to give it up! There is not much point in trying to sort out your health problems while continuing to bombard your body with highly toxic smoke.

The Pill is a more difficult issue, for it is, without doubt, the most effective and convenient form of contraception, and giving it up may not be easy. But it can easily contribute to migraine, headaches, fatigue, and a variety of other symptoms that are also attributed to food intolerance. Some doctors believe that it has more general ill effects on women's health, and that everyone with suspected food sensitivity or gut flora problems (see chapter 10) should discontinue use of the Pill, regardless of what type of symptoms they have.

You may feel perfectly happy with the Pill, because you had no problems when you first began taking it—but as the case history on page 327 shows, this can be quite misleading. Even if you have had short periods (up to six months) off the Pill before without noting any improvement, it may still be contributing to your symptoms. Nobody knows why the Pill should have these rather odd, insidious effects on some women, but they have been observed often enough to merit being taken seriously.

In general, it makes sense for any woman who is thinking about trying an elimination diet to stop taking the Pill first, and if migraines

---

Emma

Emma had first gone on the Pill when she was a student, and had experienced no problems at all. She stayed on the combined Pill throughout her twenties, later changing to the progesterone-only mini Pill, which was considered safer. During her twenties various health problems had developed, notably irritable bowel syndrome and migraines. These problems became much worse in her midthirties, which was when Emma first heard about the possible role of food in such illnesses. She discussed the idea of an elimination diet with her doctor, who suggested that she should first stop taking the Pill, to see what effect this had. Emma stayed off the Pill for two months, but her symptoms continued as before. She then tried an elimination diet, lost all her symptoms, and identified milk, chicken, and soy as the offending foods. On a diet free of these foods she felt a great deal better, and after a year of this she decided to go back on the Pill, because other methods of birth control did not suit her. She began taking the mini Pill again and within two days, to her great surprise, experienced a migraine. This was followed by a migraine the next day and the day after—three migraines in a row, the first she had had for a year. She promptly stopped taking the Pill and they did not recur. In retrospect, she wondered if the Pill had been contributing to her earlier problems, even though stopping it did not alleviate them. As this example shows, taking the Pill for a long period of time can have some rather odd and insidious effects, and stopping it does not always clear the symptoms immediately—they can persist for many months.

---

are among her symptoms the arguments for it are even stronger. Ideally, she should give the Pill up for a trial period of three months before starting the diet, to see what effect this has and to regain some sort of equilibrium. For anyone with severe symptoms, however, three months may seem like a long time to wait. So if you have tried coming off the Pill before without any obvious benefits, then you could just wait for two or three weeks before starting Stage 1.

There is fairly strong evidence that women who have been on the Pill for some years may be deficient in certain vitamins and minerals. Anyone coming off the Pill should consider taking a nutritional supplement of the type described in the next section.

Nutritional Supplements

The question of nutrition is a vexed one at present. The orthodox view is that a balanced diet provides all the nutrients we need, and common sense would suggest that our ample and very varied diet must provide more than enough—rarely have human beings been as well fed as we in the West are today. But there is a new school of thought in nutrition, which maintains that a surprisingly large number of people are deficient in certain vitamins and minerals. The proponents of this view cite many case histories in which patients with long-term health problems have been greatly helped by specific vitamin or mineral supplements.

Is there any possible explanation for this apparent paradox—an over-fed people with nutritional deficits? The suggestion is that other factors in our diet and lifestyle can cause these shortages. Some of these factors may be universal; others affect certain individuals only.

At the individual level our diets vary widely. Although we are well fed on the whole, some people still eat a very poor diet—one rich in sugars, starches, and other highly processed foods, but poor in vitamins and minerals. A recent survey by the London Food Commission found that a third of the British people buying fast food ate such food at least once a day, and for many it was their main meal. Such food provides almost no vegetables, has very low levels of vitamins, and is far richer in salt and fat than official guidelines recommend.

Even those who think they are eating healthily may in fact be under-nourished. The fashion for whole wheat everything and added bran is one factor here. Bran contains a substance called **phytate** that is known to impair the absorption of iron, zinc, calcium, and possibly magne-sium—all essential minerals. The yeasts used in making bread break down phytates, so ordinary whole wheat bread is not a problem but unleav-ened whole wheat bread (such as soda bread and chapatis), whole wheat pastries and cakes, bran-containing breakfast cereals, and other bran prod-ucts can block the absorption of these minerals.

Bran can cause serious mineral deficiencies, because iron and zinc are often lacking in Western diets. Vegetarians and vegans are particu-larly liable to iron deficiency (anemia) since vegetarian food is low in iron anyway. Children under the age of two are also at risk, as are many women, because they lose blood while menstruating and have to make good the lost iron. Drinking black tea with meals further reduces the absorption of iron and is something that all vegetarians should avoid.

Zinc deficiency is more controversial than iron deficiency and has become something of a fad, but there is fairly good evidence that it may be quite widespread. Vegetarians, pregnant women, elderly people, diabetics, and those on restricted diets are at the greatest risk, but almost anyone can be short of zinc. The processing of food may be to blame, since this appears to reduce the zinc content. In addition, viral infections seem to use up some of our stores of zinc.

The second strand of the argument is more contentious and very difficult to test scientifically. It suggests that we need more nutrients than we once did, simply because our bodies have to deal with so many more toxins—pesticide residues in food and water, air pollutants, and so on. Although this might seem rather far-fetched, it is not implausible. We protect our bodies against toxins by breaking them down with en-zymes (see page 21). Many vitamins act as coenzymes—substances that are needed by specific enzymes to help them do their work. Minerals such as zinc and magnesium are also important for enzyme function. Faced with an extra burden of toxins to destroy, perhaps we do need more vitamins and minerals than our traditional diet provides.

A related issue here is the Pill, which is said to alter the nutritional balance of some women—perhaps the majority of women who take it on a long-term basis. Zinc, magnesium, manganese, and iron may be deficient in Pill takers, while copper is often very high. Vitamin A seems to be stored in excess, while many of the B vitamins are in short supply. Some of the adverse side effects of the Pill have been linked to these changes in vitamin and mineral status. Simply stopping the Pill does not seem to put these nutritional disorders right—they may persist for three months or more and cause continuing problems.

Doctors who are concerned about possible nutritional defects suggest that anyone embarking on an elimination diet should take a nutritional supplement. They argue that many patients are likely to have deficiencies anyway, especially if they number diarrhea among their symptoms, and that the restrictions of the elimination diet will only make the situation worse. Such doctors also recommend a special type of nutritional supplement to anyone coming off the Pill—and certainly to anyone staying on it (see page 450).

It is quite easy to overdo things with both vitamins and minerals, particularly with the fat-soluble vitamins, A and D, because these are stored by the body if taken in excess. (Water-soluble vitamins, such as C, can be washed out of the body in the urine.) So grabbing a handful of ordinary vitamin pills is not the answer—they can be dangerous if the body already has an excess of vitamin A.

TABLE 11 SOME SIGNS OF NUTRITIONAL DEFICIENCY*

These are some of the physical signs of nutritional deficiencies. Bear in mind that all the signs or symptoms below can be caused by other medical conditions. If you have any of these symptoms, you should consult your doctor before taking a nutritional supplement.

Sign or Symptom	*Can be Caused by Deficiencies of*
Cracks at corners of mouth	Iron, vitamin B_2 or B_6, or folic acid
Recurrent mouth ulcers	Iron, folic acid, or vitamin B_{12}
Dry, cracked lips	Vitamin B_2
Smooth, sore tongue	Iron, vitamin B_2 or B_{12}, or folic acid
Fissured tongue	Vitamin B_3
Taste buds at tip of tongue enlarged, red and sore	Vitamin B_2 or B_6
Bruising or enlargement of veins under tongue	Vitamin C
Red, greasy skin on face, especially sides of nose	Vitamin B_2 or B_6, zinc, or essential fatty acids
Rough, pimply skin on upper arms and thighs	B vitamins, vitamin E, or essential fatty acids
Red, itchy rash on scrotum or vulva	Vitamin B_2, zinc
Dry, rough, cracked, or peeling skin	Zinc, essential fatty acids
Poor hair growth	Iron or zinc
Dandruff	Vitamin B_6 or C, zinc, or essential fatty acids
Bloodshot, gritty, sensitive eyes	Vitamin A or B_2
Poor vision after dark	Vitamin A or zinc
Dry eyes	Vitamin A or essential fatty acids
Brittle or split nails	Iron, zinc, or essential fatty acids
White spots on nails	Zinc
Pale appearance	Iron, Vitamin B_{12}, or folic acid

*Adapted from *Nutritional Medicine* by kind permission of the authors, Dr. Stephen Davies and Dr. Alan Stewart.

Ideally, everyone who is concerned about their nutritional status should have a full analysis done so that a supplement can be tailored to their specific needs. Unfortunately, testing itself is a contentious issue. The traditional method of just testing a blood sample is now considered inadequate by many doctors. It appears that some nutrients—zinc, for example—can be deficient as a whole, but show up in normal levels in the blood. The suggestion is that the blood needs the mineral more than other parts of the body, so there are mechanisms that ensure a good supply, scavenging the mineral from other tissues to keep the blood level high.

A more extensive method of testing, using hair and sweat samples as well as blood, often shows nutritional defects that are not revealed by the blood alone. This form of testing seems to be vindicated by the results in individual cases—correcting the deficiencies shown by hair or sweat tests often does wonders for patients with previously intractable health problems. This is not hard, scientific evidence, of course, and some carefully designed trials are needed to test these new approaches to nutrition.

In the meantime, what can be advised? Extensive nutritional testing is usually not covered by health insurance plans, but for those who can afford it there is little to lose. For anyone coming off the Pill, such testing is particularly valuable, and a special supplement is probably advisable (see appendix 9).

Others who may be concerned about their nutritional status but cannot afford individual testing should consult table 11 and see if they show any signs of deficiency. These are not foolproof signs, however—the same symptoms can be produced by other forms of illness, and there are several deficiencies that do not appear in the table because they produce no clear-cut signs. But if you do show some of these signs, then there is a chance that you are lacking certain nutrients, especially if your diet has not been good. The simplest and cheapest answer is to take a general supplement from a specialist supplier such as Stoke's Pharmacy (see page 457). This may be slightly more expensive than run-of-the-mill vitamin tablets, but it is free of artificial colors, unlike most commercial preparations, which come in lurid shades of red or orange as an indication of their health-giving properties! Avoiding colorings is important if you are embarking on an elimination diet.

One sign that you may notice is white spots on the fingernails. These can be an indication of zinc deficiency, and if you show no other deficiency signs and generally eat a good diet, then a zinc supplement may be all you need. Zinc is relatively safe and nontoxic, so a sensible supplement is unlikely to do any harm. For details, see appendix 9.

Sort Out Other Problems

The idea of the elimination diet is to create a period of "silence" free from symptoms in which you can listen to your body answering specific questions. Any sort of background noise is going to confuse you, so you need to eliminate other things that cause symptoms before you start. The three main items to consider are airborne allergens, hyperventilation, and chemical sensitivity.

You should suspect airborne allergens if your symptoms include asthma; hay fever; a year-round runny nose or congested nose (rhinitis); red, watery, or itchy eyes; sinusitis; or recurrent "colds." Eczema may indicate allergens in the air that land on the skin—or things that touch the skin directly. Consult pages 89–91 for likely sources of trouble. Avoidance measures are described on pages 91–94. Put these into effect for a few months before starting the diet.

Hyperventilation is suggested by dizziness, faintness, tingling in the hands and feet, numbness, spaced-out or confused feelings, shortness of breath, and a variety of other symptoms. A full list is given on page 210. It appears that hyperventilation often accompanies food intolerance, but it can sometimes be the sole cause of symptoms.

There are no typical symptoms reported for chemical sensitivity, but most people who react generally know that they do, because certain things always make them feel ill—traveling by car, smelling perfume, or swimming in chlorinated water, for example. Read chapter 9 if you are in any doubt. Complete avoidance is difficult, but try to clean up your environment as much as possible (see pages 228–34), and wait for about two weeks before starting the elimination diet, so that you can assess the effects of doing this.

If you respond to any of these avoidance measures, however slightly, they should be continued throughout Stages 1, 2, and 3 of the diet.

Planning the Diet

Timing is all-important here, because birthdays, holidays, weddings, family get-togethers, and vacations cause immense problems. Ideally, you should plan things so that the diet falls in a quiet period, or postpone celebrations until afterward. This does not matter quite so much during Stage 1 of the diet, when you can break the rules for one or two meals, if you have to. However, you should keep off alcohol, tea, and coffee, and not overdo sugar. During Stages 2 and 3 you cannot do this— *any* departure from the diet will confuse the result. Use the timing guidelines in table 12 on page 334 to plan your diet.

Obviously, you cannot abandon all social life during these diets, so you have to be flexible. If you are asked out to lunch or dinner, it is not that difficult to take your own food, and you will get over the embarrassment fairly quickly. For picnics and days out, cook the foods that you are allowed and take them in plastic boxes. Packed lunches for work, or when traveling, can be prepared in the same way. If you are following the diet during the winter months and want hot food, buy a wide-necked thermos—they are very useful and inexpensive. As an alternative to tea and coffee, take herbal tea in a thermos or carry some herbal tea bags— waitstaff in cafés and restaurants will usually give you some plain hot water if you ask for it, and watching their puzzled expressions can be quite entertaining.

You should not start the diet without planning what you are going to eat for the first few days and buying the things you need. Hunger is a very powerful urge, and unless you have plenty of allowed foods at hand you may get so famished that you raid the cookie jar or bread bin in a moment of weakness. To avoid such lapses, it is worth cooking up some meals in advance so that you can have something ready within a few minutes. A freezer is invaluable—you can cook your special meals in bulk and freeze them in individual portions. A supply of allowed snacks in a cupboard is also helpful—see page 413 for ideas.

Packaged and canned foods should be avoided if possible during these diets. You will find that most prepared foods contain excluded items anyway. It may not say "milk" or "eggs" on the ingredient label, but it could be there under another name—see appendix 3 for the synonyms used. Even if there are no prohibited ingredients you are still taking something of a gamble, because you have no idea what sort of processing methods have been used and how these might affect you. And it is not unknown for labels to omit an ingredient. So it is much better, at this stage, to stick to simple home-prepared foods because you know exactly what has gone into them. Canned foods should be avoided at first because the lining of the cans, a golden-colored phenol resin, contaminates the food slightly. Some food-intolerant people are sensitive to this.

From the point of view of food preparation, making two batches of food can be a nuisance, and some people solve the problem by putting

TABLE 12 TIMING GUIDELINES FOR PLANNING THE ELIMINATION DIET

Stage 1—the healthy-eating diet—should run for at least a month, but it can be continued for as long as you wish. Some flexibility is allowed during this stage—you can have the occasional meal off, but even then take all forbidden items in moderation, and avoid alcohol, tea, and coffee. Stage 1 will go on longer than a month if you improve substantially on this diet—but in this case you will not be proceeding to Stage 2.

If you are going on to Stage 2, you should maintain the healthy-eating diet until you are ready to start.

Stage 2 will run for about three weeks if you don't respond to the exclusion phase. If you do respond, then it will continue for two to three months. *There must be no deviation from the diet during Stage 2.*

Stage 3 will run for about three weeks if you don't respond to the exclusion phase. If you do respond, then it will continue for two to three months. *There must be no deviation from the diet during Stage 3.*

the whole family on the diet, at least for the exclusion phase. Doctors using the elimination diet have often observed unexpectedly good results in another family member as a result of this. There are numerous reports of fatigue, moodiness, headaches, runny noses, and other minor problems that had previously been taken for granted suddenly clearing up. Skeptics will claim that this could well be psychosomatic or a result of healthier eating habits, and at present there is no scientific evidence either way. But there is certainly no harm in other adults joining in Stages 1 and 2 of the diet. Children should be included only if they have some identifiable medical or behavioral problem, and prior consultation with your doctor is essential. Children may need a calcium supplement if milk is excluded.

Stage 3 of the diet is a different matter. It is unlikely that anyone with minor health problems or no acknowledged health problems would benefit from it, although a few might.

Not Making Matters Worse

For some people—though only a tiny minority—the elimination diet can go badly wrong, and they finish up with intolerance to such a wide range of foods that there is hardly anything they can eat. One reader, who recovered after following the elimination diet given in an earlier edition of this book, but then developed new sensitivities, asks us to emphasize "the dangers of choosing alternative foods, relying on them heavily, and then becoming sensitive to the new foods." The key to avoiding this problematic situation is to *never* eat any food every day, nor in very large amounts (never more than a normal portion).

During the first part of the elimination diet (the exclusion phase), it may be necessary to rely on a staple food quite heavily, and to eat it most days. But this should only last for a week or so. Once the exclusion phase is over, and certain foods have been tested and found safe, vary your diet as much as possible. If necessary introduce a few rare foods (see pages 350–51) to help ring in the changes. Be wary of food addiction—a food that you start to crave is a potential troublemaker.

You should also be wary of becoming obsessed with the idea that food is the source of your symptoms. If you have had a small improvement that seemed to be related to avoiding a food, or have had a rather variable and confusing response to the elimination diet, you may be tempted to go on cutting out more and more foods in the hope of finally hitting upon the culprit. One well-known case involved a patient who, by the time he went to see a specialist, had narrowed his diet down so much that he ate nothing but plums and sardines. Such a bizarre diet is obviously unworkable and carries a serious risk of malnutrition. In the long run you need an adequate and varied diet to maintain your health, and this should be your overriding concern. So be careful not to obsess about food, try not to worry too much, and always keep a sense of perspective. If possible, have medical supervision while carrying out an elimination diet, and don't delay seeking medical help if you feel things are not going well. A sensible friend whom you can discuss the diet with is also invaluable—being ill, and with distressing symptoms that come and go unpredictably, can make you feel rather vulnerable and confused, so it is useful to have some objective advice and suggestions.

Stage 1—The Healthy-Eating Diet

This is summarized in table 13.

CUT OUT THE FOLLOWING FOODS:
• Coffee and tea, including coffee-flavored cakes, and so on.
• Chocolate, cocoa, and all chocolate-flavored items.
• Coca-Cola, Pepsi, and other cola drinks.
• Sugar and any foods containing sugar (see the table on page 249).

Don't worry if you eat a small amount (such as in canned tomato soup) during Stage 1. During Stages 2 and 3 you'll need to be much more careful.

- Saccharin and other artificial sweeteners.
- All alcoholic drinks, including alcohol-free beers and foods cooked in wine, beer, and so forth. Don't eat too much vinegar or pickled foods—no more than a small portion twice a week.
- All colorings, preservatives, antioxidants, flavor enhancers, flavorings, thickeners, emulsifiers, stabilizers, and other additives. Some of these are natural ingredients, but that does not mean they are automatically safe, and at this stage it is easier to just avoid the lot. Read the labels on everything—don't be taken in by "natural" or "healthy" on the package. Some unlabeled food contains additives (see appendix 6). Remember that margarines contain colorings and are highly processed—any food like this should be avoided. So should bacon, ham, corned beef, and anything smoked.
- Salami-type sausages and very ripe cheeses—they are often a rich source of histamine.
- All take-out and fast food. Keep restaurant eating to a minimum, because there are a lot of unexpected additives in such meals.
- Anything that makes the gut more permeable: curries and other very spicy foods, raw pineapple and papaya, and aspirin and other NSAIDs (see pages 443–45).

At the same time, you should try to eat plenty of fresh vegetables and fruits. Green, leafy vegetables are particularly important, and salads are valuable. Choose fresh meat or fish rather than potpies, sausages, or fish sticks (even if these are additive-free).

If you have been eating bran, gradually cut this out (your bowel may need time to adjust, so don't do it suddenly). A daily intake of vegetables, potatoes, whole wheat bread, and fruits should supply all the fiber you need. Try to eat less salt, and avoid highly salted foods such as peanuts and chips. Keep your diet varied, don't eat too much at one sitting, and don't have huge amounts of a single food.

If you drink a lot of coffee or tea, cut it out gradually or you may get withdrawal symptoms. Avoid painkillers that contain caffeine. Other medicines may contain colorings—ask you doctor to prescribe uncolored equivalents.

Decaffeinated coffee and tea are not allowed. Herbal teas can be used to replace tea and coffee, but not maté (sometimes spelled *matté*), which contains some caffeine and tannin, nor redbush tea, which shares many chemical constituents with ordinary tea, even though it lacks caffeine. Jasmine, gunpowder, and other green teas are true teas, so these should not be drunk.

Stay on this diet for at least a month, unless you feel much better before then.

Possible Outcomes

Feeling Much Worse

You are probably suffering from caffeine withdrawal—or it might be the effects of cutting out alcohol. This is cold turkey—the same sort of withdrawal symptoms that a heroin addict has, though nothing like as bad. You just have to keep going in the knowledge that it will pass, and that you will then feel a great deal better than you did before. Not eating sugar might have similar effects until your body gets used to the idea.

It is most unlikely that you will still feel worse after two or three weeks. If you do, think about any other changes that have occurred. Could they be the cause? Or were you steadily getting worse anyway? If you're sure it's due to the diet, then consider any new foods you are eating, or foods eaten in greater quantity than before. It may be that you are allergic or intolerant to such foods. Consider them suspect and cut them out in the exclusion phase of Stage 2. Alternatively, if you are eating a lot more fruits and vegetables than before, and if you are sensitive to pesticide residues, then this might explain your deterioration. Read chapter 9 before going on to Stage 2.

Feeling About the Same

Proceed to Stage 2. Stay on the healthy-eating diet until you are ready to start.

Feeling Partially Better

If you are satisfied with your improvement and don't like the idea of giving up foods, you could stop here. Test tea, coffee, alcohol, and so on to see which was the problem, following the instructions given below.

If you feel you would like to be better still, go on to Stage 2 of the diet. When you have completed Stage 2 (or Stage 3), you can test your reactions to tea, coffee, alcohol, and the like.

TABLE 13 THE STAGE 1 DIET

Allowed

Whole wheat bread

Milk, butter, most types of cheese

Shredded wheat, puffed wheat, and other cereals that have no sugar or
colorings

Any fresh, unprocessed meat

Any fresh, unprocessed fish

Potatoes

Rice

Beans and lentils

Any vegetables—eat plenty of green, leafy vegetables and salads

Any fresh fruit, except pineapple and papaya

Pastry—if homemade

Any unsweetened fruit juice

Herbal teas, except maté and redbush

Not Allowed

Alcoholic drinks, including alcohol-free beers and wines

Food cooked in beer, wine, and the like

Coffee

Tea, including green tea, jasmine tea, and so on

Colas

Chocolate

Sugar and all sugar-containing foods (see page 249)

Artificial sweeteners

Vinegar and pickles (except in small quantities)

Margarine

All food additives

Smoked fish or meat

Bacon and ham

Salami-type sausages

Very ripe cheeses

Take-out food

Restaurant food (except very occasionally)

Bran

Any very salty food

Aspirin and related drugs (see pages 443–45)

Curries and other very spicy food

For further details, see pages 335–37.

Some people who feel partially better at this stage may be suffering from gut flora problems. Cutting out sugar could have improved the situation, but to get any farther may require a more stringent diet, as described in chapter 10. You could either try this diet now, or go on to the Stage 2 diet (described below) and return to the no-sugar, no-yeast diet if this does not work.

Feeling a Lot Better

Good—you can now test the various things you cut out to see which ones cause your symptoms (see the next section for instructions). Testing can begin as soon as you have been consistently well for a week. If you felt terrible at the start of the diet, then caffeine is the most likely cause. Try a fairly weak cup of coffee or tea for your first test. Bear in mind that there are dozens of other chemical componants in tea and coffee besides caffeine—you may be reacting to one of these, in which case you could be sensitive to tea but not coffee, or vice versa.

Reintroduction Phase

Reintroduce one item each week, for example:

week 1—food containing additives
week 2—tea
week 3—coffee
week 4—beer
week 5—white wine
week 6—red wine
week 7—spirits
week 8—chocolate

Take some of the test food or drink every day, starting with a small amount and continuing for a week. If there is a reaction, then stop immediately. Wait until you are better, then go on to the next item. If there is no reaction, *give it up again after a week* and test the next item. At the end of the testing period you can reintroduce all the things that produced no reaction.

If you react to food containing additives, then leave these out again for a time while you test other items. Then test them again individually—see pages 414–18 for details of the different groups of additives. If you react to one member of a group, you may well react to others in that group, too.

Try to continue your good eating habits after the diet is finished—don't go back to eating a lot of salt and sugar or drinking huge quantities of tea, coffee, or alcohol (even if these didn't cause any specific symptoms). Keep eating fresh foods, particularly green vegetables, and stay away from junk food.

Once you have established which items cause your symptoms, you will probably need to avoid these entirely for a considerable time, although you might be able to consume a small amount occasionally. Try them out from time to time, to see whether your reaction has abated.

No Reactions?

If you still feel better but did not react adversely to anything on testing, then there are various possibilities. One is that you have a genuine intolerance reaction to a component of one of these items, but that the period of abstinence has somehow corrected it. This is especially likely with things that are tested toward the end of the reintroduction phase. If you go back to taking such items every day, then the intolerance may reappear. So if you begin to get your symptoms again, you need to repeat Stage 1 and test everything in the reverse order this time.

A second possibility is that you may have gut flora problems—see chapter 10. In mild cases just cutting out sugar can clear the symptoms. If this is the explanation, you will probably begin to notice symptoms again if you start to take significant amounts of sugar or honey again. Obviously, returning to a sugar-free diet is the answer.

Stage 2—Simple Elimination Diet

You should have completed at least a month of Stage 1 before starting Stage 2, and you should still be eating the Stage 1 diet. Continue with all the Stage 1 restrictions during Stage 2. Do not begin if you have any sort of infection, especially diarrhea.

Before starting Stage 2, look at the Stage 3 diet and think about how you would do it if you had to. One possible outcome of Stage 2 is that you go straight into Stage 3—you need to be prepared to do this.

Exclusion Phase

This diet is summarized in table 14 on page 342.

CUT OUT THE FOLLOWING FOODS:

- Wheat, rye, barley, oats, corn.
- Rice (brown or white), if this is normally part of your diet and you eat it more than once or twice a week.
- Milk and all milk products, including butter.
- Eggs.
- Soy.
- Oranges, lemons, grapefruit, tangerines, limes, and all other citrus fruits.
- Yeast and yeast extract, including bouillon cubes or Vegemite.
- Mushrooms.
- Peanuts and any other nuts you eat reasonably often.
- Beef and chicken.
- Any food that you eat every day, eat in large quantities, or have a craving for.
- Any food that a member of your family reacts to, or that you suspect for any reason.
- All items disallowed during Stage 1.

As soon as you start the exclusion phase, keep a record of everything you eat, including a rough idea of how much and when. Record your symptoms, too, and continue this throughout the diet. Be very careful not to eat too much of any one food. Don't have blowouts—little and often is the best way to eat.

Stay on the exclusion phase of the diet for two weeks or until you feel better—whichever comes sooner. Those with serious problems, such as rheumatoid arthritis, may take a little longer to respond, and they should continue for three weeks. Patients with Crohn's disease *(who must have full medical supervision for such a diet)* take about nine days, on average, to respond. They may need to continue the elimination phase for longer than fourteen days.

The possible outcomes are dealt with on pages 344–46. If you do feel better, you should not delay in reintroducing foods—see pages 346–49 for instructions.

Some Special Points about the Prohibited Foods
Milk
If you are sensitive to milk, you may be able to substitute goat's or sheep's milk for it once you have completed the diet. But at this stage it is better

---

TABLE 14 THE STAGE 2 DIET

Allowed

Lamb, turkey, pork, duck, goose, rabbit (all fresh and unprocessed)

Any fresh vegetables

Potatoes

Rice, unless you usually eat this often

Any fresh fruit, other than citrus fruit (oranges, lemons, and the like),
  pineapple, and papaya

Chickpeas; also beans and lentils (but not if you have bowel symptoms)

Any nuts that you do not normally eat very often

Herbal teas, except maté and redbush

Pure vegetable oil

Not Allowed

Bread

Wheat, rye, barley, oats, corn

Rice, if you eat this regularly

Beef and chicken

Milk, butter, yogurt, and cheese

Margarine

Eggs

Soy

Pineapple and papaya

Oranges, lemons, grapefruit, and the like

Vegemite and other yeast extracts

Bouillon cubes

Mushrooms

Peanuts

Anything you normally eat every day or crave

Any suspect food

Coffee, chocolate, tea (all varieties), colas

Sugar, any sugar-containing foods, and artificial sweeteners

All additives

All alcoholic drinks, and their derivatives

Vinegar, pickles, and relishes

Bacon, ham, corned beef, and all other smoked or processed meats

Chili, curries, and other very spicy foods

Aspirin and related drugs

For further details, see pages 340–44.

to avoid these as well, because there can be cross-reactions. Soy milk is not advisable at this early stage, either; soy is found quite widely in processed foods and meat products, and some people are sensitive to it even though they are unaware of eating it.

You should be avoiding packaged and processed foods anyway, but if you do eat any, be aware that milk may be called by various synonyms on the ingredients label—see appendix 3.

Most margarines contain some milk solids, and should be avoided anyway, as they are highly processed.

Cereals

You can substitute other starchy foods such as sweet potatoes and buckwheat for some of these—see pages 403–7. Be careful to distinguish buckwheat from bulgur wheat—the latter is true wheat, but buckwheat comes from an entirely different plant. Millet is a cereal, but few people react to it. You should not eat it at first, but if you find you are unable to eat wheat, you could test it as a potential substitute.

If you are used to eating lots of bread then you may feel rather empty, and it might be tempting to stoke up on potatoes. Try to avoid this temptation by using some other, less usual foods as fillers sometimes—parsnips or turnips, for example. Acquiring a sensitivity to potatoes is not going to be helpful. Other alternatives to bread and starchy foods are given on pages 403–10.

Corn is found in the form of sweet corn, corn on the cob, cornmeal, corn syrup, cornflakes, popcorn, and grits. The Italian dish polenta is made with corn. The gum on stamps and envelopes is often made of cornstarch, and highly sensitive people may react to licking these.

Wheat is found in macaroni, spaghetti, and other forms of pasta; couscous; semolina; cookies, cakes, and pastries—as well as in bread, most breakfast cereals, and most packaged foods. When labels say "flour" they usually mean wheat flour—or corn.

If you are eliminating rice, then you should also avoid wild rice, since the two are related (though not closely). If you find you are sensitive to rice, then test wild rice later as a potential substitute.

Potato flour, rice flour, or arrowroot can be used to thicken sauces and gravies—these are available from health food stores and delicatessens. Do not use instant mashed potatoes, which contains various additives.

Eggs

This means chicken's eggs principally, but there is a strong chance of cross-reaction with other birds' eggs, so it is advisable to avoid all eggs. See appendix 3 for the synonyms that may be used on ingredients labels.

Yeast

Avoiding yeast means not eating Vegemite or other types of yeast extract, bouillon cubes, vinegar, and any food containing malt extract or "hydrolyzed protein." Also avoid overripe or moldy fruit. (Leavened bread and alcoholic drinks are also rich in yeast, but these are not allowed anyway.) Many vitamin tablets are based on yeast, and these should be discontinued—for yeast-free nutritional supplements, see page 457.

Possible Outcomes

Feeling Much Worse

This often happens during the first few days of the exclusion phase, and it is generally considered a good sign. These "withdrawal symptoms" are seen in many food-sensitive patients. They should pass by the end of the first week, if not before. Don't give up.

Feeling a Little Worse

This may be a mild version of the withdrawal symptoms, but if it persists after seven days, then it is something else. One possibility is that you were somewhat undernourished to start with and the diet has made things worse. If you think this is likely, go back to the healthy-eating diet and take a nutritional supplement—see appendix 9. Stay on this regime for a couple of months to try to recover your general health. Then try the Stage 2 diet again—or move straight on to Stage 3.

Feeling Worse, Then Much Better

Once you have felt consistently better for three or four days then you should start the reintroduction phase—see below. Don't delay doing this. Write down exactly how you feel at this point—it may be useful and encouraging to refer back to this later if you suffer a lot of reactions during food testing.

Feeling Much Better Quite Quickly

This can happen, especially in children and young people—they seem to miss out on the withdrawal symptoms. Go on to the reintroduction phase.

Feeling Much Better, but with One or Two Lingering Symptoms

It looks as if you have cut out your main offending foods but are still eating something that is a problem. If the lingering symptoms are fairly minor, then you can proceed to the reintroduction phase. Test the major foods—milk, eggs, wheat, rice, and so on—and continue eating those that cause no problems. This will help broaden your diet. Having done this, look through the food diary you kept before the diet and try to identify possible causes for your lingering symptoms—is there anything you used to eat quite frequently and have continued eating throughout the diet? Potatoes, onions, tomatoes, shellfish, and fish are likely suspects. Cut all these out and then test them.

If your lingering symptoms are fairly troublesome, or very variable from day to day, then it will not be possible to get clear results from the reintroduction phase. In this case, look back through the food diary you kept before the diet for potential culprits. Cut these out immediately. Should your symptoms clear up, then go on to the reintroduction phase immediately. If they don't, then go on to the Stage 3 diet, preferably a rare-food diet.

Before deciding which course of action to take, consider the possibility that it might be something other than food causing the residual symptoms. If you have gut flora problems, for example, the sugar-free, yeast-free diet could have helped considerably, but not removed all your symptoms. Read chapter 10 again. Or it could be that food was your main problem but something else is causing the residual symptoms— an airborne allergen or environmental chemical, perhaps. If you have not checked out these possibilities, then think about them now. Read page 332 again.

Feeling Worse, Then Much Better, Then Worse Again

If you go through the withdrawal symptoms, feel greatly improved for a while, but then begin to go downhill again, this is a rather bad sign. It does not happen to many people, but if it does happen to you then you need to think very carefully about the situation.

The most likely explanation is that you are developing a new sensitivity to something allowed on the exclusion phase—probably something you are eating a lot of. Look at your food record for the exclusion phase and try to work out what this might be—foods you ate plentifully before the diet are also suspects. Cut out any such foods and see what happens. Meanwhile, make great efforts not to eat too much of any one food. Introducing some rare foods—see appendix 5—may be the answer, but don't overindulge in these either or you may spoil your chances of following a rare-food diet later.

If you get better again and stay better for two or three days, then you can begin the reintroduction phase. Continue to vary your diet as much as possible during this period—if you can, go on to a rotation diet (see page 359). If you can't manage a four-day rotation, then three days will be some help at least.

If you are still not well, or if you have unclear results during the reintroduction phase, then the best plan is to go straight on to Stage 3, preferably a rare-food diet. As a last resort, you could try an elemental diet (see page 321), but only with medical supervision.

Feeling About the Same
You can either go back to the healthy-eating diet and think about what to do next, or you can go straight on to Stage 3.

Reintroduction Phase

Wait until you have been free of symptoms for two or three days, but don't wait any longer than this. Begin by testing foods that are probably not the cause of any trouble—things you do not eat every day. Choose items that you like—if the foods pass the test, then you can incorporate them into your menus, which will allow you to eat less of the exclusion-phase foods. Throughout the reintroduction phase it is vital that you keep your diet varied and not eat too much of any one food. In particular, do not eat any one food every day. Continue to record everything you eat, and your symptoms—if something goes wrong, this record will prove invaluable.

Test only one food at a time. Eat a normal-sized portion of the food in question, for lunch and supper. Notice any changes that occur at the time, or later in the evening, or the following day. Most symptoms will show up within this time span, although bowel symptoms may take longer—they can occur anywhere between four and forty-eight hours after the food is eaten.

If there is no reaction by the following day, eat two portions of the food again. Should you get no reaction this time, then repeat for a third day. If there is still no reaction, then the food can be considered safe, but avoid it again for four days (to offset any possible effects of eating it for three days in succession) before beginning to eat it once more.

If you get a reaction to any food, stop eating it immediately. You may be able to abort the symptoms by taking a mixture of sodium and potassium bicarbonate. It is not known how or why this works, but it appears to do so. However, it is only effective if you are clear of symptoms at the outset—it cannot be used as a general remedy for food-induced illnesses, and in any case it should not be taken too often. Mix two level teaspoons of sodium bicarbonate (bicarbonate of soda) with one level teaspoon of potassium bicarbonate, dissolve in a small glass of warm water, and drink the mixture as rapidly as is comfortable. *Never do this if you have eaten a very large meal, however—it can be dangerous in such circumstances.* Potassium bicarbonate should be obtainable from your pharmacist, although it may have to be ordered. Buy some in advance if you want to try this remedy, rather than just sweating it out when you get a reaction to a food. Do not test any more foods until the symptoms have completely subsided. Very occasionally the symptoms—which may be quite severe— persist for several days even though you have not eaten any more of the offending food. Do not feel discouraged or worried by this.

Foods to Test

Milk and **cheese** should be tested separately. Test milk first, using fresh milk, not evaporated or dried. If you react to milk you will probably react to cheese and **butter** as well, although some milk-sensitive people can eat butter. (A rare few are sensitive to butter but not milk.) Even if you can drink milk, you may react to cheese, because it contains various chemicals produced by bacteria and molds during the cheese-making process. Some people can tolerate evaporated milk, but not fresh milk. If you react to fresh milk, you could test the evaporated kind later, but wait at least a week before you do so.

Citrus fruits should be tested with **orange** first, then **lemon**. If you can eat both of these safely, then you need not test the others.

Test **yeast** before **mushrooms**. You can either use yeast extract (for example, Vegemite) or yeast vitamin tablets. Or mix half a teaspoon of baker's yeast with a cup of water, boil for ten minutes to kill the yeast, and drink when cool.

Test **wheat** before other cereals. Do not test it in the form of bread, because this contains various other ingredients as well. Certain breakfast cereals are pure wheat, notably puffed and shredded wheat, and these are good for testing—they can be moistened with fruit juice if you are not able to have milk. Alternatively, use bulgur wheat or pasta (checking first for other ingredients), or mix flour into a pancake batter with eggs (assuming you have tested eggs already and they are safe). If using flour, start with whole wheat, preferably untreated and organically grown, so you can be sure that it contains no other ingredients. You can test white flour later. Some people are intolerant of the part of the wheat grain that is lost during the production of white flour, so they only react to whole wheat flour and bread. Others are sensitive to white flour only, probably because of its additives or the chemical processes, such as bleaching, that are used in its production.

If you react to wheat, allow at least a week to pass before testing any more cereals—test something else in the meantime. **Rye** can be tested as rye crackers, but make sure they're pure rye, because some contain wheat bran. (Also bear in mind that some people who react to yeast also react to malt, which is a common ingredient in crackers and cereals.) **Oats** can be tested as oatmeal, and corn as kernels or cornmeal. **Barley** can be tested by eating pearl barley—boil about two or three tablespoons of it in plain water or homemade stock. It may seem rather pointless testing a food such as barley if you never eat it normally, but you could be sensitive to it if you drink beer regularly, or if you are sensitive to wheat. Rye, barley, and oats are all quite closely related to wheat and cross-reactions are not uncommon. Rheumatologists using elimination diets for patients with rheumatoid arthritis have found that the reaction to cereals is often very slow among their patients. They recommend more thorough and prolonged testing. In the case of wheat, you should eat a normal portion of a pure wheat cereal (see above), pasta, or bulgur wheat with all three meals for a period of up to five days—stop earlier if the symptoms reappear. Corn, rye, oats, and rice should also be tested at all meals for five full days.

Other items to be tested are: **eggs, beef, chicken,** and anything else that you decided to avoid, such as **rice** or **peanuts.**

The reintroduction phase should take about seven or eight weeks. If it takes any longer than this, there is a risk of lost sensitivity; the food-intolerant person becomes less reactive after avoiding the culprit food for a time. For some people, it may take many months or years to lose their intolerance, but for others the process can happen within two to three months.

If you have still not tested all foods eight weeks after starting the exclusion phase, then you should reintroduce all those not yet tested. Eat all of them (in normal portions) every day for a week. If, after a week, there is no reaction, then you can consider them all safe. If there is a reaction, cut them all out again, and avoid them for five days, or until your symptoms clear up if it takes longer. Then retest each of those foods in turn, using the same procedure as before.

Once you have tested all foods and established a diet on which you feel well, you can test the items that you gave up during Stage 1: tea, coffee, alcohol, and so on. Follow the procedure outlined on pages 340–41.

Incomplete Testing

If something goes wrong during the testing—you might get the flu, for example, or some other infection—then you will have to stop testing foods. All is not lost, but there is no point in trying to test foods beyond three months. Go back to the healthy-eating diet for about a month, but exclude any foods that gave a positive reaction when tested.

Keep a record of your symptoms, and see how you feel at the end of the month. If you are reasonably well, then continue with the healthy-eating diet, avoiding the incriminated foods, and see how you get on. As long as you keep your diet varied, so as not to acquire new sensitivities, you can always go through Stage 2 again later.

If after a month on the healthy-eating diet, some or all of your symptoms have returned, then you should start the exclusion phase of Stage 2 again. Any foods that you previously tested and found safe can be eaten as well, but if your symptoms have not cleared up after a week, then you should exclude these foods as well.

Assuming your symptoms clear up, you can test the excluded foods as described above. If they do not, then you should go on to Stage 3.

Stage 3—Rigorous Elimination Diet

Only a minority of those reading this book will need to try the Stage 3 diet. They will know they need to do this because they have tried Stage 2 with only partial success—or no success at all. Stage 3 is for those with multiple food sensitivities that cannot be detected by a simple elimination diet.

The Exclusion Phase

Stage 3 requires planning, even more so than the previous stages. You must decide for yourself which foods you are going to eat during the exclusion phase, because this diet has to be tailored to your own eating habits. The aim is to come up with a list of at least twelve foods that are nutritious, obtainable, and affordable, and that you have never eaten in any quantity or with any regularity before. They should include a variety of different items—some fruits, some vegetables, some meat or fish, and some starchy foods, if possible, although this is often difficult. The approach we would advocate is a combination of the few-food diet and the rare-food diet (see pages 320–21), with the exact mix of foods being chosen to suit your pocketbook and your palate.

SUGGESTED FOODS

Vegetables
- Celery, fennel, and celeriac
- Avocados
- Lettuce
- Rutabaga (can be cooked or grated raw in salads)
- Watercress
- Spinach
- Alfalfa sprouts
- Okra
- Asparagus

Meat and Fish
- Turkey
- Duck
- Goose
- Rabbit
- Pheasant or other game
- Lamb
- Fish (except smoked fish and shellfish)

Fruits
- Gooseberries
- Black currants
- Red currants
- Bananas
- Pears
- Kiwi fruit
- Mangoes
- Pomegranates
- Lychees
- Passion fruit
- Guavas

Starchy Foods
• Rice
• Millet
• Buckwheat
• Turnips
• Parsnips
• Yams (see page 405)
• Taro
• Breadfruit
• Cassava
• Sweet potatoes (see pages 405–6)
• Plantains
• Wild rice
• Tapioca
• Sago
• Chestnuts
• Chickpeas (also a good source of protein)
• Pumpkin

Oils
• Olive oil
• Sunflower oil
• Safflower oil
• Rapeseed oil
• Coconut oil and creamed coconut

Snacks
• Pumpkin seeds
• Macadamia nuts
• Pistachio nuts
• Cashew nuts
• Brazil nuts
• Pine nuts

If there are any foods on this list that you eat more than once a week—or have eaten very regularly at some time in the past—then you should exclude them. Advice on where to obtain exotic foods and how to cook them is given in appendix 5.

When deciding on your final list, bear the following points in mind: Avocados have a laxative effect on some people. If you have bowel symptoms, then you should not include these. If you have never eaten them before, try eating a couple at one sitting before you start Stage 3, to see what effect they have.

Spinach and chickpeas should not be included if you have bowel symptoms. Parsnips should be eaten in limited quantities only, and not too often, as they contain small amounts of a carcinogen.

Plantains are closely related to bananas and should not be included if you regularly eat bananas.

You should eat sunflower oil only if you have not previously eaten much margarine, nor used much sunflower oil (or vegetable oil) in cooking.

Other foods that you do not eat often can be included, but not if they are related to frequently eaten foods. Vegetables such as eggplant and cauliflower are not as safe as they might appear, because they are closely related to staple foods—tomatoes and potatoes, for eggplant, and cabbage for cauliflower. Consult appendix 5 before adding any foods to the list. Jerusalem artichokes, lentils, kidney beans, and other types of beans should not be eaten, as they all tend to affect the bacteria living in the gut.

Many nuts are potent allergens. Stop eating them immediately if you have any immediate symptoms in the mouth, such as tingling or itching.

If you are a vegetarian, then you should think carefully before going on this diet: it will be low in both calories and protein, and will be very limited in scope—which means that you may be eating too much of some foods. If you can allow yourself some fish or meat, at least for a while, then you will probably do better on the diet. Introduce these foods gradually, before starting the exclusion phase, as your body may need time to adjust to the change.

The Exclusion Phase

This is meant to be a very simple, basic diet in which you consume nothing but your allowed foods. No herbs, no spices, no flavorings, nothing canned, and no packaged foods of any sort. It is not going to be a gastronomic delight, but the diet does not last long and it may make you well again.

Eat only your allowed foods, remembering to vary your diet, not to eat any one food every day, and not to eat too much of any one food. Drink only bottled or filtered water (see appendix 6). As before, you can drink herbal teas, but avoid any that you have consumed regularly before. You should also vary them and not drink more than two or three cups a day—you can become sensitive to anything you eat or drink, and herbal teas are no exception. Check the label and avoid those containing orange, lemon, or apple extracts.

If after reading chapter 9 you think you may have chemical sensitivity, then you should try to eat only unsprayed food during this diet (as well as following the avoidance measures for synthetic chemicals on pages 228–33). Unfortunately, eating organic foods only may be very difficult, since your choice of food is limited anyway, but it is worth choosing organic produce for some of the foods even if you cannot manage it for all of them. Check a variety of sources to see what sort of organic produce is available—the range is widening all the time. Remember that friends' gardens are often the best source of unsprayed fruits and vegetables—ask around to see if you can buy surplus produce. You can test for sensitivity to pesticide residues by comparing your reactions to the same food sprayed and unsprayed.

Continue the exclusion phase for at least three weeks. If you are not substantially better by then, it is highly unlikely that you have food sensitivity. Keep a record of everything you eat and all your symptoms.

You should also weigh yourself regularly during this diet, especially if you are not overweight at the outset. Anyone who is underweight should not embark on the diet without medical advice. If you find you are losing weight rapidly, then you should discuss the matter with your doctor. Elemental diets can sometimes be useful in these circumstances as a nutritional supplement.

Possible Outcomes
Feeling Much Worse
This often happens during the first few days of the exclusion phase, and it is generally considered a good sign. These withdrawal symptoms are seen in many food-sensitive patients and seem to be caused by suddenly cutting out the offending food. They should pass by the end of the first week.

If you continue to feel worse after about eight days, then it may be that one of the rare or unusual foods you have included in your diet is affecting you. If you are eating buckwheat, cut this out for a few days— it can cause both food allergy and false food allergy in susceptible people. If this produces no improvement, then cut out all other rare foods at once, and see how you are. Should you continue to have symptoms, go back to the healthy-eating diet and reconsider other possibilities: see under Feeling About the Same on page 355.

Feeling a Little Worse
This may be a mild version of the withdrawal symptoms, but if it persists after seven days, then it is something else. One possibility is that you were somewhat undernourished to start with and the diet has made things worse. If you think this is likely, go back to the healthy-eating diet and take a nutrional supplement—see appendix 9. Stay on this regime for a couple of months to try to recover your general health. Then try the Stage 3 diet again.

Feeling Worse, Then Much Better
Once you have felt consistently better for three or four days then you should start the reintroduction phase—see page 356. Don't delay doing this. Write down exactly how you feel at this point—it may be useful and encouraging to refer back to this later if you suffer a lot of reactions during food testing.

Feeling Much Better Quite Quickly
This can happen, especially in children and young people—they seem to miss out on the withdrawal symptoms. Go on to the reintroduction phase.

Feeling Much Better, but with One or Two Lingering Symptoms
It looks as if you have cut out your main offending foods, but are still eating something that is a problem (assuming that you have ruled out all other problems, such as airborne allergens, hyperventilation, and environmental chemicals; see page 332). Think again about your previous eating habits—is there anything you used to eat quite frequently and are still eating? Cut all these out.

If your symptoms clear up, then go on to the reintroduction phase immediately. If they don't, then the best option is to go on to a full rare-food diet that includes only foods you have never eaten before. See appendix 5 for suitable foods.

If the remaining symptoms are mild and fairly constant from day to day, then you could go on to the reintroduction phase—you may get some sort of useful result from testing. If you can discover which foods are the main source of trouble and establish a diet on which you are reasonably well, then you are in a good position to investigate further. It could be that the remaining symptoms are due to some other problem— see Feeling About the Same, below, for a list of possibilities.

Feeling Worse, Then Much Better, Then Worse Again

If you go through the withdrawal symptoms, feel greatly improved for a while, but then begin to go downhill again, this is a rather bad sign. It does not happen to many people, but if it does happen to you then you need to think very carefully about the situation.

The most likely explanation is that you are developing a new sensitivity to something allowed on the exclusion phase—probably something you are eating a lot of. Look at your food record for the exclusion phase, and try to work out what this might be—foods you ate before the diet, rather than entirely novel ones, are the obvious suspects. Cut out any such foods and see what happens. Meanwhile, make great efforts not to eat too much of any one food.

If you get better again and stay better for two or three days, then you can begin the reintroduction phase. Continue to vary your diet as much as possible during this period—if you can, go on to a rotation diet (see page 359). If you can't manage a four-day rotation, then three days will be some help at least.

If you are still not well, or if you have unclear results during the reintroduction phase, then one possible solution is an elemental diet (see page 321), but you should consult your doctor about this and take his or her advice.

Feeling About the Same

It seems unlikely that food sensitivity is your problem. If possible, progress to a full rare-food diet composed only of foods that are new to you—just to check that none of the foods in the exclusion phase is the source of the trouble. If this has no effect then you should go back to the healthy-eating diet and reconsider other possibilities, such as *Giardia* (see pages 249–50), gut flora problems (chapter 10), airborne allergens (see pages 85–88), hyperventilation (see page 210–12), chemical sensitivity (chapter 9), psychosomatic problems (see pages 196–98) and nutritional deficiencies (see page 330).

Reintroduction Phase

Wait until you have been free of symptoms for two or three days, but don't wait any longer than this. Begin by testing foods that are probably not the cause of any trouble—things you do not eat very often. Choose items that you like—if the foods pass the test, then you can incorporate them into your menus, which will allow you to eat less of the exclusion-phase foods. Throughout the reintroduction phase it is vital that you keep your diet varied and not eat too much of any one food. In particular, do not eat any one food every day. Continue to record everything you eat, and your symptoms—if something goes wrong, this record will prove invaluable.

Test only one food at a time. Eat a normal-sized portion of the food in question, preferably with your evening meal. Notice any changes that occur at the time, or later in the evening, or the following day. During the first five weeks of testing, test each food for one day only. (Although eating the food for three days in succession is preferable, it takes so much time that you cannot test enough foods—there are far more to test than during Stage 2.) If you think you may have reacted slightly but are unsure, then test the same food again the next day. After five weeks, your sensitivity may be declining, so you need to test each food more thoroughly, by eating it for three days in succession. If you get no reaction by the fourth day, then the food can be considered safe, but avoid it again for four days (to offset any possible effects of eating it for three days in succession) before beginning to eat it once more.

If you get a reaction to any food, stop eating it immediately. Allow the symptoms to subside before testing any more foods. Sometimes the symptoms—which may be quite severe—persist for several days even though you have not eaten any more of the offending food. Do not feel discouraged or worried by this, but persevere with the diet.

The reintroduction phase should take about seven or eight weeks. If it takes any longer than this, there is a risk of lost sensitivity: the food-intolerant person becomes less reactive after avoiding the culprit food for a time. If you are still testing foods eight weeks after starting the exclusion phase, then you need to test the foods more rigorously still. This means eating each reintroduced food every day for a week before declaring it safe.

If there are some foods that you have still not tested after twelve weeks, then you have two options. One is to reintroduce all those foods for three to four weeks and see if any symptoms return. If they do, cut all those foods out again, wait until you feel better, then reintroduce them one at a time. Use three-day testing for preference, or one-day testing if you have a lot to get through.

The second option is to reintroduce each of the foods in turn, one per day. If there is no reaction, continue eating the food, but only on a once-every-four-days basis, for about six months. After that time, you should have become much less sensitive and be able to eat all these foods more freely.

If you suspect that you are sensitive to pesticide residues, you should be eating mainly unsprayed food during the exclusion phase of the diet. When you start to test foods, you should test unsprayed versions first, then a sprayed version of the same food, to see the difference. Leave a gap of at least four days between tests—try some other food in the meantime.

No Reaction to Testing

In either Stage 2 or Stage 3, there is the remote possibility that you will recover during the exclusion phase of the diet, and show no reactions when foods are tested. It seems that this happens more often with younger patients, but it is unusual even among children.

There are two likely explanations for this outcome. One is that the diet has had a placebo effect (see pages 199–201). The other is that the sensitivity has been greatly reduced by simply avoiding the food for a month or two. Further dietary restrictions do not seem to be needed, but it is advisable to keep the diet varied to avoid a recurrence of the problem.

FIFTEEN

After the Elimination Diet—
Treating Food Intolerance

The simplest and most effective method of treating food intolerance is to avoid the culprit foods. Assuming that you have successfully identified your culprit foods by following an elimination diet, the next step is to establish an adequate menu that excludes those foods. Make a list of the foods you cannot eat, and a list of those that you can. Talk to your doctor about your proposed diet, and ask for advice on its nutritional value.

After about six months you can retest each of the incriminated foods to see if you still react to them. If you do react, then try again six months later. If not, then you can begin eating them once in every four days. After a year of this, you can increase the frequency cautiously, but you should never go back to eating the food every day, or in large amounts. If symptoms recur, cut out the culprit foods again for a couple of months.

If you are not fully well, even after the elimination diet, then it is worth considering other possibilities—it could be that you have other problems in addition to food intolerance. Nutritional deficiencies (see page 330) or chemical sensitivity (chapter 9) are possible candidates. A continuing tendency to diarrhea and gas may indicate gut flora disturbances. The treatments currently available for this are to eat plenty of live yogurt or take a bacterial replacer (see pages 250–51).

Rotation Diets

For people who acquire new sensitivities easily, eating all foods on a four-day rotation basis may be advisable. This is known as a **rotation diet**. Items from the list of allowed foods are allocated to four separate lists, one for each day of the rotation. Ideally, food relationships should be taken into account, and foods from the same family (such as potatoes and tomatoes) eaten on only one day in the four. This does make the rotation diet quite restrictive, but it may be necessary for some people. See appendix 4 for information on related foods.

The restrictions imposed by the rotation diet are quite harsh—not only are foods disallowed, but particular foods have to be eaten on particular days. An occasional departure from the regime is acceptable, but even with such allowances eating away from home is very difficult indeed, and many social events become impossible. Some doctors recommend rotation diets to almost anyone recovering from food sensitivity, but the costs have to be weighed against the benefits. Loneliness and isolation can be as damaging to the health as eating the wrong sort of food.

Other Methods of Treating Food Intolerance

For those with multiple food sensitivities, avoiding all their culprit foods can be very difficult. And it may mean that they eat too much of other foods, with the attendant risk of developing new sensitivities. Even those who are intolerant of just one or two foods may find it difficult to avoid them, especially if they eat away from home a lot. So there have been many attempts to develop alternative methods of treatment.

Given the lack of knowledge about how food intolerance arises, these attempts are largely a try-it-and-see exercise. No treatment has yet been devised that is 100 percent effective for all patients, and some that are offered by alternative practitioners are quite ineffective and even potentially dangerous (urine therapy, for instance). However, two methods currently being tried out by some doctors, known as neutralization or desensitization treatments, are worthy of further investigation.

In some studies these treatments have performed quite well, but in others they have been less successful. Consequently, such techniques are controversial, and many doctors feel that they should not be used until there is more evidence that they work. But given the complex nature of food intolerance, and the evidence suggesting that it is caused in several different ways (see chapter 12), perhaps it is not surprising if a treatment gives varying results—it might be expected to work for some patients and not for others. Our own experience suggests that such methods are effective for a proportion of people with food intolerance. But they are probably not worth trying unless there is no reasonable dietary alternative. Other uses claimed for these techniques include desensitization to environmental chemicals, such as exhaust fumes.

Provocation-Neutralization Technique

This is also known as intradermal neutralization therapy, or the Miller technique, after Dr. Joseph Miller of Alabama, who has spent many years developing it and investigating its potential. The treatment can be applied in two ways—either using injections of food extracts under the skin (**subcutaneous injections**) or giving food extract drops under the tongue (**sublingual drops**). In both cases the doctor establishes a particular dose of the food extract that will turn off or neutralize the symptoms caused by that food.

To test for the correct dose, **intradermal injections**, which put food extracts into the skin, should be used. Intradermal injections place food extracts deeper in the skin than skin-prick tests (see page 34). A tiny amount of food extract is used—0.05 milliliters. If the body does not react to this extract it simply produces a small raised area, known as a wheal, which begins to go down soon afterward. If the body does react, then the wheal grows slightly and takes on a characteristic appearance—it is white, hard, and raised, with a sharp edge. This is known as a *positive wheal*. At the same time, the patient may experience symptoms similar to those normally produced by the food—this is the *provocation* part of the test.

The *neutralization* part of the technique is based on the finding that a particular concentration of the same food extract will put a stop to those symptoms. Such a dose also produces a *negative wheal*—one that is white, hard, and raised, but does not grow larger. It is usually the same size ten minutes after the injection.

The neutralization dose is usually the strongest solution that fails to produce a positive wheal, so it is determined by starting with a solution that does produce a positive wheal and then working gradually downward. Using this method the neutralizing dose can be determined, even though the patient has no symptoms at the time—the wheals alone show when the right dose has been reached.

The claim that the neutralizing dose turns off symptoms that have already begun sounds implausible, but this has regularly been observed, and many skeptics have been convinced by such a demonstration. How it might work is not known. Dr. Miller has speculated that when the neutralizing dose is used, the food extract is "bound" inside the wheal for a prolonged period, which allows it to exert a particular influence on the immune system. He suggests that it stimulates suppressor cells, which damp down the immune response to the food. This assumes, of course, that an immune reaction is the main cause of food intolerance, which is far from certain. Assuming enzyme deficiencies are at the root of food intolerance, then the neutralizing dose might stimulate the body to produce more detoxification enzymes.

In practical terms, neutralization therapy involves a long session of testing (usually one to three days) with different concentrations of foods—all the foods that have been incriminated by the elimination diet. The extracts are injected into the skin of the upper arm, a process that is only slightly painful. Once neutralizing doses have been determined for each of these foods, a mixture of the extracts is prepared for use. The patient is taught to carry out the subcutaneous injections, which are needed every two days at first, but only twice a week or even less frequently once the treatment has been under way for some months. Some people eventually find that they can discontinue the injections without ill effects.

Sublingual therapy should be approached in exactly the same way, the offending foods being identified by an elimination diet and the neutralizing dose being determined by a series of injections. But the mixture of extracts for home use is supplied as drops, one of which is placed under the tongue. There is rapid absorption into the bloodstream from this area, and it bypasses the liver, so the extract is not broken down rapidly. The effect of drops is not as long lasting as that of a subcutaneous injection—the treatment has to be repeated every few hours. However, they are useful for inhalant allergies or reactions to substances that are only encountered occasionally, because the drops can be used only when needed. Sublingual therapy has been successfully used to treat patients with allergic reactions to house dust mite and pollen. It is also claimed to be effective for patients sensitive to synthetic chemicals, where industrial alcohol is used instead of an extract (but see page 222).

The question of using mixtures of extracts for neutralization is a difficult one. The trials of this technique have all involved solutions containing single food extracts. Yet some practitioners use up to seventy food extracts in a mixture. Whether the method still works under these conditions is uncertain.

There is also concern over the possible dangers of this technique to patients with violent allergic reactions. It is theoretically possible for such people to suffer anaphylactic shock when injected intradermally with their allergen, and this could be fatal. However, this technique has now been widely used for many years, and no fatal (or even near-fatal) reactions have occurred. Nevertheless, anyone who has experienced immediate and violent allergic reactions to food (or other allergens) should be carefully assessed before such treatment begins.

Finally, it is claimed that the provocation-neutralization method can be used as a diagnostic test to determine which foods are the culprits, avoiding the need for an elimination diet. These claims are rejected by the majority of doctors, who feel the test is too unreliable. Detailed trials show that there are often positive reactions to extracts of foods that do not provoke symptoms when eaten (**false positives**). Occasionally foods that cause symptoms will not produce a positive wheal (**false negatives**).

Enzyme-Potentiated Desensitization

This method is less widely practiced than provocation-neutralization therapy. It depends on the ability of the enzyme, ß-glucuronidase to enhance the desensitizing effect of a food antigen. The food extract is applied to a scrape on the skin, along with the enzyme. Because the extract is not injected into the skin, it is safer for people with violent allergic reactions, and this method has been successfully used to treat food-allergic reactions involving a range of foods (see page 72).

In practice, the skin is scratched and the food extracts plus enzyme applied to it in a small plastic cup. Alternatively, it can be given by intradermal injection. The same dose is given to all patients, and a comprehensive mixture of food extracts is generally used—not just those to which the patient is sensitive. This is said to work, and it obviously means that an elimination diet is less important. One drawback of such "blanket therapy" is that there may be a worsening of the symptoms in the early stages because the patient becomes sensitized to some of the foods in the extract that were not a problem previously. Subsequent treatments apparently cancel out these effects.

An advantage of this technique over neutralization therapy is that the treatments are only needed about once every three months, and the frequency falls to once a year after a time. However, there have been far fewer trials of the method, and it is difficult to say what proportion of patients might be helped by it.

Janet

Janet was forty years old and had been ill in various ways since she was twelve, with rhinitis, severe migraine, urinary problems, and pain in the region of her kidneys. During her thirties she had also developed depression, which led to two suicide attempts and resulted in electroconvulsive therapy. Over the past six years she had made more than a hundred visits to her family doctor, spent sixty-three days in the hospital, visited outpatient clinics forty-nine times, and taken thirty-four courses of drugs.

Janet was then tried on an elimination diet that excluded all commonly eaten foods. This provoked the worst migraine she had ever experienced at first, but then left her feeling a great deal better. On testing, a glass of milk produced sneezing, rhinitis, and headache, whereas wheat left her depressed with a severe migraine. Eggs produced a headache, nausea, and pain around the kidneys. Eating corn resulted in nausea and fatigue. By avoiding these four foods, Janet has remained very well. In the six years since her treatment she has visited her doctor five times, spent only two days in the hospital, and not required any drugs—a striking contrast to her previous six years.

Conventional Allergy Shots

The two methods described above have also had some success in treating classical allergies, and in this context are safer than the traditional "allergy shots," more correctly called **hyposensitization, or incremental immunotherapy** (IIT). This method, widely used for hay fever, allergy to insect stings, and other allergies, involves injecting minute, but gradually increasing, doses of the allergen over a period of many months. There is a risk of collapse due to anaphylactic shock, especially for those with asthma, and patients have died as a result. Thus it is necessary to remain at the doctor's office after the injection for at least thirty minutes or for a full hour if asthmatic. Resuscitation equipment must be readily available. This type of immunotherapy is not currently used for food intolerance because it is unlikely to be effective. Nor is it used for true food allergy because the dangers of anaphylactic shock are too great.

Staying Well

Once you have established a workable diet or other form of treatment, you need to take care of your health generally so as to guard against becoming ill again. The most important thing is to avoid slipping back into food addiction—if you find yourself eating one sort of food very regularly, take a week off from it and then eat it on a three-day or four-day rotation basis for a while. Continue to eat healthily, with plenty of green vegetables and not too much processed food.

Exercise is very valuable, and does not have to be very strenuous or time consuming. Walking briskly, running, cycling, or swimming for half an hour is adequate. If you can do this two or three times a week, you will feel a great deal healthier—every day is even better. Just running upstairs instead of taking the elevator is beneficial.

Anyone who has had food intolerance should keep their exposure to synthetic chemicals to a minimum. Despite the rising level of air pollution and agrochemical use, the worst problems are still to be found in the home, especially the well-insulated aerosol-ridden home. Read chapter 9, even if you don't have chemical sensitivities at present, and consider ways to reduce your exposure.

Avoid anything that irritates the gut lining and makes it more permeable; see page 336. Look at the general health measures suggested on pages 316–17 and follow these if they seem appropriate.

APPENDIX 1

Foods That May Release
Sulfur Dioxide

Sulfur (or sulphur) dioxide is a gas that can irritate the airways of asthmatics and provoke an asthma attack. Some preservatives give off this gas in small amounts, and it is inhaled during eating. There is no need to avoid these preservatives unless you are sure they trigger attacks.

Most dried fruits are treated with sulfur dioxide and give off the gas when chewed. If the label does not list sulfur dioxide, but the fruit has a bright, fresh appearance, then it has been treated. Dried fruit that has not been treated will be darker in color and will usually be labeled "unsulfured."

OTHER PRESERVATIVES THAT GIVE OFF SULFUR DIOXIDE
• Sodium sulfite.
• Sodium bisulfite.
• Sodium metabisulfite.
• Potassium metabisulfite.
• Potassium bisulfite.

These preservatives are widely used in wine, beer, cocktail mixes, and cider. At one time additives used in alcoholic drinks did not have to be declared on the label. Under FDA regulations, all American wine bottled after July 9, 1987, has to be labeled if it contains sulfiting agents, but there may still be wine on the market that is sulfited and unlabeled.

Such strict regulations do not exist in most other parts of the world. Wine usually contains higher levels of sulfite than beer or spirits. Homemade wine may also be sulfited: campden tablets, sold to winemakers, contain potassium metabisulfite.

When shopping for food, note that shrimp, scallops, clams, frozen lobster, and dried cod can be treated with sodium hydrogen sulfite to preserve them. They are supposed to be labeled if the residue is more than 10 ppm (parts per million). Although sulfites are not allowed on meat, they are occasionally used illegally on old meat to give it a "fresh" red color. In all these cases, the greater part of the sulfur dioxide will be driven off by the high temperatures used in cooking. New FDA regulations prevent use on fresh fruits or vegetables that are usually eaten raw, with the exception of grapes. The residue must be less than 10 ppm (parts per million) for the grapes to be sold. Packaged foods often contain sulfites and metabisulfites, but these are easier to avoid as they are declared on the label. Look for the names given above. Bakery products could be sulfited so ask about the ingredients.

A major hidden source of sulfur dioxide is restaurant, take-out, and cafeteria food. There are no regulations requiring restaurants to disclose the presence of sulfites as yet, but you can ask the manager to check the ingredients label on the original bulk container of products, if you are concerned. French fries used in the food-service trade have usually been dipped in a metabisulfite solution and give off significant amounts of sulfur dioxide. When eating out, choose a baked potato because it is the only form of potato that you can be sure is sulfite-free. Prepared salads, avocado dip, and shellfish are also likely to be sulfited. Fresh or canned fruit, fruit salad, glacé and maraschino cherries, fruit juices, fruit pie fillings, dried vegetables and soup, pickled onions, jam, fruit jello, and custard are other possible sources of sulfur dioxide in the food-service trade. It is not worthwhile avoiding these foods unless you know they trigger your asthma attacks.

Some nebulizer solutions, used for severe asthma, contain sulfur preservatives.

APPENDIX 2

Foods Containing Salicylates

Avoiding foods containing salicylates is unlikely to be of benefit in most cases. But if you show a pronounced reaction to aspirin yet are still not well after avoiding it, a low-salicylate diet may be worth trying. Be sure to take a vitamin C supplement while on the diet. For further information, see pages 443–45. Do not follow this diet for more than two weeks without the advice of your health care practitioner.

FOODS HIGH IN SALICYLATES
- Most herbs, particularly mint, thyme, tarragon, rosemary, dill, sage, oregano, marjoram, and basil. Also celery seeds and sesame seeds.
- Most spices, particularly aniseed, cayenne, cinnamon, cumin, curry powder, fenugreek, mace, mustard, paprika, and turmeric.
- Most fruits, with the exception of bananas, peeled pears, pomegranates, mangoes, and papaya.
- Most vegetables, with the exception of cabbage, brussels sprouts, bean sprouts, celery, leeks, lettuce, and peas. Cucumbers, gherkins, olives, and endive are particularly rich in salicylates.
- Potato skins, but not potatoes themselves. Sweet corn, sweet potatoes.
- Almonds, Brazil nuts, macadamia nuts, peanuts, pine nuts, pistachios, and walnuts. Also coconut and water chestnuts.
- Coffee, tea, colas, and peppermint tea.
- Fruit juices, most alcoholic drinks (but not gin or vodka), honey, licorice, peppermints.

- Bouillon cubes, Vegemite, and other yeast-rich products.
- Tomato sauce and Worcestershire sauce.
- Many processed foods and instant meals.

FOODS LOW IN SALICYLATES
- Meat, fish, and shellfish.
- Milk, cheese, and eggs.
- Wheat, rye, oats, barley, and rice.
- Some fruits and vegetables, as listed above.

Synonyms for Food Ingredients

SYNONYMS USED ON FOOD LABELS	
Arachis oil	Peanut
Baking powder	May contain corn or wheat
Caramel	May contain traces of gluten
Casein, caseinate	Milk
Cereal binder	Usually wheat
Cereal filler	Usually wheat
Cereal protein	Usually wheat
Cereal starch	Usually wheat or corn
Citric acid	Made from corn if U.S.-produced but will not affect anyone with corn intolerance. Some citric acid made elsewhere is derived from wheat and could contain traces of gluten.
Dextrin	May contain gluten
Dextrose	A type of sugar derived from corn
Diglycerides	May contain gluten
Edible starch	Usually wheat or corn
Flour	Usually wheat flour
Food starch	Usually wheat or corn
Fructose	A type of sugar found naturally in fruit
Glucose syrup	A type of sugar, usually derived from corn
Groundnut oil	Peanut
Gum base	Could contain gluten

Hydrolyzed protein, hydrolyzed vegetable protein	Usually yeast, corn, or soy, occasionally mixed with wheat; new FDA regulations require the source of the protein to be specified
Lactalbumin	Milk
Lactose	Milk sugar
Leavening	Yeast
Lecithin	Usually egg or soy but, very rarely, peanut
Malt, malt flavoring	Usually barley so can contain gluten, but sometimes made from corn
Maltodextrin	Could contain gluten in countries outside U.S.
Maltose	A type of sugar
Miso	Soy
Modified starch, modified food starch	Usually wheat or corn or both
Monoglycerides	Could contain gluten
Monosodium glutamate (MSG)	Could contain traces of gluten if made outside U.S.
Natural flavorings	Could contain traces of wheat or milk
Ovalbumin	Egg
Starch	Usually wheat or corn
Sucrose	Sugar
Textured vegetable protein	Usually soy, sometimes corn, occasionally contains some wheat
Tofu	Soy
Vegetable gum	Can be oats, soy, or corn; could contain gluten
Vegetable oil	Usually a mixture of oils, often including corn oil
Vegetable protein	Usually soy, but could be corn, wheat, or other cereals
Vegetable starch	Can be soy, corn, or wheat
Whey	Milk

In some foods labeled "no added sugar," highly concentrated apple juice has been used to sweeten the product. It is a mistake to think of such foods as sugar-free or low in sugar.

Related Foods

The relevance of food relationships to food sensitivity is explained on pages 323–25. Briefly, a person who is sensitive to one plant food (such as oranges) may react badly to other foods from related plants (such as lemons and grapefruit). The same holds true for foods from animal sources.

In the past a great deal of emphasis has been placed on food families by those treating food intolerance. Most doctors have automatically looked at the **family** of plants and animals to predict cross-reactions. But the family is just one sort of group in biological classification and it is not always the most relevant group to consider. Sometimes we need to consider higher or lower levels of classification. The overemphasis on food families can create problems. For example, it can lead food-sensitive people to eat too much of some potentially troublesome foods (such as fish) while avoiding many plant foods unnecessarily.

In general, the problem of cross-reactions has probably been exaggerated in food intolerance. The only groups where cross-reactions are at all common are the cereals, shellfish, fish, and tree nuts. (Cross-reactions between certain foods and pollens or latex are common, however, and these are described on pages 377–78.)

The following listed relationships seem to be relevant to food sensitivity. Herbs and spices are only included where they are likely to be eaten in quantity and have the potential to cause a cross-reaction.

PLANT FOODS
  1. **Grass family, Gramineae:** Wheat, rye, triticale, barley, oats, corn, rice, wild rice, millet, sorghum, bamboo, sugarcane.

TAXONOMIC GROUPS IN CLASSIFICATION

A group of very similar individuals makes up a species.
Related species are grouped together in a **genus** (plural **genera**).
Related genera are sometimes grouped together in **tribes** and
   subfamilies.
Related genera (or tribes or subfamilies) are grouped together in a
   family.
Related families are grouped together in an **order.**
Related orders are grouped together in a **class.**
Related classes are grouped together in a **phylum** (plural **phyla**).
Related phyla are grouped together in a **kingdom.**

Some people react to all members of the family, but most are
sensitive to wheat and its close relatives, or corn or rice. The
subfamilies are more relevant here (see pages 323–25). They are:

Pooidae: Wheat, rye, barley, oats

Panicoideae: Corn, sorghum, sugarcane, bulrush or pearl
millet

Bambusoideae: Rice, wild rice

Chloridoideae: Finger millet

2. **Potato family, Solanaceae:** Potato (but not sweet potato),
   tomato, eggplant, sweet peppers (green, red, and yellow
   peppers), paprika, chile peppers, tobacco, cape gooseberry.

3. **Bean and pea family, Leguminosae:** Peas, haricot beans
   (kidney beans, whether white, red, brown, or black skinned;
   also baked beans and flageolets), peanuts, soybeans, lentils,
   split peas, broad beans, butter beans, mung beans, lima beans,
   chickpeas, black-eyed peas, carob, runner beans, green beans,
   snap beans, string beans, mangetout peas, and lupin. Different
   kinds of haricot beans and their green forms (snap beans,
   string beans, and green beans, including those sold as frozen
   vegetables) are all the same species and should be regarded as
   the same food. Peanuts belong to a separate tribe from other
   members of the family, and experience with patients who are
   allergic to peanuts suggests that cross-reactivity with other
   legumes is generally low, but peanut-sensitive people may react
   to soybeans. Patients sensitive to soybeans are likely to react to
   a wide range of legumes. Anyone with these sensitivities
   should avoid unrefined peanut and soybean oils as well, but

this may not be necessary—such oils contain no detectable protein, and tests with allergic individuals showed no reaction to the relevant oil.

4. **Cabbage family, Cruciferae:** Several members of this family are actually part of the same species, which means that they are very closely related indeed. They are: cabbage, cauliflower, brussels sprouts, broccoli, kohlrabi, and kale. These should all be regarded as the *same food* for rotation purposes. Other members of the family are: turnip, rapeseed oil, Chinese cabbage, horseradish, radish, rutabaga, cress, watercress, and mustard. Rapeseed oil might cross-react with other cabbage family foods, but this is relatively unlikely.

5. **Carrot family, Umbelliferae:** Carrot, parsnip, celery, celeriac, fennel, parsley, aniseed, caraway, dill, cumin, coriander.

6. **Cucumber family, Cucurbitaceae:** Cucumber, melon, watermelon, zucchini, squash, pumpkin.

7. **Onion family, Liliaceae:** Onion, leek, shallot, garlic, chives, asparagus.

8. **Daisy family, Compositae:** Lettuce, chicory, endive, globe artichoke, Jerusalem artichoke, salsify, sunflower, safflower, chamomile. No specific tests have been carried out on sunflower oil or safflower oil, but it seems unlikely that they would cross-react with other members of this family.

9. **Spinach family, Chenopodiaceae:** Spinach, spinach beet, chard, beetroot, sugar beet.

10. **Walnut family, Juglandaceae:** Walnut, pecan, butternut. See also the general section on nuts on page 376.

11. **Palm family, Palmaceae:** Coconut, dates, sago, palm oil.

12. **Banana family, Musaceae:** Banana, plantain, one form of arrowroot (Musa arrowroot).

13. **Mulberry family, Moraceae:** Mulberry, fig, hops.

14. **Buckwheat family, Polygonaceae:** Buckwheat, rhubarb.

15. **Currant family, Saxifragaceae:** Blackcurrant, redcurrant, whitecurrant, gooseberry. Note that the "currants" used in rolls and cakes are dried grapes.

16. **Rose family, Rosaceae:** The groups most relevant to cross-reactions are the subfamilies:
    Rosoideae: Blackberry, raspberry, wineberry, cloudberry, loganberry (all in the same genus, so quite closely related); also strawberry and rose hip.

Prunoideae: Plum, prune, apricot, greengage, cherry, peach, nectarine, sloe (all the same genus, so quite closely related); also almond.

Maloideae: Apple, pear, quince, loquat.

17. **Citrus family, Rutaceae:** Orange, lemon, tangerine, clementine, grapefruit, lime, citron, ugli. These are all members of the same genus, and therefore very closely related, so cross-reactions are likely. Kumquats are also members of the citrus family.

18. **Cashew family, Anacardiaceae:** Cashew, pistachio, mango.

19. **Grape family, Vitaceae:** Grapes, muscatels, raisins, currants (the dried fruits—not blackcurrants or redcurrants).

20. **Bilberry family, Ericaceae:** Blueberry, cranberry, cowberry.

21. **Mint family, Labiatae:** Mint, basil, marjoram, oregano, rosemary, sage, thyme, savory.

22. **Fungi kingdom:** Mushrooms, puffballs, truffles, morels, chanterelles, yeast, mycoprotein, Quorn.

POULTRY AND EGGS

Recent research suggests that people sensitized to one type of poultry may well react to all others, including game birds, making the family group irrelevant here.

23. **Pheasant subfamily, Phasianinae:** Chicken, pheasant, quail, partridge.

24. **Grouse subfamily, Tetraoninae:** Grouse, turkey, guinea fowl.

25. **Duck family, Anatidae:** All types of duck and goose.

26. **Pigeon family, Columbidae:** Pigeon, squab, dove.

27. **Snipe family, Scolopacidae:** Snipe, woodcock.

28. **Eggs:** All birds' eggs are very similar in the proteins they contain, and are best regarded as a single food item.

FISH AND SHELLFISH

29. **Fish:** The family concept is irrelevant when it comes to fish, because all the fish in the main group eaten (the bony fish) share a special type of protein known as a parvalbumin. The parvalbumins are known to provoke allergic reactions, and they probably account for the fact that many people are

sensitive to all the types of fish they have tried. It is uncertain whether parvalbumins are found in the other main group of fish, the sharks, rays, skates, and dogfish (cartilaginous fish). The two groups are only very distantly related, and it is possible that people sensitive to bony fish could tolerate cartilaginous fish.

30. **Crustaceans, Phylum Crustacea:** Crab, lobster, crayfish, shrimp, prawn. A very large group, including many different families. Many patients react to all forms of crustacea, so the family concept is rarely relevant here. Indeed, they mostly react to molluscan shellfish as well (see the section on unexpected reactions, below).

31. **Mollusks, Phylum Mollusca:** Mussels, cockles, winkles, oysters, clams, scallops, squid, cuttlefish, octopus, snails (escargots). Again, this is a very broad group, and the family concept is rarely relevant because people who are sensitive to one type are usually sensitive to them all as well as to crustacean shellfish (see the section on unexpected reactions, below).

MEAT AND MILK

32. **Cattle family, Bovidae:** Cows (beef, veal), sheep (lamb, mutton), goats. The sheep and goats are grouped in one subfamily, the cows in another, so cross-reactions are most likely between lamb/mutton and goat meat. Cross-reactions among the milks of these three species defy the taxonomic groups: those sensitive to cow's milk quite often react to goat's milk but less often to sheep's milk. Why this should be is unknown. With sufficient early exposure to goat's cheese or milk, it is possible to become sensitized to these and show a cross-reaction to cheese or milk of sheep, but no reaction to cow's milk, cheese, or other cow's-milk products. For those who are sensitive to cow's milk, the milk of other domestic animals that do not belong to the cattle family (for example, donkeys, see page 386), is far less likely to provoke reactions.

33. **Pig family, Suidae:** Pig (pork, ham, bacon).

34. **Deer family, Cervidae:** Venison.

35. **Rabbit family, Leporidae:** Rabbit, hare.

UNEXPECTED CROSS-REACTIONS

1. **Nuts:** These deserve a special note, because people who are allergic to one type of nut are often allergic to others, despite the fact that most nuts are not at all closely related. Apart from those in the walnut family (10) and the cashew family (18) every nut is an individualist—in all, there are at least eight families of plant that supply us with edible nuts. So why should there be these apparent cross-reactions among them? We can only assume that their common way of life requires certain chemical constituents (to prevent rotting, for example—most nuts have evolved to be carried off and buried by animals). Perhaps the different nuts have evolved similar chemicals for this purpose.

   Whether cross-reactions among different types of nut occurs in food intolerance as well is unknown. One problem here is that both doctors and patients tend to refer to them rather vaguely as "nuts," instead of specifying which type.

   People who are sensitive to peanuts may not be affected by other types of nut, but if they have ever had a serious allergic reaction to peanuts they should try other nuts with great caution.

2. **Cross-reactions among plant products:** Some people with hay fever find they are affected by foods. The table on page 377 shows the known cross-reactions, with the most commonly implicated foods listed first for each pollen.

   There are a number of other fruits and vegetables that may cause symptoms in people with hay fever, but these are not strongly linked with any particular pollen.

   Two further examples of cross-reactions do not involve a pollen. One is the cross-reaction between house dust mite and kiwi fruit. This is a true cross-reaction due to an entirely coincidental similarity in the allergens. Occasionally people with house dust mite sensitivity react badly to kiwi fruit the very first time they eat it. There are reports of the same cross-reaction between dust mite and papaya.

   People who are allergic to latex (see page 89) often show a cross-reaction to various plant-derived foods, particularly

PRIMARY ALLERGEN	FOOD
Birch Pollen	Apple
	Carrot
	Celery
	Cherry
	Pear
	Peach
	Plum
	Fennel
	Hazelnut
	Walnut
	Potato
	Spinach
	Wheat
	Buckwheat
	Peanut
	Honey
Mugwort Pollen	Celery
	Carrot
	Spices
	Melon
	Watermelon
	Apple
	Chamomile tea
Grass Pollen	Melon
	Tomato
	Watermelon
	Orange
	Swiss chard
	Wheat
Pellitory Pollen	Cherry
	Melon
Ragweed Pollen	Melon
	Chamomile tea
	Honey
	Bananas
	Sunflower seeds
Pine Pollen	Pine nuts
Hazel Pollen	Hazelnuts, filberts

bananas, chestnuts, figs, and avocado pears. Other foods implicated are kiwi fruit, buckwheat, oregano, dill, sage, cherries, pear, papaya, passion fruit, melon, mango, pineapple, peach, tomato, orange, and carrot. In many of these cross-reactions, the shared allergen is a protective enzyme, called a *chitinase*, which attacks chitin, the hard outer skin of insects. This enzyme fends off plant-eating and fruit-eating insects by weakening their mouthparts. However, cross-reactions between latex and both milk and egg white have also been reported—these are currently unexplained.

3. **Shellfish:** Many people are sensitive to both crustacean shellfish and molluskan shellfish, and to snails (see above, 30 and 31 on page 375).

For certain people, it may be something other than the shellfish themselves causing the problem. Toxins acquired from their food, or the preservatives that are liberally added to shellfish (see page 66) might be to blame. In other cases, there is a genuine cross-reaction. Recent research has revealed that the shared allergen is a muscle protein called tropomyosin. New research shows that, in the test tube at least, antibodies to these proteins will also bind to proteins from dust mites, various insects (including cockroaches, silverfish, and chironomid midges) and nematode worms. The reverse is also true, and in some individuals there may even be positive skin-prick tests and actual symptoms. So someone who has never eaten shrimp (an Orthodox Jew, for example) can have a positive skin-prick test to shrimp, having been sensitized by mite or cockroach allergens. Evidence is now accumulating that long courses of allergy shots against house dust mite could be responsible for some sensitivity to foods such as shrimp and snails by inducing cross-reactions.

Index of Foods

Please read the introduction to this appendix before using this list.

A number following the food shows the group it belongs to in the list on pages 371–76. An *S* shows that it is the only commonly eaten member of its family. A *U* shows that it may be involved in some unexpected cross-reactions.

alfalfa 3
almond 16
aniseed 5
apple 16, U
apricot 16
arrowroot (Musa) 12
  arrowroot S
asparagus 7
avocado S
bacon 33
baked beans 3
bamboo 1
banana 12, U
barley 1
basil 21
beans 3
beef 32
beet sugar 9
beetroot 9
black-eyed peas 3
blackberry 16
blackcurrant 15
blueberry 20
Brazil nut S
broad beans 3
broccoli 4
brussels sprouts 4
buckwheat 14
butter beans 3
cabbage 4
cane sugar 1

cape gooseberry 2
caraway 5
carob 3
carrot 5
cashew 18
cassava (tapioca) S
cauliflower 4
celeriac 5
celery 5, U
chamomile 8
chanterelles 22
chard 9
cherry 16, U
chestnut S, U
chicken 23
chickpeas 3
chicory 8
chile peppers 2
Chinese gooseberry S
Chinese cabbage 4
chives 7
chocolate S
citron 17
clams 31
clementine 17
cloudberry 16
cockles 31
coconut 11
coriander 5
corn 1
cowberry 20

crab 30
cranberry 20
crayfish 30
cress 4
cucumber 6
cumin 5
currants 15, 19
cuttlefish 31
dates 11
dill 5
duck 25
eggplant 2
eggs 28
elderberry S
endive 8
escargots 31
fennel 5
fish 29
fig 13
flageolets 3
frogs S
garlic 7
gelatin 32
globe artichoke 8
goat 32
goose 25
gooseberry 15
grapefruit 17
grapes 19
green peppers 2
greengage 16

green beans 3
grouse 24
guava S
guinea fowl 24
ham 33
hare 35
haricot beans 3
hazelnut S, U
hops 13
horseradish 4
Jerusalem artichoke 8
kale 4
kidney beans 3
kiwi fruit S
kohlrabi 4
kumquat 17
lamb 32
leek 7
lemon 17
lentils 3
lettuce 8
lima beans 3
lime 17
lobster 30
loganberry 16
loquat 16
lupin 3
lychee S
macadamia nut S, U
mangetout peas 3
mango 18
maple syrup S
marjoram 21
maté or matté S
melon 6, U
milk 32
millet 1
mint 21
morels 22

mulberry 13
mung beans 3
muscatels 19
mushrooms 22
mussels 31
mustard 4
mutton 32
mycoprotein 22
nectarine 16
New Zealand
    spinach S
oats 1
octopus 31
okra S
olive S
onion 7
orange 17
oregano 21
oysters 31
palm oil 11
papaya S
parsley 5
parsnip 5
partridge 23
passion fruit S
pawpaw S
peach 16, U
peanuts 3
pear 16, U
peas 3
pecans 10
pepper (black/
    white) S
persimmon S
pheasant 23
pigeon 26
pine nut S, U
pineapple S
pistachio 18

plantain 12
plum 16, U
pomegranate
    (grenadine) S
pork 33
potato 2, U
prawn 30
prickly pear S
prune 16
puffballs 22
pumpkin 6
quail 23
quince 16
Quorn 22
rabbit 35
radish 4
raisins 19
rape 4
raspberry 16
redcurrant 15
red peppers 2
rhubarb 14
rice 1
rose hip 16
rosemary 21
runner beans 3
rutabaga 4
rye 1
safflower 8
sage 21
sago 11
salsify 8
savory 21
scallops 31
sesame S
shallot 7
shrimp 30
sloe 16
snails 31

APPENDIX 5

Food Avoidance and Alternatives to

Common Foods

With some foods avoidance is relatively easy, but others, such as wheat, corn, milk, egg, and soy, are so widely used in ready-made foods that you have to always be on guard against eating them inadvertently. Look up the ingredient you are avoiding and familiarize yourself with all the foods where it could be a hidden ingredient. Learn the synonyms used on food labels so that you can detect it in packaged food.

If you have a true allergy to any food, as indicated by symptoms such as tingling or swollen lips, tingling in the mouth, hives, or breathing difficulties after eating, you need to be especially careful about reading labels. Subsequent exposure to the food can provoke a violent reaction known as anaphylactic shock, which is sometimes fatal. Read the section on pages 58–62 in full. Remember that these lists are *not comprehensive*—they are only intended as a guide. You must always be cautious about all foods, and not assume they are safe because they are not listed here. If you are allergic to an ingredient that can appear in disguised form then calling the manufacturer may be the only answer. The telephone number should appear somewhere on the packaging.

Finding substitutes for staple foods such as wheat and milk can be difficult. In each list here you will find a guide to substitutes for the particular food you are avoiding. Any words shown in boldface type can be looked up in the second part of this appendix (starting on page 400), where there is information on how to cook the more unfamiliar foods, and some useful recipes.

Be alert to the possibility of cross-reactions to related foods and eat these sparingly. However, you should not worry excessively about cross-reactions. They do not occur for many people, and worrying about a food can provoke a psychogenic reaction to it.

Common Foods

CORN
Rarely a cause of true food allergy, but a frequent offender in food intolerance.

Sources
Corn on the cob, sweet corn, cornflakes, Cheerios, Corn Pops, some other **breakfast cereals** (see page 407), some muesli

Soups, soup mixes

Cornmeal, custard powder

Gravy and gravy mixes, white sauce, béchamel sauce, parsley sauce, and many other sauces (see **Thickeners**, pages 404–405, for substitutes)

Some packaged snacks, such as Doritos

Many ready-made meals and sauces

Tortilla chips

Corn bread, polenta

May Be a Hidden Ingredient In
Some **baking powder** (see page 411)

Many ready-made foods—read labels with great care

Gum on stamps and envelopes

Many tablets

Food Labeling
May be described as: cornmeal, cornstarch, corn syrup, dextrose, cereal starch, edible starch, food starch, glucose syrup, hydrolysed protein, hydrolysed vegetable protein, modified starch, starch, vegetable protein and textured vegetable protein (occasionally includes corn), vegetable gum, vegetable oil, or vegetable starch.

Some additive may be made from corn (see appendix 3) but corn sensitive people are very unlikely to be affected by these.

Substitutes
Any entries marked in boldface type above can be looked up in the second part of this appendix on page 400.

Other Foods That May Cross-React
Other cereals, such as wheat, rye, barley, oats, rice, or millet, could start to cause reactions if you eat too much of them.

Essential Nutrients
You will not be short of any nutrients if avoiding corn.

EGGS
Sometimes a cause of true food allergy in children; often the culprit in food intolerance.

Sources
If you have a severe allergy to eggs, bear in mind that this cannot possibly be an exhaustive list; always be cautious.
Quiche, soufflé
Meringues (these use egg white only)
Batter, pancakes, waffles
Yorkshire pudding
Rich piecrust
Créme caramel, mousses, egg custard, custard tarts, many different desserts
Sponge cake, Madeira cake
Brioche and some other rich breads
Danish pastries, éclairs
Marzipan
Egg noodles, egg pasta

May Be a Hidden Ingredient In
A very wide range of ready-made foods—always read labels
Egg glazes on pastry
Some margarine (as lecithin)
Some ice cream

Food Labeling
May be described as: ovalbumin or lecithin (but lecithin could also be soy).

Substitutes

Nothing really tastes like eggs themselves, but there are substitutes for baking that reproduce their cooking qualities (see page 402).

Other Foods That May Cross-React

The eggs of other birds are very likely to cross-react.

People with a true allergy to eggs sometimes react to vaccines if they have been cultivated in eggs. They may also react to bird feathers (see page 93).

Essential Nutrients

You are unlikely to be lacking in nutrients if you avoid eggs, but check that you have other sources of B vitamins, such as whole grains, meat, fish or milk, green vegetables, nuts and seeds, or yeast extract. Note that only animal-derived foods can supply vitamin B_{12}. Ensure that you either get enough sunlight to make vitamin D for yourself or eat some foods rich in this vitamin, such as margarine or cod liver oil.

MILK

Sometimes a cause of true food allergy in children; often the culprit in food intolerance.

Sources

If you have a severe allergy to milk, bear in mind that this cannot possibly be an exhaustive list; always be cautious.

Cream, butter

Cheese, cottage cheese, cream cheese

Yogurt, crème fraîche

White sauce, béchamel sauce, parsley sauce, and so on

Custard, rice pudding, semolina, tapioca, and sago pudding

May Be a Hidden Ingredient In

Most margarines

A great many packaged foods—always read labels and know your synonyms (see appendix 3)

Pastries, rolls, cakes, cookies, scones

Homemade pastry

Those with true allergy to milk should also look out for labels that list "spices" or "natural flavoring," which could indicate many white breads.

Some medicines contain lactose, or milk sugar, as a filler. This does not necessarily affect everyone who is sensitive to milk (since most are reacting to milk proteins, not lactose), but it may cause problems for some. Diarrhea and flatulence are the usual reactions. There are claims that trace amounts of milk protein persist in lactose and can affect the highly allergic. Some asthma inhalers (the dry-powder kind) contain lactose and, possibly, minute traces of milk protein.

One milk protein (casein) is used in some manufacturing processes, and is found, for example, in several brands of latex rubber gloves. Enough is present to provoke marked skin reactions in some milk-allergic people.

Food Labeling
May be described as: whey, casein, caseinate, lactalbumin, or lactose.

Substitutes
See Milk Substitutes, Butter Substitutes, Cheese Substitutes (pages 400–2).
Look for items labeled "dairy-free" or "suitable for vegans."
See Cookies (pages 410–411) and Cakes (page 411) for milk-free recipes.

Researchers have shown that whereas 70 to 90 percent of those with cow's-milk allergy also react to milk from sheep and goats, only 10 percent develop a reaction to that of donkeys (the Biblical ass's milk, as used for royal baths). The donkey, of course, belongs not to the cattle family but to the horse family, Equidae. Unfortunately, we can offer no advice on how to milk one.

Other Foods That May Cross-React
Some people cross-react to beef, but this is highly unusual. A cross-reaction to goat's milk or sheep's milk is more common.

Essential Nutrients
If you avoid milk and other dairy products, you run a risk of calcium deficiency, and this is especially serious for growing children. Infants and toddlers should be given hydrolysate formula as a substitute—ask your doctor or pharmacist about this. (There is a high risk of soy allergy or intolerance developing if soy milk is used as a substitute. Cross-reactions are common with milk from goats or sheep; other animal milks are hard to obtain.) For older children and adults, it is possible to get enough calcium from fish such as sardines, eaten whole including the bones, but you would need to eat a good portion of such fish every day. It is also possible to get enough calcium from purely vegetable

sources, and vegans successfully do this, but it requires a high consumption of calcium-containing vegetable foods such as soybeans, tofu, or soy cheese (choose a brand with added calcium), fortified soy milk, almonds, and purple broccoli. This demands a very disciplined approach to eating, which is difficult for most people. A calcium supplement may be the best option for some people. A supplement that also contains magnesium in the correct ratio (about 2:1) is probably a good idea, unless you have a very high intake of green, leafy vegetables (which are magnesium-rich).

Apart from calcium, milk also supplies protein, some of the B vitamins, and some vitamin D. You are unlikely to run short of protein, unless you eat very little fish, meat, or eggs; beans and lentils can then supply you with protein.

If you eat a good mixed diet you should be getting adequate amounts of B vitamins. Sources of B vitamins include whole grains, meat, fish or eggs, green vegetables, nuts and seeds. Note that only animal-derived foods can supply vitamin B_{12}.

Ensure that you either get enough sunlight to make vitamin D for yourself or eat some foods rich in this vitamin, such as margarine or cod liver oil.

Nuts

Sources

If you have a severe allergy to nuts, bear in mind that this cannot possibly be an exhaustive list; always be cautious.

Nougat, marzipan, praline, and many other sweets and chocolate products

See also Peanuts (pages 389–90).

May Be a Hidden Ingredient In

Many bakery products, such as cakes, cookies, savory pastries, and desserts

Other bakery products may have traces of nut picked up from mixing equipment

Stuffing mixes

Special vegetarian foods

Gluten-free breads (ground almonds)

If you are sensitive to peanuts as well as other nuts, the range of food to be cautious about is even wide (see pages 389–90).

Should you have any symptoms of true allergy (see pages 58–62) in response to nuts, beware of all unlabeled foods, and restaurant food; ask before you taste.

Beware of oil in a deep-fat fryer that has been used to fry nut-containing food, and then reused. Some nut allergens may have leached out into the oil, and may then stick to any food that is fried in the same oil later.

Food Labeling

There are no synonyms for most nuts, but there are some for peanuts (see appendix 3).

Food manufacturers and supermarkets have suddenly become very nut conscious because of fatal reactions to nuts by people with a true allergy to them; notices about the presence of nuts have sprung up everywhere. If you have such an allergy, do not be lulled into a false sense of security by this. There will still be many producers and many shops that fail to prevent contamination by traces of nuts and do not apply warning labels.

Substitutes

Seeds are a good substitute nutritionally, for their value as snacks, and in vegetarian cooking.

Other Foods That May Cross-React

All nuts are potentially capable of cross-reacting one with another, even if they are from unrelated plant families. Those that are related to each other (such as pecan and walnut) are the most likely to cross-react. Reactions with peanuts are also likely, even though these are not true nuts.

Nutmeg is not a nut, and is not normally a problem, but on rare occasions there have been allergic reactions to it. Coconut rarely causes allergic reactions, and when these do occur they are usually mild. However, if you are very nut sensitive you should be cautious with nutmeg and coconut, and do a three-stage test: first, put a small amount on the skin (the cheek is a good place). If this does not react, then rub a piece against the inner lip—first making sure you are prepared to deal with what might be a severe reaction. Should this test pass uneventfully, then try eating a tiny amount. These tests are suggested for nutmeg and coconut only. *Never* try these tests with nuts or peanuts if you have any nut allergy—the risks are much too great.

Essential Nutrients

Almonds and hazelnuts are a good source of vitamin E. Sunflower seeds are an alternative source, as are sunflower spread and sunflower oil. If you're not eating plenty of these, then a supplement of vitamin E may be advisable. Nuts are also a good source of many B vitamins (but not B_{12}). Again, seeds can act as a replacement source.

PEANUTS

Sources

If you have a severe allergy to peanuts, bear in mind that this cannot possibly be an exhaustive list; always be cautious.

Peanut butter

Satay sauce (as in chicken satay); many other Thai and Malaysian dishes; occasionally in Chinese food

May Be a Hidden Ingredient In

A wide range of foods, especially crackers, cakes, cookies, savory snacks, and desserts

Bakery products sold loose, without ingredient labels, should always be suspected of containing peanuts

Even bakery products not intended to contain peanuts may have traces of peanut picked up from mixing equipment

Many curry sauces

Some Chinese egg rolls

Some brands of Worcestershire sauce

If you have any symptoms of a true allergy to peanuts (such as tingling or swollen lips, hives, or difficulty in breathing), then you must also be very cautious about eating in restaurants and cafés and religiously read the labels on packaged food. Also be cautious about party and barroom snacks.

Most peanut-allergic individuals do not react to refined peanut oil (groundnut oil), but if you have ever had a serious near-fatal reaction to peanuts it is best to be careful about the oil. Chips and other fried food may be fried in peanut oil; you should ask the chef about this. Vitamin tablets and drops sometimes contain traces of peanut oil, as do some candies.

Riskier than peanut oil itself is oil in a deep-fat fryer that has been used to fry peanut-containing food (for example, vegetarian burgers or cutlets), and then reused. Some peanut allergens will have leached out into the oil, and can then stick to the food fried in the same oil later.

Almond powder and chopped almonds imported from Asia sometimes contain powdered or chopped peanuts as a filler. Since this powder may be used for Indian sweetmeats or for curries prepared in restaurants, it is wise to be cautious about such items. Marzipan might also be affected.

The Food Allergy Network (see pages 451–452) can be a useful source of advice. See also pages 58–62.

Food Labeling

May be described as: groundnuts, groundnut oil, peanut oil, vegetable oil, or arachis oil.

Note that arachis oil (the term is usually used of creams, soaps, and cosmetics) is used in many prescribed products, including eczema creams, as well as in many over-the-counter remedies (see page 74). Where it is used in nipple creams, a breast-feeding baby is likely to consume small amounts. Pharmacists can advise on brands that are free of peanut oil. These are recommended to prevent sensitization of babies to peanut.

And see the Food Labeling section for Nuts (page 388).

Substitutes

See Nuts (page 387).

Other Foods That May Cross-React

All other nuts, even though they belong to different plant families. Nuts seem to share some common constituents that trigger allergy and intolerance.

Cross-reactions to legumes are also possible, because peanuts belong to the same plant family. Fortunately, they are rare. The members of this family include: soybeans, kidney beans (also called haricot beans, navy beans, white beans, and baked beans), lima beans, broad beans, butter beans, black-eyed peas, chickpeas, lentils, and mung beans. Carob is also a legume, as is lupin, now being grown for flour.

Essential Nutrients

See Nuts, page 389.

POTATOES

Rarely a cause of true food allergy, but a frequent offender in food intolerance.

Sources
Chips, french fries, and many other snack foods
Many ready-made meals, soups
Turnovers and pastries, many vegetarian pastries

May Be a Hidden Ingredient In
Some Indian dishes
Some ready-made foods

Food Labeling
No unfamiliar synonyms for this food, but look for potato flour.

Substitutes
There are many different starchy foods that can stand in for potatoes; see pages 405–7.

Other Foods That May Cross-React
Very occasionally there are reactions to other vegetable foods from the same plant family: tomatoes, eggplant, sweet peppers, chili peppers, paprika, and cape gooseberry *(Physalis)*.

The sweet potato belongs to an entirely different family and should not cross-react.

Essential Nutrients
Potatoes supply vitamin C, but most people get their supplies of this vitamin from fruits and green vegetables.

RICE

Rarely a cause of true food allergy, at least in the West, but an occasional offender in food intolerance. May cause both allergy and intolerance when eaten very regularly from an early age as in most parts of Asia.

May Be a Hidden Ingredient In
Many Indian and Japanese sweetmeats, which are made with rice flour

Spring rolls (the pastry is made with rice flour)
Some noodles (rice noodles are very white, unlike wheat pasta)

Food Labeling
There are no unfamiliar synonyms for this food, but look for rice flour.

Substitutes
Wild rice, sorghum, millet, quinoa, cornmeal, buckwheat, barley (see pages 407–10).

Other Foods That May Cross-React
Wild rice
Occasionally, other grains such as wheat or corn

Essential Nutrients
You are unlikely to run short of any nutrients if avoiding rice.

SESAME
An increasingly common source of true food allergy, especially among adults; not often implicated in food intolerance.

Sources
If you have a severe allergy to sesame, bear in mind that this cannot possibly be an exhaustive list; always be cautious.
Halvah (a Mediterranean and Middle Eastern sweetmeat)
Tahini (often used in vegetarian cooking)
Sesame oil
Rolls, burger buns, bread, bagels, breadsticks, and crackers may contain sesame seeds
Some snack bars—check all labels
Veggie burgers
Some rice cakes

May Be a Hidden Ingredient In
Sometimes an ingredient in hummus
Stir-fries and other Oriental foods often contain sesame oil
Bread that is not intended to contain sesame may have traces of sesame picked up from mixing equipment
Crackers may be contaminated with traces of sesame

Anything bought from a delicatessan should be viewed with caution, as sesame seeds that have dropped off bread rolls are sometimes scattered about the counter and may contaminate other food

Some mixed spices; these may be used in processed meats, sausages, sauces, chutneys, salad dressing, cakes, cookies, and beverages

Some drug preparations contain sesame oil, as do some cosmetics

Food Labeling

No specific synonyms; could feasibly be described as vegetable oil, but this is unlikely.

On imported foods look for benne, teel or till, simsim, anjoli, cingili.

Other Foods That May Cross-React

None.

Essential Nutrients

None.

SOY

Sometimes a cause of true food allergy, although this is rare; a frequent offender in food intolerance.

Sources

If you have a severe allergy to soy, bear in mind that this cannot possibly be an exhaustive list; always be cautious.

Soybeans, soy meal, soy flour

Soy sauce, miso

Textured vegetable protein (TVP)

Vegetarian burgers, risottos, sausage rolls, and most other meat substitutes

Soy milk, soy yogurt, soy cheese

Many gluten-free breads and other gluten-free products

May Be a Hidden Ingredient In

Many packaged foods: always read the labels

Food Labeling

May be described as: lecithin, vegetable gum, vegetable protein, textured vegetable protein, or vegetable starch.

Substitutes

Toasted sesame oil makes a reasonable substitute for soy sauce.

For alternatives to soy milk, see **Milk Substitutes** (page 400).

For wheat-free, soy-free bread you can bake your own or try one of the substitutes, such as rice cakes, listed under **bread** (pages 403–4).

Other Foods That May Cross-React

Some people who become sensitive to soy later react to other legumes (members of the bean family). These include kidney beans (also called haricot beans, navy beans, white beans, and baked beans), lima beans, broad beans, butter beans, black-eyed peas, chickpeas, lentils, and mung beans.

Carob is also a legume, as is lupin, now being grown for flour.

Bean sprouts could well cross-react. Peanuts are also members of this family, and cross-reactions to peanuts are possible.

Essential Nutrients

Soybeans are an important source of protein for vegetarians and vegans. Vegetarians can fulfill their protein needs by using eggs or dairy produce, assuming they can tolerate these. Vegans should ensure that they eat protein-rich vegetable foods such as nuts, seeds, and peas. Although other beans, chickpeas, and lentils are also a rich source of protein, they should be eaten in moderation to reduce the risk of cross-reactions. Quorn may be useful.

Soybeans also supply some B vitamins, but there are many other sources for these.

WHEAT

The main offender in celiac disease, an occasional cause of true, IgE-mediated food allergy, and a frequent culprit in food intolerance.

Sources

If you are celiac, or have a severe allergy to wheat, bear in mind that this cannot possibly be an exhaustive list; always be cautious.

Bread (see pages 403–4), pita bread, nan bread, pizza, some poppadoms, chapatis

Bread crumb coatings (such as that on fish sticks)

Flour (see pages 404–5)

Cookies, Cakes (see pages 410–11), rolls, scones, crackers, muffins, and the like

Pancakes (see page 404) (unless made with pure buckwheat flour)
Semolina
Pastry (see page 404) of all kinds, pies
Sauces and gravy may contain wheat flour rather than cornmeal (see
Thickeners on pages 404–405 for substitutes)
Pasta (see page 404): spaghetti, tagliatelle, macaroni, egg noodles,
pasta shells and bows, vermicelli
Many kinds of **breakfast cereals** (see page 407) even if "wheat" does
not appear in the brand name: check all labels
Many kinds of muesli
Samosas may contain some wheat flour (check the label)
Couscous, bulgur wheat

May Be a Hidden Ingredient In
Most kinds of rye bread (unless guaranteed 100 percent rye)
Some rye crackers and oat cakes
Many ready-made foods; read labels with care
Sausages, hot dogs, luncheon meats
Baking powder

Food Labeling
Look out for: flour, cereal binder, cereal filler, filler, cereal protein,
cereal starch, edible starch, food starch, modified starch, vegetable
starch, or starch.

Hydrolyzed protein, hydrolyzed plant protein, and hydrolyzed
vegetable protein occasionally contain wheat, but the source should
now be stated on U.S.-brand foods. Textured vegetable protein and
vegetable protein sometimes contain wheat.

Note that the following flours are all made from wheat: bread flour,
brown flour, graham flour, granary flour, hard flour, strong flour, and
wholemeal flour.

Bulgur wheat, bran, chilton, couscous, dinkel, durum, einkorn,
farro, fu, germ, kamut, pasta, spelt, semolina, triticum, triticale, and
udon noodles are all wheat or wheat products. Buckwheat is not and
does not contain gluten (see below).

Gluten-free products are usually wheat-free but some contain pure
wheat starch (see below).

Avoiding gluten
As well as avoiding all the forms of wheat listed here, those with
celiac disease or dermatitis herpetiformis (see pages 104–7) must be
very careful about even the tiniest trace of gluten. Items to be avoided

include all rye and barley products (for example, beer and malt). Debate continues about the safety of oats for celiacs (see page 106). Consult a doctor before deciding to include oats in your diet, and follow the safety guidelines, keeping portion sizes small.

Label reading should become a compulsion—and know your synonyms (see above). Celiacs who are particularly sensitive may also need to avoid additives made from wheat or barley, which could contain traces of gluten: caramel and caramel color, citric acid (unless made in United States), dextrin, diglycerides, gum base, malt, malt flavoring, maltodextrin, maltose, monoglycerides, monosodium glutamate (MSG) (unless made in United States), natural flavorings and spices. Stablizers or thickeners sometimes contain very tiny traces of gluten (see below). Vegetable gum and gum base can be made from oats and might affect the most sensitive. Gum tragacanth, xanthan gum, gum arabic, gum acacia, and cellulose gum should be safe.

Vitamins and medicinal drugs may have to be bought from a special pharmacy to ensure they are wheat-free (see page 457).

Unlabeled sources of gluten can be a hazard. Blue cheese can contain a little gluten since bread is used to innoculate the cheese with blue molds. Ground spices and mustard powder may have very small amounts of wheat flour added. So may icing sugar, in some countries, including Canada. Gravy powder, gravy, or stock cubes can all contain gluten traces. For more details phone the manufacturer or ask your celiac support group.

The highly sensitive celiac must also be wary of wheat flour used in food processing (see page 60) which may leave traces of gluten in food but will not be mentioned on the label. Barley enzymes are used in the production of various items including rice milk and some soy milk, soy sauce, and miso. Ice cream, candies, soup, sauces, salad dressings, cream cheese, and cottage cheese may contain stablizers or thickeners derived from wheat or other cereals and containing tiny traces of gluten.

Spirits brewed from grain, including whiskey and gin, may contain minute amounts of gluten. The same is true of distilled white vinegar.

"Gluten-free" products such as bread and cookies may not be suitable for the most sensitive celiacs. There is no way to test accurately for very small amounts of gluten, so the standard set for gluten-free foods by the Codex Alimentarius of the Food and Agriculture Organization/World Health Organization is dictated in part by what can be accurately measured. The current regulations state that such foods should not contain more than 200 parts per million (PPM), equivalent to 200 mg/kg of dry food weight. Many countries feel the level should be lower (and some, such as Sweden, have legislated for a lower limit) but the lack of a precise test means that a lower limit is difficult to police effectively. This does not mean food cannot be produced with lower levels of gluten—it is just a question of being more rigorous about the starting ingredients to keep gluten out of the process.

Wheat starch is a controversial area. Some very pure forms of wheat starch are probably safe for most celiacs, and it is permitted in gluten-free foods in many European countries where high-quality wheat starch is used. The wheat starch widely used in the United States is generally less purified and contains enough gluten to affect some celiacs.

If you live with nonceliacs, crumbs from toasters, or picked up from butter or jam, can cause trouble. Contamination can also occur in stores, especially where grains or flour are sold loose—these should be avoided. Grills and fryers in restaurants can become contaminated with gluten, but the amounts are tiny and will only affect the most sensitive. Avoid licking envelopes and gummed labels.

There is plenty of help available for celiacs from support groups and on the Internet (see pages 452–53) including a database that shows if specific products are gluten-free. It is designed to be used on the new ultraportable palm-top computers that can be taken on shopping trips.

Rare individuals with an extreme IgE-mediated allergy to wheat may benefit from following the same restrictions as celiacs.

Substitutes

Any entries marked in boldface type above can be looked up in the second part of this appendix on page 400. and see millet (pages 407–408) for a sandwich substitute. Rice, potatoes, and some of the starchy substitutes for **potato** (see pages 405–7) may prove useful in keeping your diet as varied and filling as possible while avoiding wheat and other grains.

Other Foods That May Cross-React

Rye, barley, and oats are closely related to wheat and could well cause cross-reactions for those with wheat allergy or intolerance. If you can tolerate them, you should still be cautious and not eat too much of them in order to avoid becoming sensitive. Rye is the most likely to cause problems; oats the least. Celiacs should not eat rye or barley; some can eat oats (see page 106).

Corn, rice, and millet are also grains, although less likely to cross-react. Again, eat these in moderation. These are safe for celiacs since they do not contain gluten. The same is true of amaranth, buckwheat, quinoa, sorghum (milo), and teff. Some celiacs have reported a bad reaction to one or more of these grains, but these are either due to contamination with wheat or they are individual reactions, due to a separate allergic or intolerant response, not an effect of gluten.

Essential Nutrients
If you are not replacing wheat bread with other whole grains, take care to eat other foods that supply B vitamins, zinc, and iron. A good mixed diet (with plenty of fresh green vegetables, meat, fish, milk or eggs, nuts and seeds) will include all these.

YEAST
Rarely a cause of true food allergy, but a frequent offender in food intolerance.

Sources
Yeast extract

May Be a Hidden Ingredient In
Bouillon cubes (see page 412) and other meat extracts

Bread, including sourdough bread, but excluding soda bread, most brands of pita bread, chapatis, most nan bread

Danish pastries, doughnuts, coffee cake, and any other cake with a breadlike texture

Pizza

Rolls, croissants

Beer, wine, cider (other alcoholic drinks such as whiskey and gin also contain some yeast but not as much)

Vinegar (salad dressing, pickles, chutney, and so forth)

Many vitamin tablets, especially B vitamins

Many ready-made meals and packaged foods—read the labels

Any food that is fermented or has a long processing time, (including sour cream, buttermilk, cheeses, sauerkraut, dried fruit, soy sauce, miso, and black tea); test these individually to see if you react

Very ripe fruit

Juice or jam that has been opened and kept for a while

Food Labeling
Look out for: hydrolyzed protein, hydrolyzed vegetable protein, or leavening.

Citric acid may be derived from yeast, as may monosodium glutamate (MSG).

Mycoprotein is another name for Quorn (see below).

Secondary Sources of Yeast

Dried fruit

Overripe fruit

Any unpeeled fruit

Commercial fruit juices

Anything labeled "malt"

Yogurt, buttermilk, and sour cream

Imitation cream

Soy sauce

Tofu

Any leftover food, unless eaten within twenty-four hours, or forty-eight hours if refrigerated

Whiskey, vodka, gin, brandy, and other spirits

Yeasts and molds in the air: damp houses, greenhouses (unless very dry and clean), compost heaps, rotting leaves (avoid for a while, then test whether such exposure makes you ill)

Substitutes

Any entries marked in boldface type above can be looked up in the second part of this appendix on page 400.

Try spirits instead of beer and wine. Toasted sesame oil is a good substitute for soy sauce.

Other Foods That May Cross-React

You might react to mushrooms or other edible fungi (puffballs, truffles, chanterelles)—either to the items themselves or to molds and yeasts growing on them. Quorn, a protein-rich food derived from fungi, could also cause problems. Many cheeses are rich in fungi, especially Brie and Camembert.

Essential Nutrients

If you eat a lot of bread made without yeast you may run the risk of certain mineral deficiencies, because unleavened bread contains substances that block the absorption of calcium, magnesium, iron, zinc, manganese, and copper. Make sure to eat plenty of the foods that are rich in these minerals or take a multimineral supplement.

Yeast is a good source of most B vitamins, but if you eat a good mixed diet you should be getting adequate amounts of these. Sources of B vitamins include whole grains, meat, fish or eggs, green vegetables, nuts, and seeds. If you need to take a supplement, make sure it is a *yeast-free* B-complex tablet.

Alternatives to Commonly Eaten Foods

For sources of the more unusual foods, and addresses for mail-order purchases, see appendix 10.

Milk Substitutes

Goat's milk can be bought in some health food shops, and goat's-milk powder is available by mail. There are two drawbacks to this product: it has a very rank "goaty" taste that takes quite a bit of getting used to, and it often provokes reactions in people who are already sensitive to cow's milk.

Sheep's milk is available in health food shops in some areas. It has a much less powerful taste than goat's milk and is pleasantly creamy. Unlike cow's milk, it freezes well, so you can buy it in frozen form. This milk may provoke cross-reactions in those sensitive to cow's milk, but it is less likely to do so than goat's milk.

Soy milk is made from pulverized soybeans, and its origin is evident in the flavor. Most brands have some sugar added. It is obtainable from most health food shops. To make your own, mix 5 ounces of soy flour to a paste with a few spoonfuls of water, then slowly add 3 cups of water. Bring slowly to a boil, stirring continuously, then simmer for 20 minutes, stirring from time to time. Add a teaspoon of honey; store in the refrigerator. Soy can readily provoke allergic or intolerant reactions, so it is not advisable to eat too much of any soy product. Soy desserts and soy yogurt are also available. Sugar-free forms of soy milk, and concentrated soy milk, are both available by mail order.

Creamed coconut is obtainable from Indian or West Indian groceries, and some health food shops. It can be used as a substitute for cream, if mixed with a small amount of warm water. Or you can just grate it directly onto fruit salad, chopped bananas, and the like.

Ground almonds can also be made into a cream substitute. Mix to form a paste with water and a little honey, then add more water until you get the right consistency.

Cashew nuts (unroasted) can be ground in a blender and mixed with water to form a cream substitute. Add honey and vanilla extract to taste. Dilute further to make cashew "milk."

Butter Substitutes

Margarine is the obvious substitute for butter, but some brands contain small amounts of milk solids—read all labels. The brands that do not are mainly available from health food shops.

If you hate the taste of margarine, there are other possibilities. One is **tahini,** or ground sesame seeds—quite a strong taste, but a pleasant one. Sesame can readily provoke allergy or intolerance, however, so it should not be eaten too often. **Sunflower spread** is similar. Both are available from health food shops.

Another alternative is **clarified butter,** which can be tolerated by most milk-sensitive people. Make it by melting a pound of butter over gentle heat, allowing it to cool a little, and then pouring it carefully into a glass jar. The proteins in the butter will have settled to the bottom of the pan, and are visible as white granules; by pouring very slowly you leave these behind in the pan. Any that do get into the glass jar will settle to the bottom, and since you can see them through the side of the jar you can avoid eating them. Keep clarified butter in the fridge—it is semiliquid at room temperature. You can also buy it at Indian groceries under the name **ghee.**

Clarified butter should only be used once you have completed the elimination diet, and know that you have to avoid milk. It should not be used during the elimination diet, as it still contains traces of milk protein and may confuse the result.

In sauces, **creamed coconut** makes an interesting substitute for butter, although it only suits certain foods. Try melting creamed coconut in orange juice over a low heat then adding ground almonds to thicken the mixture, plus salt and garlic—this makes a delicious rich sauce to accompany pork or chicken.

Cheese Substitutes

Goat and sheep cheeses are available from good delicatessens, and health food shops. You can also buy them by mail order. See the remarks above on cross-reactivity.

Soy-based cheese spreads are available in some health food shops.

Tofu is a more traditional soy product that can act as a substitute for soft cheese. See the remarks above about soy.

The following foods are not like cheese in taste, but are useful substitutes for cheese in filling sandwiches or making quick snacks:

Hummus, if made to a thick consistency, is a very good sandwich filling or spread. Mash 10 ounces of cooked, drained chickpeas with a potato masher, add 3 tablespoons of olive oil, 1 tablespoons of lemon juice, 2 pinches of salt, and a clove of garlic if you like. If you use canned chickpeas, this only takes a few minutes to make. Or you can cook the chickpeas yourself (see page 410), to make a larger quantity, and freeze some.

Paté is useful, although most contains preservatives. Making your own is not difficult, especially if you use a blender.

Taramasalata is a Greek dish made with smoked fish roe, olive oil, lemon juice, and garlic. Combined with tomatoes, cucumber, or watercress, it makes a good sandwich filling. Most taramasalata also contains bread crumbs and preservatives, and the majority are tinted a bright pink with artificial colorings.

Gjetost (pronounced *yay-turst*) or Norwegian brown cheese is made from milk whey, not milk solids. Specialist cheese stores and supermarkets with a cheese counter sometimes sell it. Since most milk-sensitive people are reacting to the protein casein, which forms the milk solids, they may be able to tolerate whey, the liquid part of the milk. This does contain proteins, but different ones, not casein. The thorough cooking of the whey to produce gjetost may also make it less allergenic. Unfortunately, gjetost does not taste much like ordinary cheese. It is rather sweet with a nutty, caramelized flavor that seems strange at first, but is delicious once you are used to it. It goes well with whole wheat bread and apples.

Egg Substitutes

The eggs of other birds, such as ducks or quail, may be a useful substitute for some people, but they are likely to cross-react with chicken's eggs (see page 374) and should be tested alone before being used in recipes. Anyone who has a true allergy to eggs should be *very cautious* about testing other types of eggs.

Nothing can reproduce the taste of eggs, but some other foods can mimic their cooking qualities. In puddings, where they are used to set a liquid, gelatin is a useful substitute. You will have to experiment with each recipe, but 1 teaspoon of gelatin is roughly equal to 1 egg. Dissolve the gelatin in water before adding to the other ingredients. In cookie recipes, 1 egg can be replaced by 2 tablespoons of water, 1 tablespoon of vegetable oil, and 1/2 teaspoon of baking powder. Commercial egg replacers and egg-white replacers are also available (see appendix 10). See also Cakes (page 411).

Wheat Flour for Bread

If you have an intolerance of wheat (rather than food allergy or celiac disease), it is worth checking that it is all types of wheat you must avoid. It may be the proteins in the wheat germ that affect you, or something in the outer coat of the wheat grain. If this is the case, you will be able to eat white bread and white flour, but should avoid whole wheat bread, granary bread, and any product (such as crackers) with wheat germ in it.

The proteins in wheat flour—which include gluten—are what makes wheat good for bread making. Trying to make bread without wheat involves finding a substitute for this protein.

Gluten-free bread is available in some health food stores—at a price. Or you can buy a gluten-free flour and make your own.

Gluten-free flours are made from a mixture of different flours, including cornmeal, potato flour, soy flour, split pea flour, rice flour, rice bran, carob flour, cornstarch, and ground almonds. You can improvise with simple mixtures of your own, try 1 part rice flour to 1 part soy flour and 1 part potato flour. The mixture must always include at least one type of high-protein flour, such as soy or lentil. Use yeast and make in the ordinary way, but without kneading the bread. It will have a heavier texture than ordinary bread, and may taste better toasted. If you have to avoid yeast as well, it is possible to make soda bread using gluten-free flour. The manufacturers of gluten-free flour usually supply recipes for use with their particular flour mix, and these should be followed for good results.

Bear in mind that most gluten-free mixes contain soy flour or other bean-derived flours. Make sure you are not eating soy and related foods (see pages 372–373) too regularly, especially if you are vegetarian—they are featured in most commercial meat substitutes, veggie burgers, and instant meals.

Rye bread may be a useful substitute for some people, because rye is also rich in protein, though it cannot rival wheat. Because the two are closely related, those who are sensitive to wheat quite often react to rye as well. If you buy rye bread from a local bakery, be sure to check that it is 100 percent rye—speak to the manager, and ask to be notified if they change the composition of the bread. Rye flour often contains some wheat anyway, because wheat grows as a weed in fields of rye.

Rye crackers can be eaten as long as they're pure rye—some now have wheat bran added.

Oat cakes are available from most good supermarkets, delicatessens, and health food stores. Oats are preferable to rye, since they are less likely to cross-react with wheat. Check the label, as some contain milk or sugar.

Rice cakes and rice crackers are available from health food shops. The "cakes" are actually savory—something like a cracker, but made from puffed grains of rice. They taste much nicer than they look.

Wheat Flour for Other Uses

Pastry, pancakes, and waffles can be made with rye flour, although the results are heavier than with wheat, partly because rye flour is only available in whole-grain form. Putting the rye flour through a fine sieve first improves the quality by removing the larger pieces of husk from the flour; adding some baking powder helps, too. Pancakes can also be made with cornmeal or barley flour, and taste pleasant although they are slightly rubbery—beat plenty of air into the mixture just before frying to improve the texture. Buckwheat flour is fairly protein rich and makes a good pancake batter, but should be mixed with other flours to dilute the strong taste. Gluten-free mixes for pastry and pancakes can be bought by mail order and generally give excellent results.

Pasta made with gluten-free flour is obtainable by post. Or you can try rice noodles, obtainable in Chinese groceries, or buckwheat spaghetti, from health food stores.

Soy flour and lentil flour are rich in protein as well as carbohydrates. They can be used in baking or combined with other flours (see above under Gluten-Free Flours), and tend to improve the texture of pastry and pancakes.

Rice flour, potato flour, banana flour, chestnut flour, yam flour, and other exotic flours are mostly low in protein. They are useful for making puddings and cookies, or for thickening sauces (see below). Chestnut flour tastes sweet and nutty and is pleasant in shortbread or in a crumble topping for fruit, although it is rather heavy.

Thickeners

Sago flour can be used to thicken soups, sauces, and stews. Pearl sago and pearl tapioca can be made into puddings with milk, or a milk substitute.

Arrowroot is an excellent thickener.

Rice flour, potato flour, barley flour, and rye flour are sold in some health food shops and can all be used as thickeners, although they need to be used with care, as they tend to go lumpy more readily than corn-meal. Any of the exotic flours listed in the previous section can also be used.

Potato Substitutes

Yams are probably the best potato substitute. By *yams* we mean the very large roots that have a rough brown outer skin and very solid white flesh that is starchy, dry, and not at all sweet. Yams are usually cylindrical, with the diameter of a small drainpipe, but some misshapen ones look like yeti's feet. These crops originated in West Africa and Asia, and their botanical name is *Dioscorea species*. Unfortunately, the term *yam* has been appropriated by United States growers to describe orange-fleshed sweet potatoes (see below). Yams sold in the United States are mostly im-ported from the Caribbean, unlike sweet potatoes, which are home-grown. Firmer and more fibrous than potatoes, yams are very similar in taste but with an interesting, slightly bitter aftertaste. They are best if prepared like sautéed potatoes—boiled and then fried. Boil for about 20 minutes or until they are tender. If you buy a large piece of yam and boil it, you can then pack the cooked pieces in individual portions and freeze them. You can fry them from frozen in oil—fry slowly over a low heat for best results. You need a sharp knife and a strong hand to peel them and cut them into cubes. If you find this too difficult, try baking the root whole in a moderate oven—it will take at least an hour—then peel and cut it when cool.

Sweet potatoes are found in supermarkets. There are many different sorts, with flesh ranging from white to deep yellow in color. Those with orange flesh are often described as yams in the United States, which is confusing. They belong to the same South American species, *Ipomoea batata*, as white-fleshed sweet potatoes, a point you should remember when planning your menus. Keeping your diet varied is important, and you should not eat too much of any one species. Peel and dice them, keeping them underwater as much as possible to prevent discoloration. Alternatively, you can bake them and serve them with butter (if allowed), or slice and deep-fry them. They have a very sweet, slightly sticky flesh that goes well in soups, or with meat casseroles, but is rather cloying on its own.

Serving sweet potatoes with sharp fruit is a good idea, as the acidity offsets their stickiness. Try frying them over a low heat for 20 minutes (after boiling), adding slices of apple and walnuts for the last 5 minutes.

This makes a good breakfast dish. Like yams, sweet potatoes can be peeled and boiled in a large batch, then stored in individual portions in the freezer, and fried when still frozen.

The Chinese make a soup by boiling sweet potatoes in water or stock until they disintegrate and flavoring the liquid with gingerroot. They also make a delicious snack called deep-fried sweet potato balls. To make these, boil some sweet potatoes until soft. Mash them and add rice flour (or wheat flour) to make a stiff dough. Take a small piece of the dough, press it down flat, and put 1/2 teaspoon of peanut butter (or another nut butter) in the center, then seal the dough around it. Roll in sesame seeds and deep-fry in vegetable oil.

Breadfruit is a truly exotic food, from the islands of the Pacific. It makes an excellent substitute for potatoes or other starchy foods. Breadfruit is only sold in a few specialized Indian and Chinese groceries, but is well worth looking out for. It is a large, green, spherical fruit with a delicate honeycomb-like pattern on the surface. Pierce the skin to allow steam to escape, then bake it whole at 375°F for 1 1/2 to 2 hours. The white flesh is firm, with a subtle flavor and creamy texture. Meal-sized portions can be frozen after cooking. Because it can be sliced and eaten straight from the skin (like a slice of melon), breadfruit is useful for packed lunches.

Cassava is a starchy root that makes a good substitute for potatoes or rice, with excellent flavor, texture, and color. It is not widely sold, but you may find it in Indian or West Indian stores. Boiling in plenty of water is essential for this root crop, to remove toxic compounds; it should not be baked. Peel, dice, and boil for about 15 minutes, or until soft. (There is no need to soak before cooking for the types of cassava that are sold in the United States, but this may be necessary for cassava bought elsewhere: some types contain larger amounts of toxin and need special treatment.) Cassava is easily recognized, being a regular cylindrical root, but much more slender than yams, with a light brown skin; they are often dipped in wax to preserve them.

Taro, a starchy root, is two different species, but they are closely related. One has pink flesh, the other white, and they differ in size and shape, being either symmetrical and bulbous or rather knobby and irregular. They make a very acceptable substitute for potatoes and other starchy foods. The texture is agreeable and the flavor similar to potatoes but slightly nutty. The pink-fleshed kind do turn a rather dismal blue-gray color when cooked, but they taste just as good. To cook taro, peel and dice them, then boil in salted water for about 15 minutes. They can also be baked whole, at 375°F for about 1 to 1½ hours. The flavor is stronger when cooked in this way, rather like baked potato.

Breakfast Cereals

If you are sensitive to wheat, choose cornflakes or crisped rice. Always check labels before trying a new product; a little wheat is often added to cereals based on oats, corn, or rice.

Plain porridge oats or rolled oats can be used raw as a breakfast cereal, and they are far more filling (and cheaper) than most packaged cereals. If you allow the milk to soak in for a few minutes before eating they will be more digestible. Raisins and chopped apple make a tasty addition.

If you react to wheat, oats, and corn, then you could try rice flakes or millet flakes, both available from good health food stores. Serve as for oats (see above). Do not eat too much of any grain, as you risk acquiring a new sensitivity: have something other than cereal for breakfast several times a week.

Packaged breakfast cereals are usually reinforced with several different B vitamins. However, if you eat a good mixed diet, the loss of the added vitamins in a daily bowl of cornflakes is unlikely to cause any deficiency.

Hot Cereal

A hot breakfast cereal based on cornmeal can be bought in some health food shops. Alternatively, millet can be made into a hot cereal—see the next section.

Other Substitutes for Traditional Starchy Foods

Millet can be bought at some health food shops. There are at least seven different species of plant that produce a crop called *millet* belonging to three different botanical families. All that *millet* means is "a grass crop with small, usually spherical seeds." This is good news for anyone trying to keep their diet varied—if you can find a different type of millet, you can treat it as a separate food. Some go under other names, such as teff *(Eragrostis abyssinica)* and the relatively large-seeded adlay or Job's tears *(Coix lachryma-jobi)*. Be careful with the latter, because pearl barley is sometimes sold under the name Job's tears—compare the grains with those of pearl barley and don't risk it if you are in doubt.

To cook millet, measure out 1 cup of the grains and wash thoroughly before leaving them to soak overnight. Throw away the soaking water and replace with 2 cups of fresh water. Add ½ teaspoon of salt and bring to a boil. Allow to simmer over a low heat for 20 minutes. The water should all be absorbed at the end of this time.

This oatmeal-like mix can be eaten with milk or a milk substitute as a breakfast dish. However, it is more appetizing if treated as follows:

Prepare and cook 1 cup of millet as above, but use 1 level teaspoon of salt. While still hot, add ½ cup peanut butter (or another nut butter— see page 412), and 1 level teaspoon of sesame seeds, already toasted (see page 412). Mix the ingredients together well, using a potato masher to break up the millet. Take a lump of the mixture—about the size of a small egg—roll it between your palms, and squash flat, pressing hard, to make a hamburger shape. It is important to do this while the millet is still warm, as it becomes very uncooperative when cold. These quantities make about 30 burgers.

Fry the "millet burgers" in oil over low heat, turning them twice and allowing at least 20 minutes total frying time—this gives the outside a lovely crunchy texture. Use a nonstick pan and plenty of oil, or they may stick. The burgers can be made in bulk and frozen unfried; they do not need to be defrosted before frying. Although making a large batch is fairly time consuming, it is well worth it, as they are both delicious and filling. Four or five make a good meal: eat them for breakfast, with some grated apple, or for lunch, with a salad. Cooked millet can also be added to soups and casseroles to thicken them.

Sorghum is usually grown for animal feed in the United States, but is regarded as perfectly good for human beings in many other parts of the world. It is usually sold as sorghum meal, which can be cooked in the same ways as millet (see above). To make cookies or bread, sieve the sorghum meal to get a fine flour. The larger particles can be used like oatmeal for making hot cereal.

To make waffles or pancakes, wash some sorghum meal and soak it overnight. Drain off the surplus liquid and use a blender to turn the meal into a smooth, thick paste. You can now add eggs, flavorings, salt, sugar, and so forth to make a pancake mixture.

Wild rice is only available from a few health food shops and delicatessans and is rather expensive. It has long, dark brown grains and a distinctive nutty-earthy taste that goes very well with some foods, no- tably fish, poultry, and stir-fried vegetables. To cook, wash thoroughly, place in a large saucepan, cover with cold salted water, and bring to a boil. Simmer for 45 minutes, then turn off the heat, stir the rice, and let it stand for 15 minutes. Pour off any excess water, but do not rinse. The cooked grains freeze perfectly, and can be defrosted quickly by boiling in water or stock without becoming glutinous. A mixture of orange or lemon juice and melted butter (if you are allowed these) improves its taste. For breakfast, defrost some wild rice by boiling in fruit juice, and add dried apricots and nuts.

Cornmeal can be prepared as polenta and used as an accompaniment to stews or casseroles. Combine ½ cup cornmeal with 1 level teaspoon each of salt and mild paprika, and a tiny pinch of cayenne. Mix in 1 cup of water, adding it slowly to prevent lumps from forming. Steam in a double boiler, or put a small pan (containing the cornmeal) inside a larger one, containing an inch or two of water, to get the same effect as a double boiler. After 30 minutes, turn out into a medium-sized greased baking dish and bake for 10 to 15 minutes at 350°F. Pour a few spoons of juice from the casserole over the top with a layer of grated cheese, then put under the grill to brown. This also goes well with fish.

Buckwheat or kasha can be bought in most health food stores. It consists of brown triangular grains whose strong, earthy flavor is something of an acquired taste. Wash the grains thoroughly under the tap, then cook in twice the quantity of salted water. You can make the taste less powerful by pouring off the first batch of water, after it comes to a boil, and replacing it with the same amount of fresh salted water. Simmer for about 15 minutes, or until all the water is absorbed and the grains are soft. It needs to be served with a sauce or casserole that has an equally powerful taste—beef and tomatoes with plenty of herbs, for example. Buckwheat spaghetti is also available, but check that it does not contain any wheat. It is not advisable to eat too much buckwheat because it often causes sensitivity reactions.

Chestnuts are useful as a snack or a breakfast dish. They can also be used to stuff a chicken or turkey, in the traditional manner, and eaten with the poultry as a substitute for potatoes. Dried chestnuts are the cheapest—they can be found in some health food shops and Chinese groceries. Soak them overnight, discard the water, and wash them thoroughly. Boil for about an hour or until tender all the way through but not disintegrating. You can cook a large quantity and freeze them in individual portions. They can be fried gently in oil to make a light breakfast—serve with grated apple or a salad. Alternatively, you can make chestnuts into a soup, preferably with oranges or some other fruit. For chestnut flour, see page 404.

Pumpkin is sweet and slightly sticky—not unlike sweet potato. Prepare and use it in the same way.

Chickpeas are more floury than other beans, with a less "beany" taste, and fewer unpleasant aftereffects. They make a good filler if you cannot eat wheat or potatoes. Soak them overnight, pick out any discolored ones, and boil for 1 to 1 1/2 hours. If you do find that they give you gas, try removing the skins—they rub off very easily. Canned chickpeas are not expensive if you buy supermarket brands. Add to soups and casseroles. You can also mash them to make hummus (see pages 401–2). Other beans and lentils are also useful fillers for those who cannot eat wheat or potatoes.

Pearl barley is sold in most large supermarkets, and in health food stores. Add it to stews, casseroles, and soups to make them more filling. The barley needs about 1 to 1 1/2 hours cooking time.

Plantains look like very large green bananas. They are starchy and less banana-like in flavor than you might expect. Peel them (quite difficult—needs a sharp knife) and then fry in oil, or boil and mash. They can also be baked in their skins.

Poppadoms are obtainable in some Indian groceries and can be eaten as an accompaniment to a meal. Check that they do not contain wheat flour. This is a traditional Indian recipe for gram-flour bread: mix 2 cups of gram flour with a small, finely chopped onion, 1/2 teaspoon cumin seeds, 1/2 teaspoon salt, and a pinch of chili powder. Rub in 1 tablespoon of clarified butter (see page 401). Add a little water—enough to make a stiff doughy mixture. Take small balls of this and press down lightly with your hand on a floured surface. Fry on a griddle or hot plate, turning once.

Cookies

If you must avoid wheat, but can eat oats, flapjacks are a good substitute for cookies, and easily made. Heat 1/2 cup of margarine or butter with 1/4 cup honey. When melted, add 2 cups rolled oats and 2 to 3 heaping tablespoons chopped nuts. Mix well, spoon into a shallow greased pan, and bake at 350°F for 20 to 30 minutes. Cut into fingers while still warm, but do not remove from the pan until cool.

Your favorite cookie recipes can be used with nonwheat flours, such as rye flour, rice flour, or carob flour (see flour, pages 404–5). If the flour of your choice is low in protein, an egg is a useful addition to the mixture: reduce the quantities of the other added liquids and the butter or margarine a little, to compensate for the extra fluid and fat in the egg.

Gluten-free cookies can be bought at most health food shops, and these should be free of wheat protein. Milk-free cookies can easily be made using margarine, and most store-bought cookies are milk-free, but check the label. See also Egg Substitutes (page 402).

Cakes

A typical cake includes egg, wheat flour, and milk. If you are avoiding wheat, you should be able to find gluten-free cakes in a health food shop, or you can make your own substituting an alternative **flour**, or mixture of flours, for wheat. You need some high-protein flour, or the result will be rather heavy. An extra egg can help to give better texture to cakes made from low-protein flour; obviously, you must decrease the milk or other liquid to compensate for the additional liquid. Making a cake without milk is not difficult: use any **milk substitute** (page 400), or just use water, or a mixture of water and a little beaten egg. Replace the butter in your recipe with milk-free margarine (see pages 400–401).

Making a cake without eggs is difficult. The best answer is egg replacer, available in grocery stores. Recipes are usually supplied with such products. The replacer is designed to reproduce the baking qualities of eggs and give the cake its characteristic lightness and texture—it does not replace the flavor of eggs. To simulate that rich eggy taste, try adding some vanilla essence. In fruit cakes and tea breads, where lightness is not essential, a mashed avocado can enrich the mixture. Mashed bananas also give richness: look in any good cookbook for a recipe for banana bread (actually a cake rather than a bread).

Baking Powder

Most commercial baking powder contains a small amount of wheat flour, and those who are very sensitive to wheat should buy a wheat-free brand or make their own. Combine one part sodium bicarbonate with two parts cream of tartar. Add one part potato flour, rice flour, or some other flour that you are allowed. Put through a sieve twice and then store in an airtight jar.

Yeast

The main sources of yeast are bread, bouillon cubes, yeast extract, and alcoholic drinks.

Soda bread, pita bread, and **chapatis** are good substitutes for yeast-leavened bread, although some pita breads do contain yeast, so check before eating. Soda bread is made using baking powder.

Bouillon cubes are very difficult to replace, and stews and casseroles do taste rather insipid without them, although your taste buds adapt to this eventually. If you have the time, you can make your own stock using bones and waste meat, or the remains of a roast chicken for poultry stock. Add some bay leaves or other herbs, and boil for about 20 minutes. Skim off the fat when cool, remove the bones, and then add salt to taste. The stock can be frozen for future use.

When cooking beef casseroles, try frying the beef thoroughly before stewing it, making sure all the juices in the frying pan are subsequently transferred to the casserole. This creates a rich meaty taste, which can be enhanced by adding thoroughly browned onions.

Instant stocks often contain yeast. You may be able to find a yeast-free vegetable bouillon at some health food shops.

Toasted sesame seeds (spread them on aluminum foil and toast under the broiler using low heat) or toasted sesame seed oil (available at Chinese groceries) can also be used to give a stocklike flavor to casseroles, but be careful not to eat too much sesame.

Peanut Butter

Almond butter and **cashew butter** are both delicious. They are sold by some health food shops. Be careful not to eat too much of either, as nuts are frequently implicated as allergens. **Hazelnut butter** is another useful alternative, along with **tahini** (ground sesame seeds) and **sunflower spread.**

Chocolate

Carob makes a reasonable substitute. Health food stores stock various carob products, and you can also buy carob powder for cake making.

Coffee and Tea

Redbush tea tastes very similar to the real thing. It contains no caffeine and little tannin, but may still provoke symptoms in people who are sensitive to tea. Caffeine-free coffee substitutes abound, including **dan-**

delion coffee based on the roasted root, and other beverages based on roasted barley and chicory. Any coffee substitute may irritate the stomach lining of those who are already sensitive to coffee. Herbal teas are much less likely to cause problems.

Snacks

Pumpkin seeds and sunflower seeds make excellent snacks, and both are sold by most health food stores. Such stores also sell most kinds of nut, including some of the more unusual varieties, such as cashews, pistachios, Brazil nuts, and pecans—these can be useful for keeping the diet varied. Macadamia nuts are very filling, although rather expensive. Potato chips without additives can be bought at health food stores and make a good snack. Corn chips, also without additives, and popcorn are useful for those not sensitive to corn. Dried fruit, dessicated coconut, and roasted chickpeas (sold in most Indian groceries) are other useful snack items.

Fruits and Vegetables

Some people who are allergic to a type of fruit find they can eat the same fruit if it has been canned, cooked, or even just frozen and defrosted. The allergens would appear to be modified by these processes, but the modification does not help everyone. The same is true of some allergies to vegetables that are eaten either raw or cooked, such as tomatoes.

Indian and West Indian grocery stores sell many exotic fruits that can be substituted for common ones. Some of the larger supermarkets also stock a wide range of unusual fruits, such as mangoes, papayas, star fruit, and lychees. These can be useful during the first phase of an elimination diet, although they tend to be expensive.

Synthetic Chemicals in
Food and Water

This appendix summarizes the main groups of synthetic chemicals to be found in our food and drinking water. The general comments on safety and toxicity refer to the "average" healthy person, rather than someone who is unduly sensitive to one or more synthetic chemicals.

Food Additives

About 3,500 additives are in use, but not all of these are synthetic compounds. Some are natural products, or synthetic versions of natural chemicals, although this may not mean that they are things we would normally eat. The average American eats about 20 pounds dry weight of additives each year. This is ten times the amount used forty years ago. Those who eat a lot of packaged, processed or take-out foods may eat twice the average amount or more. Children, in particular, have a very high intake because many of the manufactured foods that appeal to them are rich in additives.

Having said that, it is important to keep the risks of additives in proportion. As with pesticide residues and other synthetic chemicals that are found in food, most people can break down the small quantities of food additives eaten each day and render them harmless. Indeed, we use the same detoxification enzymes for this as we use for natural toxins in food (see pages 287–98). For the vast majority of people, therefore, although there may be some justifiable concern about undetected long-term effects of additives or "cocktail effects," there is not a huge amount to worry about when it comes to additives. Compared to the health risks from smoking, for example, or eating a diet with hardly any fruit and vegetables, consuming food additives is probably a minor risk.

Those with some kind of chemical sensitivity, especially if severe, may be in a different position, probably because their detoxification enzymes are not working as well (see pages 226–27). However, there is no reason to avoid food additives unless you are really certain they affect you or your child. An additive-free diet is a difficult one in our modern world, particularly for children. The mistaken idea (see pages 267–68) that hyperkinetic syndrome is primarily (and invariably) due to food additives has gained such widespread currency that many children are put on such diets without any proof of the need for them. It is important to be sure that food additives are playing a role, by means of an elimination diet and careful observation (see pages 271-75).

Most foods and drinks have to be labeled, with all additives (apart from flavorings) listed. Certain items are exempt, including food or drink served in restaurants and food that is sold unwrapped, but these, too, are likely to contain additives. Dried fruit is usually treated with sulfur dioxide, but this may not appear on the label (see also appendix 1).

Another source of hidden additives is medicinal drugs. They may contain colors, preservatives, and antioxidants. These do not have to be declared on the label, and some people have reacted adversely to the additives in drugs.

Food additives include:

Preservatives prevent bacteria and fungi from decaying the food. Those most dangerous to health are the nitrates and nitrites, which have been used for hundreds of years to make bacon and ham—they are potentially carcinogenic. Because of the long tradition of use, and the fact that the characteristic flavor of bacon cannot be produced in any other way, these preservatives are difficult to outlaw.

Preservatives are also used in almost all wines. One group of preservatives, the sulfites, metabisulfites, and sulfur dioxide, can trigger asthmatic attacks (see appendix 1) because they have an irritant effect on the airways.

Antioxidants stop fats and oils from going rancid. These are restricted to certain foods and the amount used is limited by law. Those most likely to cause health problems are BHA and BHT. One study showed

BHT to cause behavior disorders in animals.

Emulsifiers, stabilizers, and **thickeners** improve texture. The amount that can be used is not limited, but they are restricted to certain foods.

Colorings include both natural colorings and synthetic ones. Some of the "natural" colors are extracted from grass, nettles, and other plants, or produced by a chemical process. There is a new trend toward colors produced by fungal cells or plant cells in culture—because these too can be labeled "natural," even though we would not consider eating the items from which they are derived. Such colors are being sought as a replacement for the synthetic colors known as azo-dyes, which have caused much concern. Azo-dyes include colors such as tartrazine, sunset yellow, and amaranth—a complete list is given at the end of this section. Any colorings in foods or medicines must now be listed on the label in the United States. Regulations may be less strict in other countries, especially regarding medicines.

Flavor enhancers can affect some people. The most important of these are monosodium glutamate, or MSG, and its relatives. Eating large amounts of MSG is said to produce a set of symptoms known as "Chinese restaurant syndrome." The symptoms described for this condition vary considerably: "tightness, pain, and tingling in the front of the chest, radiating to the arms, often associated with palpitations and faintness" according to one authority, but "flushing, sweating, loss of coordination, headache, and hypotension [low blood pressure]" according to another. Some studies have failed to confirm the existence of a reaction, but it has been suggested that the source from which the MSG is manufactured is important.

Flavorings do not have to be listed separately on food labels, unlike the other additives. There are over three thousand of these, and most have never been properly tested for safety. However, they are used in extremely small quantities and are assumed to be nonharmful for this reason. Although this may be true for the majority, there are doubts over some flavorings, particularly a group known as the allyl alcohols, which are potent toxins. The average person only receives small amounts of these, but anyone eating large amounts of sweets, potato chips, and soft drinks would get a much higher dose.

Testing Additives

New additives are all tested very thoroughly, although there are rarely tests on humans—rats, mice, bacteria and human cells cultured in a test tube are the main subjects used for testing. There are quite a few reports of illness among food workers handling certain additives, which raises the question of whether humans might react differently from these test animals. There has also been some concern about how well tests are carried out.

Concern has also been expressed over the possibility of "cocktail effects"—the unknown impact of eating two or more additives together. A single meal can contain as many as sixty different additives, yet, surprisingly, the effect of additives in combination is never taken into account when setting safety standards. Very few tests have been carried out in this area due to lack of resources. One test, in which two preservatives were tested together, showed that they had a much greater effect in combination than when eaten separately. A public health specialist, writing in a book on additives published by the European Commission, comments: "It is not scaremongering to say that the possibility cannot be ruled out of two substances, both harmless by themselves, interacting to yield a product which is toxic."

Pesticides

There are three main types of pesticide used on food crops: insecticides to kill insect pests, fungicides to kill fungal diseases, and herbicides to kill weeds. The vast majority of these pesticides leave residues on the crops, but there are time limits between when the crop is last sprayed and when it is harvested—this allows time for the residue to break down. Unfortunately, it is difficult to ensure that growers observe the safe period between the last spraying and the harvest—and no official means of checking if they do so. The only checks that take place are routine tests of foods for pesticide residues.

The U.S. Department of Agriculture tests ten to twelve fruit/vegetable foods for pesticide residues each year, usually including five hundred to seven hundred samples of each of the chosen foods. A different set of foods is tested the following year. Because most foods are not tested in successive years, the data is somewhat limited and cannot show trends over time.

Each sample consists of about five pounds of the fruit and vegetable concerned. Because the samples are made up in this way, individual high readings—an apple with a particularly high level of pesticides, for example—will not be picked up. In other words, there is a leveling off effect in the procedure, which concerns some observers (see below).

In February 1999, the Consumers Union of United States published

THE AZO-DYES

Tartrazine, F D & C Yellow No. 5—Banned in Austria and Norway.

Quinoline yellow—Banned in Australia, Japan, Norway, and the USA.

Yellow 2G—Not approved by EC and used only in Britain. Also banned in Austria, Japan, Norway, Sweden, Switzerland, and the USA.

Sunset yellow FCF/orange yellow S—Banned in Finland and Norway.

Carmoisine/azorubine—Banned in Japan, Norway, Sweden, and the USA.

Amaranth—Banned in France and Italy (except in caviar), Norway, and the USA.

Ponceau 4R/cochineal red A—Banned in Norway and the USA.

Erythrosine BS—Banned in Norway and the USA.

Red 2G—Not approved by the EC, and used only in Britain. Also banned in Australia, Austria, Canada, Finland, Japan, Norway, Sweden, and the USA.

Allura red AC—Not approved by the EC.

Patent blue V

Indigo carmine/indigotine—Banned in Norway.

Brilliant blue FCF—Not approved by EC, but permitted in some countries, including Britain. Banned in Austria, Norway, Sweden, and Switzerland.

Green S/ acid brilliant green S/ lissamine green—Banned in Canada, Finland, Japan, Norway, Sweden, and the USA.

Brilliant black PN—Banned in Canada, Finland, Japan, Norway, and the USA.

Brown FK—Only used in Britain and Ireland. Banned by Austria, Australia, Canada, Finland, Japan, Norway, Sweden, and the USA.

Chocolate brown HT—Banned in most of Europe, Australia, Norway, Sweden, and the USA.

Pigment rubine/lithol rubine BK—Only used for coloring the rind of Edam cheese.

an excellent analysis of the USDA data on pesticide residues for 1994–97. The report, prepared by Edward Groth III, Charles M. Benbrook, and Karen Lutz, is written in nontechnical language and is admirably succinct and clear. If you want to read the whole report you can find it on the Internet at http://www.consumersunion.org/food/ do_you_know1.html. The following information is based very largely on that report.

To give a single measure of pesticide risk, the amounts of pesticide residue found and the toxicity of that pesticide were combined to give a toxicity index or TI. This allowed direct comparisons to be made.

Some foods tested had very low levels of pesticides, notably frozen and canned corn, broccoli, and orange juice produced in the United States, bananas, canned peaches, and apple juice. Other foods had high levels, the worst offenders being fresh peaches and U.S. winter squash (fresh). Apples, grapes, spinach, and pears also had high TIs. The worst TIs were found on U.S. fresh peaches (largely due to one insecticide, methyl parathion, which is a nerve toxin) and fresh winter squash (due to dieldrin, a carcinogenic and highly toxic insecticide, banned in the 1970s, but persisting in the soil and absorbed through the roots by certain crops). Spinach had residues of pesticides that were not licensed for use on this crop, suggesting illegal spraying.

Could these pesticide residues be damaging to health? The Consumers Union report points out that the residues are mostly within the legal limits, but that these legal limits do not define safety. The residues found on some foods, such as fresh U.S. peaches, would frequently expose a small child to a dose greater than the "safe" daily intake as defined by the U.S. government. For example, a child weighing 44 pounds (safe intakes depend on the body weight of the consumer) eating a medium-sized peach with just an *average* level of methyl parathion would be consuming a dose fourteen times higher than the government-defined "safe" daily dose. Bearing in mind that the child will be consuming other pesticides from the same peach (as many as twenty) and more from other foods eaten during the day, this is alarming.

Even a peach with the lowest methyl parathion residue level would deliver a dose above the "safe" daily intake for a child.

The Food Quality Protection Act, passed in 1996, was intended to protect children's health against pesticide residues. If implemented, this law would require the EPA to severely restrict many of the most toxic pesticides (such as methyl parathion), or ban them entirely. The process of implementing this law is very slow, partly due to powerful objections from vested interests, such as the chemical companies that make the pesticides.

Given the lack of official protection, the Consumers Union makes the following recommendations to the public:

- Don't restrict your intake of fruits and vegetables—the risks to health from eating a poor diet are much worse than those from eating pesticide residues.
- Peel (preferably) or wash fresh food, particularly apples, peaches, and pears. Most of the residue is on the outside. Always peel these fruits before children eat them.
- Buy organically grown food where you can, especially peaches, apples, pears, grapes, winter squash, spinach, and green beans. You could also ask your local store to look for growers and suppliers who avoid the really high-risk pesticides such as methyl parathion, azinphos-methyl, methomyl, methamidophos, and aldicarb—pesticides such as these are banned by many canning and freezing companies (hence the lower TIs on processed food), and the same ban could be applied to fresh produce if consumer pressure were applied.
- Keep you choice of fruit and vegetable varied: don't eat a lot of any one type. Go very easy on those that have high TI values (see above).
- Processed foods are often safer than fresh. For example, canned peaches are much less contaminated by pesticides than fresh peaches, and apple juice is much safer than fresh apples. Unfortunately, canned foods lack many of the vitamins found in fresh food, but freezing preserves most vitamins.

Contrary to popular myth (and the frequent claims of agribusiness representatives) U.S.-grown food is no safer than imported food. As the Consumers Union report observes, "Foods that might fairly be characterized as 'loaded' with pesticide residues, based on our Toxicity Index, are almost all 'Made in the USA.'"

This advice from the Consumers Union is, of course, intended for the average consumer in relatively good health. It is based, ultimately, on toxicity studies carried out with animals. There are safety factors built into the calculations that (it is hoped) cover the possibility that humans react differently than animals. However, we believe there is still justifiable concern about toxicity estimates. In particular, pesticides are never tested in combination for any possible "cocktail effects." Such effects are not unlikely. Some insecticides affect the liver, for example, making it less able to break down other chemicals.

The experience of doctors working with people affected by chemical sensitivity suggested that they may, in some cases, be much more sensitive to pesticide residues than the average person. Such individuals need to be even more careful to avoid pesticides. But you should not assume that this is the case for you without comparing organic and nonorganic produce. If you can, arrange for this to be done blind—the food being prepared by someone else, so that you do not know if you are eating organic food or ordinary food. Have four days exclusively on one and four days exclusively on the other, while keeping your surroundings and activities fairly constant so that food is the only thing varying. Repeat this three times, without being told which food you are (or have been) eating. You should be in the dark until the very end of the testing period. See if there is a real difference in your health by keeping a symptom diary and try to guess which days were which. If you were right 80 percent of the time, then you probably are reacting to pesticide residues and would benefit from a fully organic diet.

Heavy exposure to pesticides, as from a spray plane, a chemical spill, or severely contaminated food or water, can sometimes be the starting point for chemical sensitivity and a general (often very debilitating) state of allergy or intolerance to various foods. For those who already have allergies or food intolerance heavy pesticide exposure could make matters considerably worse. Do whatever you can to avoid such accidents—staying well away from agricultural fields during spraying for example.

In addition to pesticide residues, some foods contain hormones and antibiotics that are routinely fed to farm animals. Meat, poultry, milk, cheese, and eggs are the main sources of these chemicals, but fish from fish farms may also contain some antibiotics. Some individuals are allergic to minute amounts of certain antibiotics, and they may react to traces of antibiotic in food (see page 68).

Water Pollution

The level of pollutants in drinking water has been steadily rising in recent years. Pollutants run off the land into rivers or seep down through the soil into groundwater. Various purification measures are taken before the water reaches our taps, but these are never 100 percent effective. Well water is also likely to be contaminated these days, even in apparently unpolluted areas. Most of the pollutants are tasteless and colorless, so you can have no idea what you are drinking without laboratory tests.

Agriculture makes a major contribution to water pollution because nitrates, used as fertilizers, run off from the fields. Although nitrates have received a lot of publicity, they are not as worrying as some of the other water pollutants. There are no clear signs that the nitrate levels found in drinking water are damaging to health, except in newborn babies. As far as chemical-sensitive patients are concerned, nitrates are unlikely to be a problem.

Small amounts of pesticides also get into the water supply from farm use. In addition, there have been accidents in which large amounts of highly toxic pesticides have been emptied into drains or soakaways close to boreholes, causing major pollution of the groundwater below.

Oil from spillages may find its way into drinking water, but usually this is only in minute amounts. Gasoline can leak from underground storage tanks and pollute groundwater. Organic solvents (see page 221, table 3) also turn up in water supplies, usually as a result of factories discharging their waste solvents into drains or ditches. Some of the chemicals used for purification also leave a residue in the water.

Chlorine is added to water to kill bacteria and viruses, and while chlorine itself is relatively harmless to most people, it does react with certain organic molecules to produce trihalomethanes and other chlorinated hydrocarbons (chlorinated organics). (The organic molecules may themselves be pollutants, or they may be produced by leaves or waterweed rotting in reservoirs.) Some of these chlorinated hydrocarbons are carcinogenic, and they have occasionally turned up in drinking water.

For details of water filtration systems that can remove some of these pollutants, see pages 424–30.

Other Synthetic Chemicals That Can Contaminate Food

A variety of other synthetic chemicals may find their way into our food, including droplets from aerosol sprays, and plasticizers from cling-film and some other soft plastics. These plasticizers are used to give such items their flexibility, but they are soluble in oil and fat, and will migrate into the food if used to wrap fatty foods such as cheese or paté. In general, little is known about the safety of these substances, but there are unconfirmed reports that plasticizers can accumulate in the eye, leading to a form of blindness known as macular eye disease. Some insecticidal strips, which are not safe for use near food (for example, Vapona), are often hung in kitchens of restaurants.

Bottled Water and Water Filters

Bottled Water

There is some confusion about the meaning of *mineral water*, which complicates the issue of bottled water. All tap water, and any water from a spring or well, contains some mineral salts (calcium, magnesium, sodium, iron, and so on) dissolved in it. The composition of the water is affected by the sort of rock it percolates through, and some springwaters contain large amounts of minerals. At one time, it was believed that these waters had health-giving properties and they were marketed as "mineral waters." (In fact, mineral-rich water is of no special benefit to health, and some can be injurious to those with kidney problems.) Today's bottled waters often come from the same springs and may well be sold under the name "mineral water" because this denotes that they are high-quality waters from a natural source. However, the most richly mineral-laden waters are not marketed, and those that are on sale have low to moderate levels of minerals. A few brands are rich in sodium and should be avoided by those on low-sodium diets.

FDA regulations state that mineral water must contain at least 250 ppm of natural minerals. *Springwater* is the term used for water from a contained underground source that flows to the surface naturally but has levels of minerals lower than 250 ppm. A third category is artesian water, which comes from a confined aquifer, but is pumped to the surface. Finally, there is sparkling water, which is mineral or springwater that is naturally carbonated.

The main reason for buying bottled water now is not what it contains, but what it doesn't contain. Because of the locations of the springs, good-quality water from a reliable source is unlikely to be contaminated significantly by pesticides, industrial solvents, and other pollutants. Unlike most tap water, bottled waters should not contain chlorine and, for the most part, should contain lower levels of nitrates. (Perrier is an exception. Its nitrate content is almost as high as the maximum nitrite level permitted for tap water in many countries, and twice as high as other mineral waters.)

Any of the four kinds of water described above (mineral, spring, artesian, or sparkling) should be reasonably good for those with chemical sensivity, as long as a reputable brand is chosen. The label should clearly state the geographical location of the source and an address or telephone number for obtaining testing and treatment information. Water from another state is covered by FDA regulations, but water bottled and sold within a state is exempt, so you have greater guarantees of safety when buying an out-of-state water.

Just because it's in a bottle, don't assume it's springwater. It could be bottled tap water—yes, really! Look on the cap and label for "from a municipal source" or "from a community water system." Carbonated water, seltzer, and purified water are of no value to the person with chemical sensitivity (*purified* just means that particulates and minerals have been removed.)

Because they are not chlorinated, bottled waters can foster large numbers of bacteria. Tests have shown very high levels in some brands. However, these are not usually harmful types of bacteria and will not affect most people. (The water should be boiled for babies, and for anyone with low immunity, due to HIV infection or cancer treatment, for example.) Sparkling springwater resists bacterial growth better than still water.

Bottled water is very expensive, compared to filtered water, making it unsuitable for long-term use.

Water Filters

There are two main methods of removing synthetic chemicals from water: activated carbon filters and reverse osmosis.

Activated Carbon Filters
Activated carbon is a highly reactive surface that attracts substances such as chlorine, chloroform, carbon tetrachloride, trichloroethylene,

phenols, pesticides, PCBs, and dioxins. These and other organic molecules found in tap water stick to the carbon leaving the water much less contaminated.

There are various forms of activated carbon. The amount and quality of activated carbon in a filter determines how efficient it is at removing pollutants. Plumbed-in filters contain far more activated carbon than jug filters.

A major problem with these filters is that they are an ideal breeding ground for bacteria, including harmful forms. To combat bacterial growth, most such filters are now impregnated with silver. There have been alarming reports of silver leaching out into the water, but new production methods, such as bonding the silver to the carbon at high temperatures, have largely overcome this problem.

Reverse Osmosis

This form of filtration is only available in plumbed-in units. It uses a membrane with microscopic holes in it that, in principle, only water molecules can get through. Tap water is held in one chamber under pressure and water molecules slowly seep out into the other. It removes the vast majority of organic pollutants (but see below), and takes out fluoride, lead, aluminium, and other metals, unlike the activated carbon filters.

Unfortunately, the process is very slow (even the best filters only produce about 10 gallons a day) and uses up large amounts of tap water to produce a relatively small amount of filtered water (up to 10 gallons per filtered gallon). Many of the natural minerals in the water are removed at the same time. Without minerals, water loses its characteristic flavor, and there is also the question of whether we need minerals in our drinking water. Many experts say that we can get all the minerals we need from food by eating a good balanced diet. Others say that a mineral supplement is advisable if drinking reverse osmosis water (likewise distilled water or rainwater). A third, and much smaller group, says that the mineral supplement should actually be dissolved in the water before you drink it because there's a problem, in the long-term, with drinking mineral-free water however good other mineral sources in the diet. At present the evidence is too scarce to decide among these options, so play safe and opt for the third one.

Another problem with reverse osmosis is that a few molecules can get through the membrane along with the water, including some chlorinated compounds that are known to be injurious. These tend to concentrate in the filtered water, making the original problem worse. This difficulty is easily overcome, however, by combining the reverse osmosis unit with an activated carbon filter. Systems of this type produce a water of very high purity, which may be needed by some patients with severe chemical sensitivities.

In fact, all good water filters now combine several different treatment methods. Typically, a modern reverse osmosis (RO) unit will have one or two prefilters to take out particles, then activated carbon to reduce the chemical load on the RO unit. Next comes the RO unit itself, followed by another activated carbon filter to take out organics that bypass the osmosis membrane, and finally an ultrafine particle filter that can remove any bacteria generated from the carbon filter.

A good activated carbon filter will have fewer layers, and no RO unit, but the same sort of prefilters, and some postfilters (a "polishing system").

When you read the sales literature, be sure to distinguish activated carbon filters and RO units (both of which take out synthetic chemicals) from

- filters that take out particles,
- filters (such as ion exchange resins and electrodeionizers) that reduce calcium carbonate (scale or hardness),
- filters and other treatments that combat bacteria or parasites, (such as UV light, ozone, and mircoporous filtration).

All these have their own value, but are not the crucial thing you are looking for if you suffer from chemical sensivity. Avoid units that use ozone to kill bacteria, because they can introduce toxins.

Be aware that there are all sorts of unproven treatments now being sold as well, most of which are almost certainly a huge waste of money. Two we have come across are magnetic treatments and the "Water Wand," which "contains highly charged and special energized, positive polarizing water." This water (which just sits there sealed in its wand forever) is apparently "transferring information into the water in the Home Water Pipe, so that this water changes into positive—you will feel, smell, and taste the difference." What is mostly being transferred, of course, is dollars (two hundred of them, for a small plastic tube of water) from gullible purchasers to the manufacturer.

Some doctors report that patients with extreme sensitivity to chemicals react to water that has been in contact with plastic (including the plastic containers of water filters), because minute quantities of material leach out of the plastic into the water. This is unlikely to be true except for a tiny minority of highly sensitive patients. Where such problems are suspected, reverse osmosis units in nonleaching plastic or stainless steel housing are a possible solution. Check that plastics really are the source of the problem before pursuing this option. Drinking good-quality spring- or mineral water in glass bottles for a while should provide a good test. If you are still having problems on this type of water, write to the manufacturer to check that the water is not stored in plastic before bottling. Always bear in mind that it could be something other than water causing your symptoms.

Choosing a Filter

There are two major problems in choosing a filter. First, it is impossible to tell if the product is working properly, without chemical analyses, although if it has a serious defect, a smell of chlorine in the filtered water might be noticeable. Second, there are no standards for domestic water filters at present. As a customer, you therefore need to be well informed about what you are buying. Some of the filters at present on the market actually remove very few contaminants from the water supply. Others may work well at first, but their performance drops off sharply—long before they have filtered the number of gallons claimed by the manufacturer. There are no legally enforceable standards for domestic water filters in the United States, but the National Science Foundation (NSF) now runs an optional certification scheme. Before buying a filter, ask the manufacturer for documentation of the NSF certification. Make sure the certificate applies to the particular model being purchased and note that you are interested in standards for health effects, not for aesthetic effects. (You could, alternatively, check that a particular filter is certified by looking on the NSF Web site, at www.nsf.org. This site can also be used to find good filters and their manufacturers—there are links to manufacturers' Web sites where you can order on-line. Those without Internet access can write to the NSF at

NSF International
P.O. Box 130140
Ann Arbor, MI 48113-0140
Telephone: (734) 769-8010
Toll Free (800) NSF-MARK
Fax: (734) 769-0109
E-mail: info@nsf.org
Contact NSF Departments or Regional Offices

The NSF standards state that if a filter claims to reduce levels of VOCs (Volatile Organic Chemicals) it must be shown to reduce forty-two common standard pollutants, including, for example, benzene, toluene, styrene, carbon tetrachloride, lindane, and 2,4 D. The full list can be viewed at www.nsf.org/consumer/dwtuconsumer.html. A separate category of claim exists for chlorine and another for trihalomethanes (by-products of chlorine disinfection—see page 422).

These are the three categories of interest to people with chemical sensitivity. (There are, in addition, several other categories—such as turbidity, scale or hardness, bacteria, and parasite cysts—which are not of special importance to those with chemical sensitivity.)

Many of the water filters purchased are of the pitcher type. The advantage of these is that the initial outlay is very low. The cost per gallon is usually cheaper than bottled water.

The prime objective of the **pitcher filters** is to improve the taste and appearance of water, and to remove hardness (calcium carbonate or chalk) so that kettles do not become lined with scale. They contain an activated carbon filter to remove chlorine and another component, an ion exchange resin, which takes out the calcium carbonate. The latter component also removes lead and some other metals. Calcium carbonate is not injurious to health and cannot cause sensitivity reactions, so it is the kettle that benefits rather than the drinker.

The activated carbon also takes out some organic pollutants such as chloroform and trichloroethylene, but the majority of pitcher filters are not really designed for this task. They contain a relatively small amount of activated carbon and cannot remove all organic contaminants. In fact, most of the manufacturers do not claim that they can, but many people who buy these filters have an exaggerated idea of their abilities.

For people whose main problem is sensitivity to chlorine, and who cannot afford a plumbed-in filter, a pitcher filter would be a good choice.

Most pitcher filters contain silver to prevent bacterial growth, but even if silver is present it is important not to leave water standing in the pitcher for more than a day, as there can be a buildup of bacteria. These are not usually harmful species, but it is wise to be careful. The top part of the jug should be cleaned out once a week. Pitcher filters without silver cannot be recommended. To discover if the filters do contain silver, you will probably have to write to the manufacturer.

In areas with hard water, the filter may not last as long as the manufacturer claims. However, the activated carbon element should go on working after the ion-exchange resin is saturated with calcium carbonate. So you should continue to get chlorine removal, even if the kettle furs up slightly.

Plumbed-in filters using activated carbon are intended to remove much more from the water than pitcher filters. They contain far more carbon, and it is generally of a higher quality. Some of these filters may not contain ion-exchange resins, so they do not remove hardness from the water, nor do they necessarily take out metals such as lead. But for anyone whose main problem is chemical sensitivity, they are a good choice.

A high-quality filter of this type will be quite expensive to buy, but the filter should last for several years. The running costs usually work out a lot cheaper than the pitcher filters. Reverse osmosis units usually cost even more, but once this outlay has been made, the running cost is low.

Needless to say, the better filters are more expensive, but a high price is not an unfailing guide to quality, so you need to ask some searching questions:

- Does it contain silver? If not, what controls are there on bacterial growth?
- Is the faucet made from lead-free material?
- Is the filter certified by the NSF? If not NSF-certified, then don't buy it.
- What percentage of chlorine, trihalomethanes, and other chlorinated organic chemicals, pesticides, and organic solvents does it remove? Ask to see test results. (Should be more than 95 percent for each of these groups. The tests should have been carried out by an independent laboratory.)
- How many gallons will the filter process in total? How many gallons per day?
- What percentage removal can be expected when it is nearing the end of its life? (This is a crucial question—the manufacturer may say the filter is good for 5,000 gallons, but if it is only removing 30 percent of contaminants after 4,000 gallons you may as well drink tap water. Good filters should still be removing 90 percent or more at the end of their useful life.)
- How much does a replacement filter cost?

Given these figures, you can work out the cost per gallon. Bear in mind that the cheapest price per gallon may not be the best in terms of water quality.

The same sort of questions should be asked if you are choosing a filter that combines activated carbon with reverse osmosis (see page 425). If they do not include silver, ask about bacteriological control. Filters that work by reverse osmosis alone are not recommended.

None of the above systems remove harmful bacteria, so they are only suitable for use with tap water that has already been chlorinated or otherwise disinfected. All water used for baby feeds should be boiled before use, including bottled or filtered water.

For people who can obtain water directly, from a borehole or spring, there are large-scale devices that kill bacteria as well as removing pollutants and sediment. These are known as water purification systems and are much more expensive, but the water obtained should be of very high quality.

Firms supplying certified quality filters direct to the public can be located through NSF (see page 427).

Whatever filter you buy, do maintain it properly and replace parts as often as suggested by the manufacturer, otherwise you could be drinking water that is effectively unfiltered. (Be wary of manufacturers who suggest that you will "know" when to change the filter by the taste of your water—most of the serious pollutants are tasteless.)

Finally, whether or not you filter your own water, do your bit to take care of natural water resources—the more polluted these get, the greater the toll on everyone's health. Whenever you have to get rid of motor oil, fuel, paints, pesticides, bleach, cleaning fluids, or other household chemicals, or water containing antifreeze, find out the disposal site or method recommended for your locality. Never pour these substances into storm drains, where they can eventually reach rivers, lakes, and underground water supplies.

Water-Softeners for Eczema

In hard-water districts, children with eczema may suffer less skin irritation if the water used for washing and bathing is softened. Plumbed-in water-softeners will take out most of the calcium carbonate (limescale or chalk) from the water.

Medicinal Drugs

This appendix covers the drugs commonly used treating allergies and some of the other conditions discussed in this book. Where food plays a part in such an illness, it may often be a question of deciding whether to alter the diet or control the symptoms with drugs. Almost all drugs have some side effects and the decision to use them involves weighing their good effects against their bad ones. This is a decision that only a qualified doctor can make. The information given here is intended to help patients understand the basis for such decisions, and participate in them where this is appropriate.

Drugs are often referred to in different ways—by their proper name (or generic name), and by the trade names given them by the manufacturers. The same drug may be marketed under a number of different trade names if it is produced by different manufactures. Some medicines contain a mixture of two or more drugs. Drugs are described here under their generic names, which are given in italics, for example *albuterol*. The trade names are shown with a capital letter, for example Ventolin. To make use of this section, you need to know what type of drug it is that you are taking. For example, Ventolin *(albuterol)* is a bronchodilator and, more specifically, a B-2 bronchodilator. You can find out what type or category your particular drug belongs to by asking a pharmacist.

1 Mast-cell Stabilizers

These drugs have the effect of stabilizing mast cells so that they do not release histamine and other mediators. The main one used *cromolyn sodium,* is also called *sodium cromoglycate.* It is only effective if it reaches the mast cell before the allergen. So it can be used to prevent the symptoms of allergy, as long as the patient remembers to take the drug when they are feeling well, before they encounter the allergen.

The drug is given in inhalers (Intal) as a preventive treatment for asthma. The time from when treatment starts to when the good effects become noticeable is variable—from a few days to several weeks. The drug must be taken continuously to be effective. In some people, it can cause irritation of the throat, coughing, or, more rarely, an asthmatic attack. In rare cases there may be a true allergic reaction to the drug. In general, however, cromolyn sodium is remarkably free of side effects.

Although the main effect of cromolyn sodium is to stabilize mast cells, it appears to make the bronchi less reactive in other ways as well. Thus, it is used for exercise-induced asthma. Its long-term effect is to make the bronchi less sensitive, which is beneficial.

A related drug, *nedocromil sodium* (Tilade), is sometimes prescribed instead of cromolyn sodium for asthma. It acts in much the same way, but is a more powerful drug, and is not prescribed for children. Sometimes cromolyn sodium is combined with other drugs, as in Intal Compound, which contains *isoprenaline* (section 4A).

In cases of food allergy, taking cromolyn sodium by mouth (Nalcrom or Gastrocrom) can block the allergic reaction. But it is only used where the symptoms are not of the immediate-and-violent kind. Thus, it might be prescribed for patients with food-induced symptoms, such as diarrhea, asthma, rhinitis, eczema, or chronic hives, but not for those who suffer swelling of the mouth and tongue on eating a particular food. In such cases, the slight risk of the drug not working has to be considered, because of the serious consequences of such a failure.

Cromolyn sodium appears to block mast cell degranulation in the gut wall, which prevents the gut wall becoming inflamed and thus makes it less permeable to food molecules.

To be effective, cromolyn sodium (taken by mouth) must be taken ten or fifteen minutes before the food is eaten. The beneficial effects of the drug may not appear for several days. Occasionally, the drug may make the symptoms worse, for reasons that are not yet understood, and sometimes it has no effect, or only partially controls the symptoms. Sometimes patients experience side effects such as headaches, hives, diarrhea, or vomiting.

Because of doubts about its effectiveness if used long term, simply taking cromolyn sodium is not the best way to deal with food allergy. Its main use is in patients with reactions to a very wide range of foods, who find it difficult to avoid them all. Even though they are taking the drug, such patients must usually restrict their intake of the main offending foods as well. Babies who react to a wide range of foods on weaning have been helped by cromolyn sodium.

This drug can also be useful in giving mildly food-allergic people a "day off" from their restricted diet. Children may be given it for holidays or birthdays, to allow them to eat normally for a day. Cromolyn sodium is also used in hay fever and other forms of allergic rhinitis (Nasalcrom) and in allergic conjunctivitis (Opticrom). It can cause stinging when applied, but this wears off quickly and again there are no serious side effects.

2 Drugs That Counteract Histamine

Histamine is one of the mediators released by mast cells when they degranulate (see page 29). It is also released by various other cells in the body, since it acts as a local messenger substance, conveying instructions to neighboring cells.

The main effects of histamine are to make smooth muscles (in the bronchi, gut, bladder, and so forth) contract, to make the small blood vessels enlarge, and to make the capillaries (tiny blood vessels) become leakier. These last two effects cause a drop in blood pressure. Locally, the increased leakiness of the capillaries contributes to inflammation.

Antihistamines (more correctly referred to as *histamine H1-receptor antagonists*) block the effects of histamine. They do this by binding to the H1 receptors on cells. Histamine normally binds to these receptors triggering a reaction by the cell. So by blocking the receptors, antihistamines prevent histamine from affecting those cells.

A wide range of antihistamines is available today, including *cetirizine* (Zyrtek), *fexofenadine* (Allegra), and *loratadine* (Claritin). Some antihistimines, such as *diphenlydramine* (Benadryl) are rather unspecific and can also bind to the receptors for other messenger substances, such as epinephrine and serotonin. They tend to cause drowsiness through blocking messengers such as epinephrine, and they can also cause dizziness, nervousness, tremors, stomach upsets, dry mouth, blurred vision, and impotence. These side effects are not damaging in the long term, although they can be inconvenient. Some patients are not affected at all and others develop a tolerance of these drugs after a while, so the side effects diminish. So, if an antihistamine controls the allergic symptoms well, but causes side effects, it is worth persisting with it for a while. Sometimes the sedative effects of antihistamines can be useful, as in children with hives who tend to scratch at night. Should side effects continue, experiment with other antihistamines: they are all different and reactions are very individual.

More specific drugs, which show a stronger preference for histamine receptors and so cause less drowsiness, have now been introduced. *Astemizole* (Hismanal) and *terfenadine* (Triludan, Seldane) are the main ones, but the former is to be withdrawn from the market due to side effects. These can have some side effects but should not cause as many problems as the other antihistamines. If you are taking beta-blockers for a heart condition, ask your doctor's advice before taking *terfenadine*. *Terfenadine* should also be avoided by anyone with a heart arrhythmia (irregular heartbeat). Grapefruit juice contains a substance that blocks the breakdown of *terfenadine*, so that the concentration builds up in the body. This can cause heart arrhythmias even in normal, healthy people, so you should not drink grapefruit juice, or eat large amounts of grapefruit, while taking *terfenadine*.

Antihistamines, taken by mouth, are useful in hay fever and perennial rhinitis, where there are symptoms in both the nose and eyes, together with itching in the mouth or ears. Where there are only symptoms in the nose, a cromolyn sodium or corticosteroid spray may be more appropriate because these have fewer side effects.

Antihistamines are also effective in some cases of chronic urticaria, including cold-induced utricaria. They are not effective in asthma, because other mediators, besides histamine, play a major role in producing the symptoms.

Ketotifen (Zaditen) acts both as an antihistamine and a mast-cell stabilizer (Section 1), and is used to prevent asthma attacks. Its side effects are similar to those of most antihistamines.

Azatadine and *cyproheptadine* act both as antihistamines and serotonin antagonists (section 13A). They are used for allergic rhinitis and urticaria.

3 Sympathomimetics

These are drugs that mimic the effects of naturally produced epinephrine , the messenger of the sympathetic nervous system, which produces the "flight-or-fight" reaction. Sympathomimetics have various effects, but one local effect is to make small blood vessels (capillaries) contract. Thus, they have an opposing effect to histamine. This is exploited in some nasal sprays for hay fever and perennial rhinitis. The drugs concerned are *phenylephrine, oxymetazoline* (Afrin, Dristan, Sudafed) *xylometazoline* (Otrivine), and *neosynephrine* (Sinex).

These sprays make the capillaries in the nose contract providing immediate relief from congestion, but if used for more than two weeks they can have adverse effects. The blood vessels become "hooked" on the drug so that when the spray is discontinued they react by expanding, causing congestion again. *These sprays are for short-term use only.*

Some sprays combine sympathomimetics with antihistamines. Others combine sympathomimetics with antihistamines and antibiotics or with corticosteroids and antibiotics. Sprays containing antibiotics are only used where there are signs of infection as well as allergy.

Sympathomimetics such as *pseudoephedrine* are sometimes taken in tablet or syrup form, as in Actifed, CoTylenol, Drixoral, and Sudafed. They may also be combined with antihistamines in medicines taken by mouth, such as Allegra-D (*pseudoephedrine* and *fenofexadine*), Sudafed Plus (*pseudephedrine* and *tripolidine*), and Claritin-D (*pseudoephedrine* and *loratidine*).

When taken by mouth, the sympathomimetic helps to overcome the main side effect of the antihistamine, drowsiness. (See page 438 for side effects.)

4 Bronchodilators

These are drugs that make the bronchial muscles relax, and are therefore useful in asthma. There are three types of bronchodilators: ß2-adrenoceptor agonists, xanthines, and anticholinergics.

4A ß2-Adrenoceptor Agonists
Antagonists are drugs such as antihistamines (section 2) that bind to receptors and block the effect of the natural messenger (for example, histamine) that normally binds to the receptor. Agonists have the opposite effect. They bind to receptors and stimulate the cell, in the same way that the natural messenger would—in other words, they mimic the effects of that natural messenger.

The ß2-adrenoceptor agonists mimic the effects of epinephrine on the bronchial muscles, by binding to receptors for epinephrine. These are called ß2 adrenoceptors, hence the name of the drugs. They include: *albuterol* (Ventolin, Provertil), *pirbuterol* (Maxair), *bitolferol* (Tornalate), and *terbutaline* (Breathaire).

Of all the bronchodilators, these drugs have the most specific effects on the bronchi. They are now preferred to *isoprenaline*, which has a less specific effect, and tends to combine with epinephrine receptors in the heart muscles as well as those in the bronchi, sometimes causing irregular heartbeat, flushing, and headaches. *Isoprenaline* is combined with a sympathomimetic, *phenylephrine* (section 3) in some inhalers.

Isoetharine and *orciprenaline* (Alupent) are drugs of the same type with similar side effects. If you are taking any of these older nonspecific drugs, ask your doctor about better alternatives.

Side effects can also occur with the specific ß2-adrenoceptor agonists, such as *salbutamol*, although they are generally less of a problem. They include tremor, nervous tension, headache, flushing, and dry mouth. Taking the drugs from an inhaler reduces the side effects by targeting the drug on the bronchi—this allows a much lower dose to be used than if the drugs were taken by mouth.

The effect of these drugs lasts for up to six hours. Learning how to operate the inhaler properly is very important, or the drug can fail to reach the airways. Dry powder inhalers (Ventodisks) are easier to operate for many people than conventional inhalers.

If they are used several times a day over a period of time these drugs may increase the risk of a fatal asthma attack. They do not reduce the inflammation of the airways as corticosteroids and cromolyn sodium do so their beneficial effects are limited; all they do is suppress the symptoms of asthma.

If you need your reliever inhaler more than once a day, see your doctor about getting a preventer such as a steroid inhaler, a leukotriene antagonist, or cromolyn sodium—or about increasing the dose if you already use a preventer. These are far safer, and more valuable, than regular doses of reliever inhaler.

Long-acting B-2 relievers

The main drug of this type is *salmeterol* (Serevent). Very similar chemically to the short-acting B-2 relievers, it can produce an initial effect almost as quickly, within five to ten minutes. Where it differs is that the effect goes on building up, reaches a maximum after an hour or so, and then lasts for another nine to eleven hours. When taken regularly (twice a day) for several days, there is a gradually increasing benefit.

These drugs are especially useful for nocturnal asthma. Unfortunately, like the short-acting B-2 relievers, a drug of this type can make asthmatic airways less responsive to the benefits of the drug itself and to other B-2 relievers, which is worrying in the long term. However, it seems to be safer to take a long-acting B-2 reliever twice a day, rather than a short-acting one, four times a day.

Never take additional doses between the scheduled doses: these are not "as required" drugs. They should not be used if you have a sudden and more serious asthma attack. Do not stop taking your preventer drug, even if you feel considerable improvement: these drugs are not a substitute for preventers.

4B Xanthines

These are naturally occurring substances that are chemically similar to caffeine. They include *theophylline* (Slo-Bid, Slo-Phyllin, Theo-Dur, Uniphyl), *aminophylline,* and *choline theophyllinate.* They make the bronchial muscles relax, but affect the heart muscles as well. The dose must be exactly right, as there is only a small difference between the dose that will open up the airways, and the overdose that causes unpleasant, or even dangerous, reactions. Such side effects usually occur in the early stages, when the doctor is still trying to work out the correct dose (which varies from one person to another).

However, once asthmatics are established on a safe dose (and provided their general health and their intake of alcohol, tobacco, and other drugs is stable—see below) they can usually go on taking *theophylline* on a long-term basis without serious side effects.

Some doctors give *theophylline* at a fairly low dose—too little to relax the airway muscles. At this dose it may have a preventive effect in reducing airway inflammation. In Europe, low-dose steroids are preferred for producing this effect in mild to moderate asthma, but there is a long tradition of using *theophylline* in the United States.

When first taking *theophylline,* blood samples must be taken regularly to check the levels of the drug in the blood. Don't miss your appointments.

If you give up smoking, or cut down, tell your doctor. Your dose of *theophylline* will need to change immediately because smoking affects the breakdown of the drug. (So will any other source of nicotine, such as chewing tobacco.) Heavy drinking also changes the effects of the drug. Taking contraceptive pills, and a variety of other drugs, alters the dose needed. Check with your doctor or pharmacist before starting any new drugs, or discontinuing use of the Pill. Viral infections, flu vaccinations, heart disease, and liver disease also change the effects of *theophylline*. Watch for side effects and consult your doctor immediately if you are concerned. Simply getting older changes your reaction to this drug: your dose may need to change as you age. Be very careful never to take a double dose by mistake: if you are at all forgetful about tablets, keep a careful record of taking your *theophylline*. Always report any side effects to your doctor immediately. If you are concerned, stop taking the drug.

These drugs are usually taken by mouth. There are slow-release formulations that are taken before going to bed, for those who suffer from nocturnal early-morning attacks of asthma.

4C Anti-Cholinergics

The main drugs in this group are *ipratropium* and *oxitropium,* which are taken by inhalation. Side effects are rare except at high doses. They include dry mouth, difficulty in passing urine, and constipation. Other anti-cholinergics include *butethamate* and *atropine.* Anti-cholinergics help to reduce the amount of mucus present in the airways as well as relaxing the muscles, and may be useful where asthma and bronchitis occur together.

Sympathomimetics (section 3), such as *adrenaline* and *ephedrine,* are sometimes combined with anti-cholinergics in inhalers.

4D Other Bronchodilators

Sympathomimetics (see section 3 above) were once the main drugs used for bronchodilation, but they are much less specific for the bronchial muscles than the drugs described above. They produce side effects more easily than modern bronchodilators and are much less used now. They include *adrenaline, ephedrine,* and *phenylephrine.* Typical side effects include nervousness, anxiety, tremor, irregular heartbeat, and dry mouth.

5 Leukotriene Antagonists

These are entirely new types of drugs, specifically designed for asthma. They are particularly useful because they can be taken in tablet form rather than inhaled. They fall into two groups, the *leukotriene-receptor-antagonists* (such as *zafirlukast/*Accolate and *montelukast/*Singulaire) and the *5-lipoxygenase-inhibitors* (such as *zileuton/*Zyflo). Both groups reduce levels of inflammation by interfering with the pro-inflammatory messages carried by natural chemicals that the body produces, called leukotrienes.

These drugs work in a completely different way from either steroids or cromolyn sodium, the two main drugs previously used to reduce inflammation in asthma. The prerelease trials showed only minor side effects for these new drugs, except for the possibility of a very rare immune disorder that might not actually have been caused by the drug. However, rare or long-term side effects from new drugs do not become apparent until they have been in use for some years. If taking one of these drugs, report any unusual symptoms promptly to your doctor.

6 Corticosteroids

These drugs mimic the action of the hormones produced by the outer layer (cortex) of the adrenal glands, a pair of small glands that sit on top of the kidneys. The main hormone produced is hydrocortisone (cortisol), which has a variety of effects on the body. It controls the amount of sodium and potassium ("salts") that the kidney allows to pass into the urine, and releases glucose into the blood. Hydrocortisone also moves protein out of the muscles and bones, and influences the way fat is deposited. Finally, it suppresses inflammation. In the case of asthma, it does so by damping down late-phase reactions (see page 48), but in other inflammatory conditions the mechanism of action is probably more complex. This effect on inflammation makes corticosteroids useful in the treatment of allergic reactions, and in other diseases—such as rheumatoid arthritis, Crohn's disease, and ulcerative colitis—where inflammation plays a major role.

Because corticorsteroids have so many different functions in the body, there are various unpleasant side effects from using them as drugs. These effects mainly occur when the drugs are taken by mouth. Long-term use of these drugs at high doses can result in Cushing's Syndrome, characterized by deposits of fat around the face ("moon face"), and on the shoulders and abdomen, water retention producing puffiness, bruising, acne, muscle wasting, and weakening of the bones leading to easy breakage. In children, there is also stunted growth. All these changes are due to the effects of corticosteroids on other body processes, as described above. Some of the effects are reversible, if corticosteroids are withdrawn, but there can also be permanent damage.

In using corticosteroids to suppress allergic reactions, the trick is to persuade the drug to reduce inflammation without carrying out any of its other actions. This has been achieved, to a large extent, by modifying hydrocortisone and the other adrenal hormones chemically. Chemical tinkering with the hydrocortisone molecule has produced drugs such as *prednisolone*. This suppresses inflammation but has very little effect on the excretion of salt by the kidneys, so it will not cause water retention.

Unfortunately, these are not the only bad effects of corticosteroids. Because they suppress inflammation, which is a valuable part of the body's fight against disease, they tend to make infections more likely. Viruses and fungi, in particular, are likely to flourish.

If corticosteroids are taken over a long period of time, the adrenal glands' natural activity is suppressed. Stopping the drug leaves the body without corticosteroids, which can lead to collapse in the worst cases. This means that corticosteroids taken by mouth should never be stopped abruptly if they have been taken for more than a few weeks. The glands must be given time to recover their natural level of activity, by gradually reducing the dosage. Even after as little as two weeks, corticosteroids should be withdrawn gradually, by halving the dose each day, to avoid a flare-up of the original problem.

In general, applying corticosteroids locally (where they are needed) is preferable to taking them by mouth or injecting them, because it reduces the dose needed and thus minimizes side effects. This means applying the drug in creams or ointments for eczema, inhaling it for asthma, or injecting it directly into an affected joint for rheumatoid arthritis. Some of the drug still gets into the bloodstream, however—for example, it can be absorbed through the skin. Children with eczema who are smothered in high-dose corticosteroid cream by their parents can develop Cushing's Syndrome, although this is now very rare as doctors are more aware of the dangers.

Corticosteroids are valuable weapons in the fight against many diseases but must always be used with some caution. The doctor's instructions, as regards the amount and timing of the dose, must be followed exactly.

Corticosteroids are often used in chronic asthma to reduce the inflammation of the membranes lining the airways. Corticosteroids can be given by inhaler, in these circumstances, and this allows a very low dose to be used. Little is absorbed into the bloodstream, so it is safe to use corticosteroids in this way for many years if necessary. The main drugs used are *beclomethasone* (Beclovert, Vancenase, Vanceril), *flunisolide* (AeroBid), *triamcinolone* (Azmacort), *budesonide* (Rhinocort), and *fluticasone* (Flonasen, Flovent). In general, if the asthma is known to be provoked by an allergen, it is a good idea to try out cromolyn sodium inhalers before giving corticosteroids, as this drug alone may be effective.

The only common side effect of corticosteroid inhalers is *Candida* (thrush) infections in the throat, due to suppression of the immune response there. This can be reduced by washing the mouth out with warm water after each inhalation. If infections do develop, they can be controlled with antifungal lozenges.

Acute attacks of asthma are often dealt with by giving a short course of corticosteroid tablets. Such treatment suppresses inflammation in the airways within a few days, but is continued for about three weeks, followed by gradual withdrawl. This allows the bronchi to settle down and become less sensitive. Stopping the course of treatment before three weeks can result in a flare-up of asthma again, shortly afterward.

For some asthmatics, controlling their attacks may require treatment with three or even four different types of drugs—cromolyn sodium, a ß2 agonist, a xanthine, and a corticosteroid inhaler. By using several different drugs, good control of the symptoms can be achieved without the need for high doses of any one drug.

In hay fever and perennial rhinitis, corticosteroid sprays or drops are sometimes used. The drugs used include *beclomethasone* (Beconase), *betamethasone* (Betamethacot, Betatrex, Beta-Val), *budesonide* (Rhinocort) and *flunisolide* (AeroBid). In general, these are very effective. Relatively little corticosteroid is absorbed, and there seem to be few side effects, but overuse should be avoided. A cromolyn sodium spray would be preferable if it controls the symptoms well. Students who suffer from bad hay fever are sometimes given corticosteroid tablets to help them get through important examinations, but this is only done in exceptional circumstances.

Some doctors use short courses of corticosteroid tablets for patients with chronic urticaria, to allow the irritation to settle down before other treatments are tried. In very severe cases of rheumatoid arthritis, corticosteroid tablets are sometimes used (see section 6). A corticosteroid injection into an affected joint can reduce inflammation for some time.

In eczema, corticosteroid creams or ointments are used when other forms of treatment (see section 7) have failed. The creams, ointments, and other preparations are classified into four groups: mildly potent, moderately potent, potent, and very potent. In general, only preparations in the first two groups are prescribed for children, since there is a risk of stunting and other side effects when corticosteroids are absorbed into the bloodstream. Even in adults, the potent and very potent preparations are generally only used for a few weeks, to control an acute outbreak of skin irritation; a less potent preparation is then substituted.

The amount absorbed depends on certain other factors, besides the potency of the cream or ointment. More will be absorbed from the face and genitals, and creams should be used sparingly in these areas. Damaged skin will also absorb more.

If corticosteroids have been applied to the skin for more than a few weeks, treatment should not end abruptly, or there may be a flare-up of the eczema. The cream should be withdrawn gradually, a little less being applied each day. The corticosteroid cream can be used alternately with an emollient (see section 7) to ease withdrawal.

In general, treatment with mildly potent corticosteroid preparations can be continued for as long as necessary. Provided there is good medical supervision, such treatment can safely continue for several years if needed.

The corticosteroid most commonly used in creams and ointments for eczema is *hydrocortisone*. (See also section 6A.)

Creams and ointments used for eczema often contain other drugs, besides the corticosteroid. Some include antibiotics and/or antifungal drugs to treat secondary infections. Others contain substances that help to reduce itching, soothe the skin, or restore its water content.

Preparations containing a mixture of coal-tar (which reduces itching) and hydrocortisone are often very effective, the coal-tar helping to make the hydrocortisone effective, even at a low dosage.

7 Emollients and Related Treatments

An emollient is a substance that soothes the skin and restores water to it, thus reducing the symptoms of eczema. White soft paraffin, glycerin, and lanolin are commonly used. Most emollients and similar preparations contain several different ingredients. Urea is sometimes added to the cream or ointment because it helps the skin to bind water, but it may sting slightly and has a urinelike smell. Emollients may be applied directly to the skin or added to the bath, and some can be used instead of soap.

Crepe bandages soaked in calamine lotion, or bandages soaked in saline, are also used in eczema, to relieve the itching and prevent scratching.

Drugs that reduce itching (antipruritics) such as *crotamiton* or *antazoline* may also be used. Nonsteroidal anti-inflammatory drugs (see section 8) such as *bufexamac* are sometimes helpful.

Soothing treatments of this type are generally tried as a first step, where the eczema is not severe. They are free of side effects, although a small minority of patients may become sensitized to lanolin, so that lanolin-containing creams cannot be used thereafter.

8 Nonsteroidal Anti-Inflammatory Drugs (NSAIDs)

These are drugs that suppress inflammation but are not corticosteroids (see section 6). They work by reducing the quantities of prostaglandins produced by the body. Their main use is in rheumatoid arthritis, where they can reduce the pain and swelling in the joints.

The NSAID that everyone knows is *aspirin,* which belongs to a group of drugs called *salicylates.* There are many other NSAIDs, and they are very varied chemically, the only common factor being their effect on prostaglandin synthesis.

Because prostaglandins do a variety of different jobs in the body, a drug that interferes with their production is likely to have side effects. In particular, prostaglandins play an important role in the stomach, and NSAIDs tend to cause stomach upsets, or more serious damage to the stomach lining. Aspirin is the worst offender in this respect. Various modified forms of aspirin have been introduced in an effort to reduce its side effects on the stomach. But these may still affect the stomach, and should not be taken by anyone who has ever had a stomach ulcer.

Prostaglandins also play an important role in the kidney, and some NSAIDs affect kidney function causing water retention (edema). Long-term use of NSAIDs, without proper supervision, can lead to kidney damage, but this is rare.

Some people appear to be particularly sensitive to aspirin (see page 78) and may suffer from a deteriorization in their asthma or urticaria if they take it. Some of these people react in a similar way to other NSAIDs, and a few (about 5 percent) may be affected by acetaminophen as well.

Current recommendations are that no one with a stomach or duodenal ulcer should take NSAIDs. Other patients should start with the safest NSAID at the lowest possible dose, only increasing the dose or changing to another NSAID if this is ineffective.

No one should be taking more than one type of NSAID simultaneously. Note that *aspirin* or *ibuprofen* are found in many painkillers, cold and flu remedies, headache and migraine tablets. You should avoid taking these drugs if you are already taking NSAIDs: check the labels carefully for their ingredients. *Acetaminophen* can be taken safely if you need a painkiller.

Recent research has shown that some NSAIDs tend to speed up the breakdown of cartilage in the joints, although other NSAIDs seem to protect the cartilage. This may be something that you wish to discuss with your doctor, especially if you have osteoarthritis (the most common form of arthritis, in which the cartilage breaks down faster than it is repaired). *Misoprostol*, a drug that is sometimes given to protect the stomach lining from the harmful effects of NSAIDs, also protects cartilage from breakdown, and may be worth considering.

An important group of NSAIDs are the *propionic acid derivatives*. These do not reduce inflammation quite as well as aspirin, but they are effective painkillers and cause far fewer problems in the stomach than aspirin. However, some patients may suffer from stomach upsets or rashes, and some of the drugs can also cause headaches, drowsiness, and other minor problems. *Tiaprofenic acid* has also been associated with some cases of severe cystitis, and you should see your doctor promptly if you have any pain on urination, urgency, or increased frequency, while taking this drug. These drugs are generally used for mild forms of rheumatold arthritis, where the inflammation is not very great. Some are available as gels that are applied directly to the affected area.

The remaining NSAIDs have a powerful anti-inflammatory action, on a par with aspirin. They can all produce side effects in susceptible individuals, but are reasonably safe for long-term use. Some are available as gels, which are applied directly to the affected area.

Indomethacin is a powerful anti-inflammatory drug that has been in use for many years. It is useful for morning stiffness because it goes on acting for a long time, and a dose taken the night before will make getting up easier. This drug can cause stomach upsets, headaches, or dizziness, in which case another drug will usually be tried. When taken for a long period of time it can also affect the eyes, and it is important to have regular checkups. Anyone who is allergic to aspirin may react to this drug too. *Acemetacin* is a similar drug, chemically related to *indomethacin*.

Sulindac is a similar drug, with less anti-inflammatory effect than *indomethacin* but fewer side effects. It sometimes causes stomach upsets, rashes, dizziness, or ringing in the ears. Occasionally more serious side effects occur and should be reported to the doctor. Other NSAIDs that are similar to *indomethacin* are *etodolac* and *diclofenac*. *Diclofenac* is combined with another drug, *misoprostol*, in some medicines. *Misoprostoc* is included to protect the stomach lining from the harmful effects of the NSAID.

Piroxicam, meloxicam, and *tenoxicam* are NSAIDs with strong anti-inflammatory effects. They have the advantage of only needing to be taken once a day. These drugs can sometimes cause stomach upsets, water retention, ringing in the ears, headaches, or other side effects.

Azapropazone is another powerful anti-inflammatory. It can sometimes cause side effects in the form of stomach upsets, headache, water retention, and rashes (the skin may become more sensitive to sunlight). As with other drugs of this type, anyone taking them on a long-term basis should have regular checkups.

9 More Powerful Drugs Used in Rheumatoid Arthritis

These drugs are used where NSAIDs (see section 8) have been tried and have failed to control the symptoms. Most have some effect on the immune response within the joint. They have the advantage of checking the progress of joint destruction caused by rheumatoid arthritis, whereas NSAIDs simply suppress the immediate effects. On the other hand, they are powerful drugs that are more likely to cause serious side effects. Once they are started, they will probably have to be taken for many years. For this reason, doctors delay using them until they are sure the drugs are necessary. If taking such drugs, it is very important to have regular medical supervision and report any side effects to the doctor.

The drugs commonly used are: *penicillamine, gold salts, sulphasalazine, chloroquine, hydroxychloroquine,* and *methotrexate.*

In severe cases of rheumatoid arthritis, that do not respond to other treatments, drugs that have a general suppressive effect on the immune system may sometimes be used. The main ones are *cyclosporin* and *azathioprine*. These drugs make the body less able to fight infections, and at high doses they could make patients more susceptible to cancer. Corticosteroids (see section 6) are sometimes used where none of the above treatments are effective.

10 Painkillers

These are drugs that can block pain sensations. Our main interest in them is in connection with headache and migraine.

Aspirin and other salicylates (see section 8) reduce pain and inflammation. They also have some effects on the blood platelets, and this may help to avoid a migraine attack. Regular, prolonged use of salicylates can irritate the stomach lining and have other adverse effects, so this should be avoided.

Acetaminophen reduces pain but has very little anti-inflammatory effect. It has no ill effects on the stomach and, as long as the maximum dose is strictly observed and it is not combined with asprinlike painkillers, it is a very safe drug. However, it should not be taken long-term at the maximum dosage, nor should it be taken by anyone who has kidney or liver disease.

Ibuprofen and related drugs (see section 8) are effective painkillers and have fewer ill effects on the stomach than aspirin, although they can cause problems for some people.

Codeine is a very mild opiate (a morphinelike drug) used in some migraine preparations. It is fairly safe but can cause constipation.

Caffeine is added to some painkillers to speed up absorption and improve the effectiveness of the drug. Caffeine can also produce headaches (see page 214), so heavy use of this type of painkiller is not advisable.

11 Drugs That Reduce Nausea and Vomiting

Migraine remedies often contain a drug to reduce nausea and vomiting (anti-emetics), as well as a painkiller. One problem in migraine is that absorption from the stomach is much reduced once an attack starts, so that painkillers taken by mouth have little effect. Anti-emetics can improve the absorption of the painkiller, so they are useful for migraines, even if nausea is not a symptom. The main drugs used are *buclizine, cyclizine,* and *metoclopramide.* These are safe drugs with few side effects.

Because of the problem of nonabsorption, it is very important to take migraine treatments as soon as an attack begins—or in advance, for those patients who have advance warning of their attacks, in the form of visual disturbances, mood changes, and other signs.

12 Ergotamine

Ergotamine is a powerful drug that makes the blood vessels contract. Since it is expansion of the blood vessels that causes the pain of migraine, this drug can be useful in treating an acute attack. But if ergotamine is used regularly, the underlying problem of migraine—failure to control the expansion and contraction of blood vessels—could be made worse. Some patients who have taken ergotamine for many years find that the drug is actually causing the attacks.

Ergotamine also has various side effects, including nausea, stomach pains, and cramps. Some medicines combine *ergotamine* with *caffeine*, or with caffeine and an anti-emetic, *cyclizine*.

Because of its many drawbacks, *ergotamine* is much less used now. Most acute attacks of migraine are better treated with a mixture of painkiller, anti-emetic and sedative. If nondrug methods, such as an avoidance diet, can reduce or eliminate the need for *ergotamine*, they should definitely be implemented.

13 Drugs That Can Prevent Migraine Attacks

There are various drugs that, taken regularly, can prevent migraine attacks, or at least reduce their frequency. Beneficial effects may not be apparent until they have been taken for several weeks.

In conventional migraine treatment, these are not generally prescribed unless migraines are fairly frequent and severe, and other measures have been tried without significant success. Other measures might include reducing stress, avoiding situations that trigger migraines, and avoiding foods such as chocolate, cheese, red wine, and citrus fruits (see pages 170–72). By extension, it would seem reasonable to investigate food intolerance, using an elimination diet, before starting on (or continuing with) these drugs.

13A Serotonin Antagonists

Serotonin, or *5HT,* is a chemical messenger produced by the blood platelets that is known to play a part in migraine (see page 170). Drugs that block the receptors for *serotonin* seem to help prevent migraine. Some of these drugs also act as antihistamines (see section 2). The main drug used is *pizotifen*, which is generally safe but can cause weight gain and drowsiness in some people.

Methysergide is equally effective, but it can cause serious side effects with lasting damage. It is no longer used, except under hospital supervision.

Sumatripan is an injection, given under the skin, for acute migraine.

13B ß-Blockers

These drugs block ß-receptors for epinephrine, the hormone that produces the "flight-or-fight" reaction. Their main use is in other diseases, principally heart diseases, and it is not entirely clear how they help to prevent migraine.

Some of these drugs block the effects of epinephrine generally and they should not be taken by asthmatics, since they have the opposite effect of ß2 bronchodilators (see section 4A). The ones in question are *nadolol, propanolol,* and *timolol.* Others are more selective, only affecting ß-receptors in the heart, and they can be taken by asthmatics, although good medical supervision is needed. The principal drug of this type is *metoprolol.*

All these drugs have certain side effects, including cold hands and feet, disturbed sleep, stomach upset, and wheezing. If dry eyes or skin rash develop this should be reported to the doctor immediately, as it can indicate a severe reaction to the drug. The drugs should not be stopped abruptly, but gradually withdrawn.

13C Clonidine

Clonidine is used to lower blood pressure and when taken at low dosage (Dixarit) it can prevent migraine in some patients. It is a relatively safe drug, but some patients may suffer from drowsiness, dizziness, dry mouth, or insomnia.

13D Other Drugs

A group of drugs called *tricyclic antidepressants* can be used to prevent migraine in some patients. If taking such drugs you should not discontinue them abruptly: seek your doctor's advice. An antihistamine known as *cyproheptadine* which is also a serotonin antagonist (see section 13A), can also prevent migraine. Some patients are helped by drugs known as calcium-channel blockers, for example, *nifedipine* or *verapamil.*

APPENDIX 9

Nutritional Supplements

A general vitamin and mineral supplement is not suitable for everyone, and if you have been eating a very inadequate diet, or have serious symptoms that you think might be due to nutritional deficiencies, then you should seek professional help. For some patients a full nutritional analysis may be needed (see page 332) to identify the particular nutrients that are in short supply. Where there are serious deficiencies, treatment should be carried out by a nutritional specialist, because the level of one vitamin or mineral can affect the level or absorption of another. Specialist treatment includes repeated monitoring of nutrient levels to see how they respond to the supplement and making the appropriate adjustments.

Zinc Supplements

If you think you may be deficient in zinc (see page 330), it is worth trying a zinc supplement to see if this produces an improvement. A dose of 20 to 40 mg of elemental zinc per day is recommended, and even if you are not deficient this dose is most unlikely to do any harm. Zinc sulfate tablets are widely obtainable from chemists. The amount of elemental zinc per tablet should be given on the label.

Take the supplement last thing at night, preferably without any late-night snacks or milky drinks, as zinc supplements are not well absorbed if taken with food. You may need to take the supplement for a month or more before any good effects are obvious.

Supplements and the Pill

A special type of supplement is recommended for anyone currently taking the Pill, or stopping the Pill (see page 329).

Recommended Supplement*

The supplement described below is designed for those who have minor health problems. Some women experience more serious nutritional deficiencies as a result of taking the Pill, and they will need professional help of the kind described above. Women coming off the Pill usually need to take the supplement for two to three months. You should consult your doctor before taking the supplement.

This supplement is not obtainable in a single combined tablet, but the different vitamins and minerals can all be purchased from specialist suppliers (see appendix 10).

Vitamin B$_1$	10–50 mg
Vitamin B$_2$	10–50 mg
Vitamin B$_3$	10–50 mg
Vitamin B$_5$	50–100 mg
Vitamin B$_6$	50–100 mg
Vitamin B$_{12}$	200–400 mcg (mg)
Folic acid	400 mcg–2mg
Inositol	50–75 mg
Vitamin C	250–2000 mg (or more)
Vitamin E	50–200 IUs
Magnesium	100–200 mg (or more)
Zinc	5–15 mg (or more)
Manganese	3–5 mg

The supplement should not contain vitamin A or copper. Iron should be included only if a blood test indicates anemia.

---

*Adapted from *Nutritional Medicine* by Dr. Stephen Davies and Dr. Alan Stewart, with permission.

Useful Addresses

Inclusion of an organization in this list does not necessarily mean that the authors agree with all the policies or opinions advanced by that organization. In the same way, we give no general endorsement of the commercial companies included—they may sell other items, besides those for which they are listed here, which we believe to be ineffectual or even damaging if used wrongly. Readers are advised to be skeptical about the claims made for some products, such as nutritional supplements and herbal medicines. Buying from a reputable company is advisable.

Certain commercial companies now quote from this book, or from other materials written by one or both of us, in their sales material (which may masquerade as "general information"). We would like to make it clear that such quotes are made without our permission and do not necessarily endorse their products or agree with their views.

Information of Food Allergies

Food Allergy Network (FAN)
10400 Eaton Place, Suite 107
Fairfax, VA 22030-2208
Tel: 703-691-3179
Fax: 703-691-2713

Becoming a member is highly recommended if you have true food allergy, especially life-threatening reactions. Emergency alerts go out to members when a packaged food is found to have an allergenic ingredient such as peanut, milk, or egg not listed on the label. In 1999 there were also special alerts about a defective batch of epinephrine injectors. All this is information that could save your life!

FAN deals with classic IgE-mediated food allergies and is identified with a conventional medical view of the field. For those who have multiple food allergies, or complex and unusual reactions, it might be useful to belong to another group, such as FAST (see below), in addition to FAN. Those with food intolerance (reactions that do not give positive skin-prick tests or RASTs—see page 111) should look for other groups.

Food Allergy Survivors Together (FAST)

A very useful chat/forum/support group geared to those with multiple true allergies, unusual reactions, non-IgE food allergy, and so on. This organization can only be contacted via the Internet at www.angelfire.com/ mi/FAST.

Support Groups for Celiacs

Celiac Disease Foundation Newsletter
c/o Elaine Monarch
13251 Ventura Blvd., Suite 3
Studio City, CA 91604-1838
Tel: 818-990-2379 or 990-2345
E-mail: CDFoundtn@aol.com

The informative newsletter costs $35 per year.

For news and views on celiac disease, www.celiac.com/misc.html is useful.

The University of Maryland's Center for Celiac Research now has a Web site on www.celiaccenter.org.

There is some useful information on www.csaceliacs.org/basics.html the Web site of the Celiac Sprue Association. However, it could be confusing and a little alarming for the beginner, so start somewhere else. For example, it does not distinguish between foods that are risky because they contain gluten, and those that might be risky for other reasons, such as raw eggs. Some of the information is not correct: for example, millet, buckwheat, and quinoa do not contain gluten, and European "gluten-free" foods do not contain up to 3 percent gluten.

The Canadian Celiac Association
190 Britannia Road East
Unit #11
Mississauga, Ontario
Canada L4Z 1W6

Their website at www.celiac.ca is a good source of information, and they produce pamphlets for teachers, a handbook for celiac children, and helpful cards for use in restaurants explaining celiac food requirements. These are available in all major languages.

The celiac UPC database, designed for use at home or on a palm-top computer while shopping, can be found on www.brandtbeach.com/celiac/upc.

Support Groups for Atopic Dermatitis

National Eczema Association for Science and Education
1220 SW Morrison, Suite 433
Portland, OR 97205
Tel: 503-228-4430
Fax: 503-224-3363
E-mail: nease@teleport.com
Web site: www.eczema-assn.org

An excellent organization, committed to a scientific-medicine approach to eczema, but open-minded about the range of possible causes and treatments, including diagnostic diets for eczema. Their leaflets and Web site offer useful and very detailed advice about moisturizing, avoiding eczema triggers, the causes of eczema, and choosing a physician. They can help you find a doctor who is experienced in treating eczema and has been recommended by other eczema sufferers (or their parents).

Emergency Alert Bracelets

Anyone who suffers from anaphylactic shock, or has very severe and sudden asthma attacks, or is allergic to latex or penicillin, should wear an emergency alert bracelet or pendant. Key medical information is engraved on the bracelet, and there is also a telephone number that gives medical staff access to a computer database where essential medical data about you is available. These useful items are sold by a nonprofit company, Medic Alert.

MedicAlert Foundation
2323 Colorado Avenue
Turlock, CA 95382-2018
Tel: 800-IDALERT (800-432-5378)
Fax: 209-669-2495
Web site: www.medicalert.org
(In Canada, telephone 416-696-0142.)

Pollen Counts and Forecasts

You can call a toll-free line: 1-800-9-POLLEN for pollen counts and forecasts.

There is also detailed information available on the Internet at: www.aaaai.org. This site is valuable because it provides separate counts for trees, grasses, weeds, and mold spores, and specificies the predominant allergen at the time for different regions of the USA.

Breast-Feeding Support Organizations

La Leche League International
9616 Minneapolis Avenue
Franklin Park, IL 60131
Tel: 312-455-7730
Hotline: 800-LALECHE (open 9 A.M.–3 P.M. Central Standard Time, for advice, and so forth)
Web site: www.lalecheleague.org/LLLICatMain96.html

International Lactation Consultant Organization
4101 Lake Boone Trail
Raleigh, NC 27607
Tel: 919-787-5181
Web site: www.ilca.org/jhl.html

Magazines on Breast Feeding
La Leche League's *New Beginnings*
1400 N. Meacham Road
Schaumburg, IL 60173
Tel: 847-519-7730
Web site: www.lalecheleague.org

Mothering
The Magazine of Natural Family Living
P.O. Box 1690
Sante Fe, NM 87504
Tel: 800-984-8116
Web site: www.mothering.com

Nurturing Magazine
Magazine of Natural Parenting
#373, 918 Sixteenth Avenue NW
Calgary, Alberta
Canada T2M OK3
Web site: www.nurturing.ca

Co-counseling

If you have access to the Internet, you can contact the United States Co-counseling Circle at http://users.multipro.com/circle.

Otherwise, try the following coordinators:

Judy Hartling: 413-747-3924 or judy_a_hartling@spfdcol.edu

Bob Sawyer: 860-423-6292 or bobsawyer7@aol.com

Jlynn Silvers: 860-523-8665 or jlynnalive@aol.com

Lactose Intolerance

One solution for those with lactose intolerance is to replace the missing enzyme—**lactase** (see page 259). You can take lactase in pill form, and there are several different brands available. It is important to take a large enough dose to "cover" the amount of lactose you are eating: more for a meal with high dairy content. The dose on the package may be given in milligrams (mg) or FCC Lactase Units. Fifteen Lactase Units equals 1 mg. If you have a severe lactase deficiency you need pills that contain 3000 Lactase Units or 200 mg of lactose. Many of the widely available lactase pills contain only 25 mg of lactose, an amount that is unlikely to help most sufferers unless they take large numbers of the pills.

There will be other ingredients in most lactase pills. Some contain mannitol, which might be a problem for some people: there are claims that it can act as a laxative and cause abdominal cramps. If you are very sensitive to gluten and the pills contain dextrose or maltodextrin, check with the manufacturer for an assurance that the pills are gluten-free.

Taking too much lactase is unlikely to do any harm, but large amounts of some of the other ingredients, such as magnesium, might be a problem long term if you are taking a lot of pills. Choose a pill with a minimum of other ingredients.

Lactase drops are also available. Add them to milk and leave it to stand for about twenty-four hours stirring occasionally. You can add more drops after twelve hours to increase the effect. This will reduce the lactose content considerably, but probably will not remove all lactose, so the supersensitive should test the results cautiously.

Health food stores sell lactase pills, but if you have difficulty finding them, or obtaining a suitable brand, contact the manufacturers below.

Lactaid
McNeil Consumer Products Co.
Division of McNeil-PPC, Inc.
Ft. Washington, PA 19034
Supplies pills and drops that contain dextrose and mannitol.

Nature's Way Lactase Enzyme
Nature's Way Products
10 Mountain Springs Parkway
Springville, UT 84663
Product contains maltodextrin.

Equate
Perrigo Co.
Allegan, MI 49010
Product contains dextrose and dextrates.

Dairy-Ease
Rite-Aid Corporation
Harrisburg, PA 17105
Supplies pills and drops that contain mannitol.

Food Sensitivity: Avoiding Problem Ingredients

If you have access to the Internet, you can find a huge range of suppliers catering to every possible aspect of allergy, intolerance, and chemical sensitivity at www.allallergy.net/allallergy/products.

Ener-G Foods, Inc., sells wheat-free, yeast-free, egg-free, and milk-free foods. Can be ordered on-line at www.allallergy.net/allallergy/products, or call 800-331-5222.

Those with wheat sensitivity may find gluten-free bread and bakery products useful, although these tend to be expensive and are made to a higher standard than people with wheat intolerance require. Many of the products sold by The Gluten-Free Mall are also suitable for those avoiding egg, milk, or soy. Contact them at www.glutenfreemall.com. Every ingredient used is labeled.

Vermont Nut-Free Chocolates
P.O. Box 67
Grand Isle, VT 05458
Tel: 888-4-NUT-FREE or 802-372-4654
Web site: www.vermontnutfree.com
Nut-free chocolates.

Food Ingredients in Medicinal Drugs

Many drugs and vitamin supplements contain lactose, gluten, corn, dyes, or preservatives. Those with lactose deficiency, a true allergy to wheat or corn, celiac disease, or sensitivity to additives may be badly affected by these unlisted ingredients. You can find out what is in your drugs by asking a pharmacist (small independent pharmacies are more likely to help than those in large stores).

Where there are no commercially available drugs free from your problem ingredient, you may need to buy a custom-compounded formulation. For expert advice on this contact:

Stokes Pharmacy, Inc.
639 Stokes Road
Medford, NJ 08055
Tel: 800-754-5222 or 609-654-5222
Fax: 800-440-5899
E-mail: pharmacist@stokesrx.com

Gluten-Free Foods and Medications

Before buying, it is as well to know something about the meaning of gluten-free (see pages 396–97), especially if you are highly sensitive to gluten.

The Gluten-Free Mall is run by a celiac and can be found on www.glutenfreemall.com. It buys products from all over the world, and implements its own labeling policy, where every ingredient used must be labeled. Many of the products are also suitable for those avoiding egg, milk, and soy—good news for the celiacs who also have food intolerance (see page 104).

If you are cooking your own gluten-free foods and want to try baking, you will benefit from buying some special ingredients, such as xanthan gum, guar gum, methylcellulose, or Clear Gel, which improve the rising qualities and crumb structure of baked foods. These can be obtained from health food stores or special gluten-free mail-order companies. Gluten-free communion wafers can be ordered from:

Meyer Vogelpohl
717 Race Street
Cincinnati, OH 45202-4304
Tel: 800-543-0264

Many celiacs are affected by wheat flour used in their medicinal drugs or vitamin supplements. The following pharmacy can make up special gluten-free formulations:

Stokes Pharmacy, Inc.
639 Stokes Road
Medford, NJ 08055
Tel: 800-754-5222 or 609-654-5222
Fax: 800-440-5899
E-mail: pharmacist@stokesrx.com

Bacterial Replacers

Bacterial replacers are often called *probiotics*. They can be valuable after a prolonged course of antibiotics, for anyone suffering yeast overgrowth in the bowel (along with other treatments), and for some other conditions. Buying by mail usually ensures more live organisms, as long as the delivery time is fast (less than three days). Stores may not have kept the product refrigerated and the number of viable organisms could be low.

CAG Functional Foods
222 South Fifteenth Street, Suite 770
Omaha, NE 68102-7315
Tel: 402-595-7315 or 888-828-4242
Fax: 402-595-4498
Web site: www.culturelle.com

Household Products for Allergen Avoidance

Many different companies sell products that can be useful for those with classical allergies, such as mattress covers for reducing dust-mite allergen exposure.

National Allergy Supply
4400 Abbott's Bridge Road
P.O. Box 1658
Duluth, GA 30096
Tel: 800-522-1448
Web site: www.nationalallergysupply.com

Allergy Control Products
96 Danbury Road
Ridgefield, CT 06877
Tel: 800-422-DUST
Web site: www.allergycontrol.com

The Allergy Store
8567 Coral Way, Suite 108
Miami, FL 33155
Tel: 305-223-2847 or 888-337-5665
Fax: 305-220-3334
Web site: www.allergystore-2.com

Allergy Supply Company
11994 Star Court
Herndon, VA 20171
Tel: 800-323-6744 or 703-391-2011 (in Washington, D.C.)
Fax: 800-681-5454
E-mail: allergy@allergysupply.com
Web site: www.allergysupply.com

American Allergy Supply
P.O. Box 722022
Houston, TX 77272-2022
Tel: 800-321-1096 or 800-221-6483
E-mail: American@neosoft.com
Web site: www.neosoft.com
Products for those with chemical sensitivity.

Nirvana Safe Haven
3441 Golden Rain Road, Suite 3
Walnut Creek, CA 94595
Tel: 800-968-9355
Fax: 925-938-9019
Web site: www.nontoxic.com
E-mail: daliya@nontoxic.com

INDEX